Quality of Care for

General
Medical Conditions

A Review of the Literature
and Quality Indicators

Eve A. Kerr • Steven M. Asch
Eric G. Hamilton • Elizabeth A. McGlynn

Editors

RAND Health

Supported by the Agency for Healthcare Research and Quality

Principal funding for this report was provided by a cooperative agreement from the Agency for Healthcare Research and Quality.

ISBN: 0-8330-2916-9

Published 2000 by RAND
1700 Main Street, P.O. Box 2138, Santa Monica, CA 90407-2138
1200 South Hayes Street, Arlington, VA 22202-5050
RAND URL: http://www.rand.org/
To order RAND documents or to obtain additional information, contact Distribution
Services: Telephone: (310) 451-7002;
Fax: (310) 451-6915; Internet: order@rand.org

PREFACE

This report is one of a series of volumes describing the QA Tools, a comprehensive, clinically based system for assessing care for children and adults. The quality indicators that comprise these Tools cover 46 clinical areas and all 4 functions of medicine—screening, diagnosis, treatment, and follow-up. The indicators also cover a variety of modes of providing care, including history, physical examination, laboratory study, medication, and other interventions and contacts.

Development of each indicator was based on a review of the literature. Each volume documents the literature on which the indicators were based, explains how the clinical areas and indicators were selected, and describes what is included in the overall system.

The QA Tools were developed with funding from public and private sponsors—the Health Care Financing Administration, the Agency for Healthcare Research and Quality, the California HealthCare Foundation, and the Robert Wood Johnson Foundation.

The other four volumes in this series are:

Quality of Care for Oncologic Conditions and HIV: A Review of the Literature and Quality Indicators. Steven M. Asch, Eve A. Kerr, Eric G. Hamilton, Jennifer L. Reifel, and Elizabeth A. McGlynn, eds. MR-1281-AHRQ, 2000.

Quality of Care for Cardiopulmonary Conditions: A Review of the Literature and Quality Indicators. Eve A. Kerr, Steven M. Asch, Eric G. Hamilton, and Elizabeth A. McGlynn, eds. MR-1282-AHRQ, 2000.

Quality of Care for Children and Adolescents: A Review of Selected Clinical Conditions and Quality Indicators. Elizabeth A. McGlynn, Cheryl L. Damberg, Eve A. Kerr, and Mark A. Schuster, eds. MR-1283-HCFA, 2000.

Quality of Care for Women: A Review of Selected Clinical Conditions and Quality Indicators. Elizabeth A. McGlynn, Eve A. Kerr, Cheryl L. Damberg, and Steven M. Asch, eds. MR-1284-HCFA, 2000.

These volumes should be of interest to clinicians, health plans, insurers, and health services researchers. At the time of publication, the QA Tools system was undergoing testing in managed care plans,

medical groups, and selected communities. For more information about the
QA Tools system, contact RAND_Health@rand.org.

CONTENTS

TABLES

FIGURES

ACKNOWLEDGEMENTS

Funding for this work was provided by a Cooperative Agreement (No. 5U18HS09463-02), "Adult Global Quality Assessment Tool") from the Agency for Healthcare Research and Quality. We appreciate the continued and enthusiastic support of our project officer, Elinor Walker.

We are indebted to our expert panelists who gave generously of their time, knowledge and wisdom:

David M. Baughan, M.D.
Vice President
Saco River Medical Group
Conway, NH

Charles E. Boult, M.D., M.P.H.
Associate Professor
Program in Geriatrics
Department of Family Practice and Community Health
University of Minnesota Medical School
Minneapolis, MN

Randall D. Cebul, M.D. (Panel Chair)
Director, Center for Health Care Research and Policy
Case Western Reserve University -
MetroHealth System Institute for Public Health Sciences
MetroHealth Medical Center
Cleveland, OH

Rebecca Elon, M.D., M.P.H.
Medical Director
North Arundel Senior Care
Severna Park, MD

Donald E. Girard, M.D.
Associate Dean, Graduate and Continuing Medical Education
Oregon Health Sciences University
Portland, OR

Charles J. Hatem, M.D.
Director of Medical Education
Program Director, Internal Medicine Training Program
Mount Auburn Hospital
Cambridge, MA

Kurt Kroenke, M.D.
Regenstrief Institute for Health Care
Regenstrief Health Center
Indiana University Medical Center
Indianapolis, IN

Wally R. Smith, M.D.
Associate Professor and Chair
Division of Quality Health Care
Department of Internal Medicine
Virginia Commonwealth University
Richmond, VA

Jeffrey L. Susman, M.D.
Associate Dean for Primary Care
Department of Family Practice
University of Nebraska Medical Center
Omaha, NE

Our thanks also go to the following experts who reviewed and provided consultation on specific chapters:

Joshua Offman, MD, Cedars-Sinai Medical Center (Dyspepsia and PUD)

Robert W. Baloh, M.D., UCLA School of Medicine, Department of Neurology (Vertigo and Dizziness)

We are also greatly indebted to the following project staff whose contributions made this document possible: Kenneth Clark, Landon Donsbach, Sandy Geschwind, Kevin Heslin, Nicole Humphrey, Amy Kilbourne, and Tammy Majeski.

INTRODUCTION

Developing and implementing a valid system of quality assessment is essential for effective functioning of the health care system. Although a number of groups have produced quality assessment tools, these tools typically suffer from a variety of limitations. Information is obtained on only a few dimensions of quality, the tools rely exclusively on administrative data, they examine quality only for users of services rather than the population, or they fail to provide a scientific basis for the quality indicators.

Under funding from public and private sponsors, including the Health Care Financing Administration (HCFA), the Agency for Healthcare Research and Quality (AHRQ), the California HealthCare Foundation, and the Robert Wood Johnson Foundation (RWJ), RAND has developed and tested a comprehensive, clinically based system for assessing quality of care for children and adults. We call this system QA Tools.

In this introduction, we discuss how the clinical areas were selected, how the indicators were chosen, and what is included in the overall system. We then describe in detail how we developed the indicators for children and adolescents.

ADVANTAGES OF THE QA TOOLS SYSTEM

QA Tools is a comprehensive, clinically based system for assessing the quality of care for children and adults. The indicators cover 46 clinical areas and all four functions of medicine including screening, diagnosis, treatment, and follow-up. The indicators also cover a variety of modes of providing care, such as history, physical examination, laboratory study, medication, and other interventions and contacts. Initial development of indicators for each clinical area was based on a review of the literature.

The QA Tools system addresses many limitations of current quality assessment tools by offering the following:

1

They are clinically detailed and require data typically found only in medical records rather than just relying exclusively on data from administrative records.

They examine quality for a population-based sample rather than for a more restricted sample of those who use care or have insurance.

They document the scientific basis for developing and choosing the indicators.

The QA Tools system is designed to target populations vulnerable to underutilization.

Because of the comprehensiveness of the system, it is difficult for health care organizations to focus on a few indicators to increase their quality scores.

- QA Tools is a system that can be effective for both internal and external quality reviews. Health care organizations can use the system in order to improve the overall quality of the care provided.

- Because of the simple summary scores that will be produced, it will be an important tool for purchasers and consumers who are making choices about health care coverage and which provider to see.

Given its comprehensiveness, the QA Tools system contrasts with *leading indicators*, the most common approach to quality measurement in use today. Under the leading indicators approach, three to five specific quality measures are selected across a few domains (for example, rates of mammography screening, prevalence of the use of beta blockers among persons who have had a heart attack, and appropriateness of hysterectomy).

Leading indicators may work well for drawing general conclusions about quality when they correlate highly with other similar but unmeasured interventions and when repeated measurement and public reporting does not change the relationship of those indicators to the related interventions. However, to date no real evaluation of the utility of leading indicators in assessing health system performance has been done. We also do not know whether the selected indicators currently in use consistently represent other unmeasured practices.

By contrast, a comprehensive system can represent different dimensions of quality of care delivery by using a large number of measures applied to a population of interest and aggregated to produce index scores to draw conclusions about quality. A comprehensive system works well when evidence exists of variability within and between the diagnosis and management of different conditions and when the question being asked is framed at a high level (for instance, how well is the health system helping the population stay healthy, or how much of a problem does underuse present?).

In the 46 clinical areas they encompass, the QA Tools adequately represent scientific and expert judgment on what constitutes quality care. However, both the science and the practice of medicine continue to evolve. For the QA Tools to remain a valid tool for quality assessment over time, the scientific evidence in each area needs to be reviewed annually to determine if new evidence warrants modifying the indicators and/or clinical areas included in the system.

SELECTING CLINICAL AREAS FOR THE QA TOOLS

We reviewed Vital Statistics, the National Health Interview Survey, the National Hospital Discharge Survey, and the National Ambulatory Medical Care Survey to identify the leading causes of morbidity and mortality and the most common reasons for physician visits in the United States. We examined statistics for different age and gender groups in the population (0-1, 1-5, 6-11, 12-17, 18-50 [men and women], 50-64, 65-75, over 75).

We selected topics that reflected these different areas of importance (death, disability, utilization of services) and that covered preventive care as well as care for acute and chronic conditions. In addition, we consulted with a variety of experts to identify areas that are important to these various populations but that may be underrepresented in national data sets (for example, mental health problems). Finally, we sought to select enough clinical areas to represent a majority of the health care delivery system.

Table I.1 lists the 46 clinical areas included in the QA Tools system by population group; 20 include indicators for children and 36 for adults. The clinical areas, broadly defined, represent about 55 percent of the reasons for ambulatory care visits among children, 50 percent of the reasons for ambulatory care visits for the entire population, and 46 percent of the reasons for hospitalization among adults.

Note: Table I.1 reflects the clinical areas that were included in the system currently being tested. Several clinical areas (for example, lung cancer and sickle cell disease) for which indicators were developed were not incorporated into the current tool due to budgetary constraints.

Table I.1

Clinical Areas in QA Tools System By Covered Population Group

Clinical Areas	Children	Adults
Acne	X	
Adolescent preventive services	X	
Adult screening and prevention		X
Alcohol dependence		X
Allergic rhinitis	X	
Asthma	X	X
Atrial fibrillation		X
Attention deficit/hyperactivity disorder	X	
Benign prostatic hyperplasia		X
Breast cancer		X
Cataracts		X
Cerebrovascular disease		X
Cervical cancer		X
Cesarean delivery	X	X
Chronic obstructive pulmonary disease		X
Colorectal cancer		X
Congestive heart failure		X
Coronary artery disease		X
Depression	X	X
Developmental screening	X	
Diabetes Mellitus	X	X
Diarrheal disease	X	
Family planning and contraception	X	X
Fever of unknown origin	X	
Headache		X
Hip fracture		X
Hormone replacement therapy		X
Human immunodeficiency virus		X
Hyperlipidemia		X
Hypertension		X
Immunizations	X	X
Low back pain		X
Orthopedic conditions		X
Osteoarthritis		X
Otitis media	X	
Pain management for cancer		X
Peptic ulcer disease & dyspepsia		X
Pneumonia		X
Prenatal care and delivery	X	X
Prostate cancer		X
Tuberculosis	X	X
Upper respiratory tract infections	X	
Urinary tract infections	X	X
Uterine bleeding and hysterectomy		X
Vaginitis and sexually transmitted diseases	X	X
Well child care	X	
Total number of clinical areas	**20**	**36**

SELECTING QUALITY INDICATORS

In this section, we describe the process by which indicators were chosen for inclusion in the QA Tools system. This process involved RAND staff drafting proposed indicators based on a review of the pertinent clinical literature and expert panel review of those indicators.

Literature Review

For each clinical area chosen, we reviewed the scientific literature for evidence that effective methods of prevention, screening, diagnosis, treatment, and follow-up existed (Asch et al., 2000; Kerr et al., 2000; McGlynn et al., 2000a; McGlynn et al., 2000b). We explicitly examined the continuum of care in each clinical area. RAND staff drafted indicators that

addressed an intervention with potential health benefits for the patient were supported by scientific evidence or formal professional consensus (guidelines, for example)

can be significantly influenced by the health care delivery system

can be assessed from available sources of information, primarily the medical record.

The literature review process varied slightly for each clinical area, but the basic strategy involved the following:

Identify general areas in which quality indicators are likely to be developed.

Review relevant textbooks and review articles.

Conduct a targeted MEDLINE search on specific topics related to the probable indicator areas.

The levels of evidence for each indicator were assigned to three categories: randomized clinical trial; nonrandomized controlled trials, cohort or case analysis, or multiple time series; and textbooks, opinions, or descriptive studies. For each proposed indicator, staff noted the highest level of evidence supporting the indicator.

Because of the breadth of topics for which we were developing indicators, some of the literature reviews relied exclusively on textbooks and review articles. Nonetheless, we believe that the reviews adequately summarize clinical opinion and key research at the time that they were conducted. The literature reviews used to develop quality indicators for children and adolescents, and for women, were conducted between January and July 1995. The reviews for general medical conditions, oncologic conditions, and cardiopulmonary conditions were conducted between November 1996 and July 1997.

For each clinical area, we wrote a summary of the scientific evidence and developed tables of the proposed indicators that included the level of evidence, specific studies in support of the indicator, and the clinical rationale for the indicator. Because the organization of care delivery is changing so rapidly, we drafted indicators that were not in most cases inextricably linked to the place where the care was provided.

Types of Indicators

Quality of care is usually determined with three types of measures: *Structural measures* include characteristics of clinicians (for instance, board certification or years of experience), organizations (for instance, staffing patterns or types of equipment available), and patients (for instance, type of insurance or severity of illness). *Process measures* include the ways in which clinicians and patients interact and the appropriateness of medical treatment for a specific patient. *Outcomes measures* include changes in patients' current and future health status, including health-related quality of life and satisfaction with care.

The indicators included in the QA Tools system are primarily process indicators. We deliberately chose such indicators because the system was designed to assess care for which we can hold providers responsible. However, we collect data on a number of intermediate outcomes measures (for example, glycosylated hemoglobin, blood pressure, and cholesterol) that could be used to construct intermediate clinical outcomes indicators.

In many instances, the measures included in the QA Tools system are used to determine whether interventions have been provided in response to poor performance on such measures (for instance, whether persons who fail to control their blood sugar on dietary therapy are offered oral hypoglycemic therapy).

The Expert Panel Process

We convened expert panels to evaluate the indicators and to make final selections using the RAND/UCLA Appropriateness Method, a modified Delphi method developed at RAND and UCLA (Brook, 1994). In general, the method quantitatively assesses the expert judgment of a group of clinicians regarding the indicators by using a scale with values ranging from 1 to 9.

The method is iterative with two rounds of anonymous ratings of the indicators by the panel and a face-to-face group discussion between rounds. Each panelist has equal weight in determining the final result: the quality indicators that will be included in the QA Tools system.

The RAND/UCLA Appropriateness Method has been shown to have a reproducibility consistent with that of well accepted diagnostic tests such as the interpretation of coronary angiography and screening mammography (Shekelle et al., 1998a). It has also been shown to have content, construct, and predictive validity in other applications (Brook, 1994; Shekelle et al., 1998b; Kravitz et al., 1995; Selby et al., 1996).

Approximately six weeks before the panel meeting, we sent panelists the reviews of the literature, the staff-proposed quality indicators, and separate rating sheets for each clinical area. We asked the panelists to examine the literature review and rate each indicator on a nine-point scale on each of two dimensions: validity and feasibility.

A quality indicator is defined as valid if:

1. Adequate scientific evidence or professional consensus exists supporting the indicator.
2. There are identifiable health benefits to patients who receive care specified by the indicator.
3. Based on the panelists' professional experience, health professionals with significantly higher rates of adherence to an indicator would be considered higher quality providers
4. The majority of factors that determine adherence to an indicator are under the control of the health professional (or are subject to influence by the health professional—for example, smoking cessation).

Ratings of 1-3 mean that the indicator is not a valid criterion for evaluating quality. Ratings of 4-6 mean that the indicator is an uncertain or equivocal criterion for evaluating quality. Ratings of 7-9 mean that the indicator is clearly a valid criterion for evaluating quality.

A quality indicator is defined as feasible if:

1. The information necessary to determine adherence is likely to be found in a typical medical record.

2. Estimates of adherence to the indicator based on medical record data are likely to be reliable and unbiased.

3. Failure to document relevant information about the indicator is itself a marker for poor quality.

Ratings of 1-3 mean that it is not feasible to use the indicator for evaluating quality. Ratings of 4-6 mean that there will be considerable variability in the feasibility of using the indicator to evaluate quality. Ratings of 7-9 mean that it is clearly feasible to use the indicator for evaluating quality.

The first round of indicators was rated by the panelists individually in their own offices. The indicators were returned to RAND staff and the results of the first round were summarized. We encouraged panelists to comment on the literature reviews, the definitions of key terms, and the indicators. We also encouraged them to suggest additions or deletions to the indicators.

At the panel meeting, participants discussed each clinical area in turn, focusing on the evidence, or lack thereof, that supports or refutes each indicator and the panelists' prior validity rankings. Panelists had before them the summary of the panel's first round ratings and a confidential reminder of their own ratings.

The summary consisted of a printout of the rating sheet with the distribution of ratings by panelists displayed above the rating line (without revealing the identity of the panelists) and a caret (^) marking the individual panelist's own rating in the first round displayed below the line. An example of the printout received by panelists is shown in Figure I.1.

Chapter 1		
ASTHMA	Validity	Feasibility

DIAGNOSIS

3. Spirometry should be measured in patients
with chronic asthma at least every 2 years.

```
                                    1   1 2 3 1 1                    3 4 2
                                    1 2 3 4 5 6 7 8 9      1 2 3 4 5 6 7 8 9   ( 1- 2)
                                                ^                            ^
```

TREATMENT

7. Patients requiring chronic treatment with
systemic corticosteroids during any 12 month
period should have been prescribed inhaled
corticosteroids during the same 12 month
period.

```
                                          1 6   2                      2 3 4
                                    1 2 3 4 5 6 7 8 9      1 2 3 4 5 6 7 8 9   ( 3- 4)
                                                ^                            ^
```

10. All patients seen for an acute asthma
exacerbation should be evaluated with a
complete history including all of the
following:

```
                                        2 2 2   3                  2 2   1 1 3
   a. time of onset                 1 2 3 4 5 6 7 8 9      1 2 3 4 5 6 7 8 9   ( 5- 6)
                                                ^                            ^
```

```
                                            4 1 4                      3 1 5
   b. all current medications       1 2 3 4 5 6 7 8 9      1 2 3 4 5 6 7 8 9   ( 7- 8)
                                                ^                            ^
```

```
   c. prior hospitalizations and emergency   5 1 3              5 1 3
      department visits for asthma   1 2 3 4 5 6 7 8 9      1 2 3 4 5 6 7 8 9   ( 9-10)
                                                ^                            ^
```

```
   d. prior episodes of respiratory      1 1 3 2 2          1   2   3 1 2
      insufficiency due to asthma    1 2 3 4 5 6 7 8 9      1 2 3 4 5 6 7 8 9   (11-12)
                                                ^                            ^
```

Scales: 1 = low validity or feasibility; 9 = high validity or feasibility

Figure I.1 - Sample Panelist Summary Rating Sheet

Panelists were encouraged to bring to the discussion any relevant published information that the literature reviews had omitted. In a few cases, they supplied this information which was, in turn, discussed. In several cases, the indicators were reworded or otherwise clarified to better fit clinical judgment.

After further discussion, all indicators in each clinical area were re-ranked for validity. These final round rankings were analyzed in a manner similar to past applications of the RAND/UCLA Appropriateness Method (Park et al., 1986; Brook, 1994). The median panel rating and measure of dispersion were used to categorize indicators on validity.

We regarded panel members as being in *disagreement* when at least three members of the panel judged an indicator as being in the highest tertile of validity (that is, having a rating of 7, 8, or 9) and three members rated it as being in the lowest tertile of validity (1, 2, or 3) (Brook, 1994). Indicators with a median validity rating of 7 or higher without disagreement were included in the system.

We also obtained ratings from the panelists about the feasibility of obtaining the data necessary to score the indicators from medical. This was done to make explicit that failure to document key variables required to score an indicator would be treated as though the recommended care was not provided.

Although we do not intend for quality assessment to impose significant additional documentation burdens, we wanted the panel to acknowledge that documentation itself is an element of quality particularly when patients are treated by a team of health professionals. Because of the variability in documentation patterns and the opportunity to empirically evaluate feasibility, indicators with a median feasibility rating of 4 and higher were accepted into the system. Indicators had to satisfy both the validity and feasibility criteria.

Five expert panels were convened on the topics of children's care, care for women 18-50, general medicine for adults, oncologic conditions and HIV, and cardiopulmonary conditions.

The dates on which the panels were conducted are shown in Table I.2.

Table I.2

Dates Expert Panels Convened

Children	October 1995
Women	November 1995
Cardiopulmonary	September 1997
Oncology/HIV	October 1997
General Medicine	November 1997

Tables I.3 through I.6 summarize the distribution of indicators by level of evidence, type of care (preventive, acute, chronic), function of medicine (screening, diagnosis, treatment, follow-up, continuity), and modality (for example, history, physical examination, laboratory test, medication) (Malin et al., 2000; Schuster et al., 1997).

The categories were selected by the research team and reflect terminology commonly used by health services researchers to describe different aspects of health service delivery. The categories also reflect the areas in which we intend to develop aggregate quality of care scores. However, a significant benefit of the QA Tools system is its adaptability to other frameworks.

Note: In the following tables, the figures in some columns may not total exactly 100 percent due to the rounding of fractional numbers.

Table I.3

Distribution of Indicators (%) by Level of Evidence

Level of Evidence	Children	Women	Cancer/HIV	Cardio-pulmonary	General Medicine
Randomized trials	11	22	22	18	23
Nonrandomized trials	6	16	37	4	17
Descriptive studies	72	59	26	71	57
Added by panel	12	4	15	7	4
Total	101	101	100	100	101

Table I.4

Distribution of Indicators (%) by Type of Care

Type of Care	Children	Women	Cancer/HIV	Cardio-pulmonary	General Medicine
Preventive	30	11	20	3	18
Acute	36	49	7	26	38
Chronic	34	41	74	71	44
Total	100	101	101	100	100

Table I.5

Distribution of Indicators (%) by Function of Medicine

Function of Medicine	Children	Women	Cancer/HIV	Cardio-pulmonary	General Medicine
Screening	23	18	9	3	12
Diagnosis	31	30	27	54	41
Treatment	36	43	53	36	41
Follow-up	10	12	10	8	6
Total	100	103	99	101	100

Table I.6

Distribution of Indicators (%) by Modality

Modality	Children	Women	Cancer/HIV	Cardio-pulmonary	General Medicine
History	19	18	4	11	23
Physical	19	10	5	21	15
Lab/Radiology	21	23	24	23	18
Medication	25	29	25	25	26
Other	17	19	42	20	17
Total	101	99	100	100	99

DEVELOPING QUALITY INDICATORS FOR GENERAL MEDICAL CONDITIONS

We now describe in more detail the process by which we developed quality indicators for general medical conditions.

Selecting Clinical Areas

We began our selection of clinical areas by examining national data sources to identify the leading causes of mortality, morbidity, and functional limitation among adult men and women. The principal data sources for this review were Vital Statistics, the National Health Interview Survey (NHIS), the National Ambulatory Medical Care Survey (NAMCS), and the National Hospital Discharge Survey (NHDS). From these data sources, we selected the conditions that represent the leading causes of mortality, morbidity, hospitalization, and outpatient visits. This process led to the selection of some areas that overlapped with an earlier panel conducted on women's care (McGlynn et al., 2000b).

To facilitate the review and rating process, we grouped the selected areas into three categories: cardiopulmonary conditions, oncologic conditions and HIV, and general medical conditions. Table I.7 lists the clinical areas covered by each of these categories. "Cancer Pain and Palliation" was not among the originally selected clinical areas, but was added during the panel process as a result of strong recommendations from several oncology panelists.

Table I.7

Clinical Areas Covered by Each Expert Panel

Cardiopulmonary (N=12)	Oncology and HIV (N=11)	General Medicine (N=22)
Asthma*	Breast Cancer Screening	Acne*
Atrial Fibrillation	Breast Cancer Diagnosis	Alcohol Dependence*
Cerebrovascular Disease	and Treatment*	Allergic Rhinitis*
Chronic Obstructive	Cervical Cancer	Benign Prostatic
Pulmonary Disease	Screening*	Hyperplasia
Cigarette Counseling*	Colorectal Cancer	Cataracts
Congestive Heart	Screening	Cholelithiasis
Failure	Colorectal Cancer	Dementia
Coronary Artery Disease	Diagnosis and	Depression*
Diagnosis and	Treatment	Diabetes Mellitus*
Screening	HIV Disease	Dyspepsia and Peptic
Coronary Artery Disease	Lung Cancer	Ulcer Disease
Prevention and	Prostate Cancer	Hormone Replacement
Treatment	Screening	Therapy
Hyperlipidemia	Prostate Cancer	Headache*
Hypertension*	Diagnosis and	Hip Fracture
Pneumonia	Treatment	Hysterectomy
Upper Respiratory	Skin Cancer Screening	Inguinal Hernia
Infections*	Cancer Pain and	Low Back Pain (Acute)*
	Palliation	Orthopedic Conditions
		Osteoarthritis
		Preventive Care*
		Urinary Tract
		Infections*
		Vaginitis and Sexually
		Transmitted Diseases*
		Vertigo and Dizziness

* Previously addressed by the panel on quality of care for women (McGlynn et al., 2000b).

Conducting Literature Reviews

The literature reviews were conducted as described earlier in this Introduction by a team of physician investigators, many of whom have clinical expertise in the conditions selected for this project. Based on the literature review, each investigator drafted a review of the literature for his or her topic area, focusing on important areas for quality measurement (as opposed to a clinical review of the literature, which would focus on clinical management) and drafted potential indicators.

Each review and set of indicators were reviewed by Drs. Asch or Kerr for content, consistency, and the likely availability of information necessary to score adherence to the indicator from the medical record. On a few occasions, when questions remained even after detailed literature review, we requested that a clinical leader in the field read and comment on the draft review and indicators.

In addition, the physician investigators updated the 16 clinical areas carried over from the women's care panel. This included reading the previous reviews and indicators, updating the supporting literature from 1995 to 1997, and modifying the pre-existing indicators as was appropriate.

In most cases, few changes were made, but indicators were deleted if the evidence changed or if our implementation experience proved that it was not feasible to collect the data necessary to score adherence to an indicator. Indicators were added if strong evidence since 1995 supported the need for a new criterion. In the clinical areas previously addressed by the women's care panel, the expert panel for general adult medicine rated only those indicators that had been added or significantly revised (indicated by bold type in the indicator tables in the chapters that follow).

This quality assessment system is designed to encompass a substantial portion of the inpatient and ambulatory care received by the population. In order to estimate the percentage of ambulatory care visits covered by this system, we aggregated applicable ICD-9 codes into the clinical areas for which we are developing quality indicators. We then calculated the number of adult visits for each condition in the 1993 National Ambulatory Medical Care Survey (NAMCS). We used the same method to estimate the percentage of inpatient admissions accounted for by each clinical area in the 1992 National Hospital Discharge Survey.

Aggregating ICD-9 codes into the clinical areas covered by this system was an imprecise task, requiring a rather broad definition of what is "included" in each clinical area. The clinical conditions covered by this quality measurement system encompass 50 percent of all ambulatory care visits and 46 percent of non-federal inpatient hospital admissions.

Developing Indicators

In each clinical area, we developed indicators defining the explicit criteria by which quality of care would be evaluated. These indicators focus on technical processes of care for the various conditions and are organized by function: screening, diagnosis, treatment and follow-up. Although we have developed indicators across the continuum of management for each condition, we have not attempted to cover every important area or every possible clinical circumstance. The indicators were designed to apply to the average patient with the specified condition who is seeing the average physician.

Our approach makes a strong distinction between indicators of quality care and practice guidelines (see Table I.8). Whereas guidelines are intended to be comprehensive in scope, indicators are meant to apply to specific clinical circumstances in which there is believed to be a strong link between a measurable health care process and patient outcomes.

Indicators are not intended to measure all possible care for a condition. Furthermore, guidelines are intended to be applied prospectively at the individual patient level, whereas indicators are applied retrospectively and scored at an aggregate level. Finally, indicators must be written precisely in order to be *operationalized* (that is, to form useful measures of quality based on medical records or administrative data).

Table I.8

Clinical Guidelines versus Quality Indicators

Guidelines	Indicators
Comprehensive: Cover virtually all aspects of care for a condition.	**Targeted**: Apply to specific clinical circumstances in which there is evidence of a process-outcome link.
Prescriptive: Intended to influence provider behavior prospectively at the individual patient level.	**Observational:** Measure past provider behavior at an aggregate level.
Flexible: Intentionally allow room for clinical judgment and interpretation.	**Operational:** Precise language that can be applied systematically to medical records or administrative data.

The indicator tables at the end of each chapter of this book

identify the population to whom the indicators apply

list the indicators themselves

provide a "grade" for the strength of the evidence that supports each indicator

list the specific literature used to support each indicator

provide a statement of the health benefits of complying with each indicator

include comments to further explain the purpose or reasoning behind each indicator.

Selecting Panel Participants

We requested nominations for potential expert panel participants from the relevant specialty societies for general medicine: the American College of Physicians, American Academy of Family Physicians, American Geriatrics Society, and the Society of General Internal Medicine. We received a total of 206 nominations for the panels on general medicine, oncology and HIV, and cardiopulmonary conditions.

We sent nominees a letter summarizing the purpose of the project and indicating which group had recommended them. Interested candidates were asked to return a curriculum vitae and calendar with dates on which they were available to participate in the panel. We received positive responses from 156 (76%) potential panelists. The quality of the recommended panelists was excellent.

We sought to ensure that each panel was diverse with respect to type of practice (academic, private practice, managed care organizational practice), geographic location, gender, and specialty. The general medicine panel included five general internists, two family physicians, and two geriatricians. Dr. Randall Cebul, a general internist, chaired the panel. (See the Acknowledgements at the front of this book for a list of panel participants.)

Selecting and Analyzing the Final Set of Indicators

A total of 386 quality indicators were reviewed by the general medicine expert panel. All 140 indicators retained by the women's care panel were accepted by the general medicine panel on the basis of the earlier panel's ratings. Fifteen newly proposed indicators were deleted before the final panel ratings in response to comments from panelists prior to or during the panel meeting. Of the remaining 231 indicators that received final ratings from the general medicine panel, 13 were added by the panel itself. This occurred either when panelists agreed that a new indicator should be written to cover an important topic, or, more frequently, as a result of splitting a staff-proposed indicator.

The panel accepted 173 (75%) of the 231 indicators it rated. Fifty-eight indicators (25%) were dropped due to low ratings: 56 for low validity scores and 2 for substantial disagreement on validity. Table I.9 summarizes the disposition of all 386 proposed general medicine indicators by the strength of their supporting evidence. The final set consists of 313 indicators (173 rated by this panel and 140 approved based on ratings by the women's care panel), or 81 percent of those proposed. Table I.9 reveals that indicators that are not based on randomized clinical trials (that is, Level II and especially Level III indicators) were much more likely to be rejected by the panel.

Table I.9

**Disposition of Proposed General Medicine Indicators
by Strength of Evidence**

Strength of Evidence	Total Proposed	Indicator Disposition			
		Accepted	Retained from Women's Panel	Drop before Rating	Drop Due to Low Rating
I. Randomized controlled trials	76 (100%)	37 (49%)	34 (45%)	2 (3%)	3 (4%)
II. Non-randomized trials	59 (100%)	45 (76%)	8 (14%)	0 (0%)	6 (10%)
III. Opinions, descriptive studies, or textbooks	238 (100%)	79 (33%)	98 (41%)	13 (5%)	48 (20%)
IV. Added by Clinical Panel	13 (100%)	12 (92%)	0 (0%)	0 (0%)	1 (8%)
Total	**386 (100%)**	**173 (45%)**	**140 (36%)**	**15 (4%)**	**58 (15%)**

The summary ratings sheets for general medical conditions are shown in Appendix A. Figure I.2 provides an example of a final summary rating sheet. The chapter number and clinical condition are shown in the top left margin. The rating bar is numbered from 1 to 9, indicating the range of possible responses. The number shown above each of the responses in the rating bar indicates how many panelists provided that particular rating for the indicator. Below the score distribution, in parentheses, the median and the mean absolute deviation from the median are listed. Each dimension is assigned an A for "Agreement", D for "Disagreement", or I for "Indeterminate" based on the score distribution.

Note: We recommend caution when reviewing the ratings for each indicator. The overall median does not tell us anything about the extent to which the indicators occur in clinical practice. To determine that, actual clinical data to assess the indicators must be collected and analyzed.

## Chapter 4

BENIGN PROSTATIC HYPERPLASIA (BPH)   Validity   Feasibility

DIAGNOSIS

1. Men age 50 and older who present for
routine care should be asked at least once a
year about recent symptoms of prostatism.

```
1      2 2 1 1 2        2    1 1 2 2 1
1 2 3 4 5 6 7 8 9  1 2 3 4 5 6 7 8 9  ( 1- 2)
  (5.0, 1.7, I)        (7.0, 1.7, I)
```

2. If the patient has recent symptoms of
prostatism, the provider should document one
of the following on the same visit:

  - AUA symptom score
  - How bothersome the patient considers the
    symptoms

```
        1 3 4 1            1 1 3 2 2
1 2 3 4 5 6 7 8 9  1 2 3 4 5 6 7 8 9  ( 3- 4)
  (8.0, 0.7, A)        (7.0, 1.0, A)
```

3. Patients with new recent symptoms of
prostatism should have the presence of
absence of at least one of the following
conditions documented:

  - Parkinson's disease
  - Diabetes mellitus
  - Stroke
  - History of urethral instrumentation

```
      2 3 1 3            1 4 2   2
1 2 3 4 5 6 7 8 9  1 2 3 4 5 6 7 8 9  ( 5- 6)
  (4.0, 1.0, A)        (4.0, 1.0, I)
```

4. Patients with new recent symptoms of
prostatism should be offered a digital rectal
examination (DRE) within one month after the
visit in which the symptoms are noted, if
they have not had a DRE in the past year.

```
  2 1   1   3 1 1          2 1 2 3 1
1 2 3 4 5 6 7 8 9  1 2 3 4 5 6 7 8 9  ( 7- 8)
  (7.0, 2.1, D)        (7.0, 1.1, I)
```

5. If a patient has new recent symptoms of
moderate prostatism the health care provider
should offer at least one of the following
within one month of the note of symptoms:

  - Uroflowometry
  - Post void residual
  - Pressure flow study

```
  1 1 4 1 2            1   5 1 1 1
1 2 3 4 5 6 7 8 9  1 2 3 4 5 6 7 8 9  ( 9-10)
  (4.0, 0.9, A)        (5.0, 0.9, I)
```

6. If a patient has new recent symptoms
prostatism, the provider should order the
following tests within one month of the note
of symptoms, unless done in the past year:

  a. Urine analysis

```
        5 2 2              3 2 4
1 2 3 4 5 6 7 8 9  1 2 3 4 5 6 7 8 9  (11-12)
  (7.0, 0.7, A)        (8.0, 0.8, A)
```

  b. Serum creatinine

```
        7 1 1              1 2 2 4
1 2 3 4 5 6 7 8 9  1 2 3 4 5 6 7 8 9  (13-14)
  (7.0, 0.3, A)        (8.0, 0.9, A)
```

TREATMENT

7. Patients diagnosed with BPH who report
recent symptoms of prostatism, and who are on
anticholinergic or sympathomimetic
medications, should have discontinuation or
dose reduction of these medications offered
or discussed within one month of the note of
symptoms.

```
        1 5 3          1 1 1   3 1 2
1 2 3 4 5 6 7 8 9  1 2 3 4 5 6 7 8 9  (15-16)
  (7.0, 0.4, A)        (7.0, 1.6, I)
```

Scales: 1 = low validity or feasibility; 9 = high validity or feasibility

Figure I.2 - Sample Rating Results Sheet

The tables in Appendix B show the changes made to each indicator during the panel process, the reasons for those changes, and the final disposition of each indicator. Wherever possible, we have tried to briefly summarize the discussion that led the panel to either modify or drop indicators. These explanations are based on extensive notes taken by RAND staff during the panel process, but should not be considered representative of the views of all of the panelists, nor of any individual.

Because the final quality assessment system will produce aggregate scores for various dimensions of health care, it is useful to examine the distribution of the final indicators across some of these dimensions. Table I.10 summarizes the distribution of quality indicators by type of care (preventive, acute, and chronic), the function of the medical care provided (screening, diagnosis, treatment, and follow-up), and the modality by which care is delivered (history, physical examination, laboratory or radiologic study, medication, other interventions,[1] and other contacts[2]).

Indicators were assigned to only one type of care, but could have up to two functions and three modalities. Indicators with more than one function or modality were allocated fractionally across categories. For example, one indicator states, "For patients who present with a complaint of sore throat, a history/physical exam should document presence or absence of: a) fever; b) tonsillar exudate; c) anterior cervical adenopathy." This indicator was allocated 50 percent to the history modality and 50 percent to the physical examination modality.

---

[1] Other interventions include counseling, education, procedures, and surgery.
[2] Other contacts include general follow-up visit or phone call, referral to subspecialist, or hospitalization.

23

Table I.10

Distribution of Final General Medicine Quality Indicators by Type of Care, Function, and Modality

	Number of Indicators	Percent of Indicators
Type		
Preventive	55	18%
Acute	120	38%
Chronic	138	44%
Function		
Screening	37	12%
Diagnosis	128	41%
Treatment	129	41%
Follow-up	19	6%
Modality		
History	71	23%
Physical Examination	48	15%
Laboratory or Radiologic Study	57	18%
Medication	82	26%
Other Intervention	45	14%
Other Contact	10	3%
Total	**313**	**100%**

CONCLUSION

This report provides the foundation for a broad set of quality indicators covering general medicine. The final indicators presented here cover a variety of clinical conditions, span a range of clinical functions and modalities, and are rated by the level of evidence in the supporting literature. When combined with the indicators approved by the women's care, child and adolescent care, cardiopulmonary, and oncology and HIV expert panels, the complete quality assessment system will be more comprehensive than any system currently in use.

The comprehensive nature of this system is demonstrated by the broad scope of the indicators. Of the 386 indicators reviewed by the general medicine expert panel, 313 (81%) were retained. These indicators cover a mix of preventive, acute, and chronic care. They address all four functions of medicine, including screening, diagnosis, treatment and follow-up. Moreover, the indicators cover a variety of modes of care provision, such as history, physical examination, laboratory study, and medication.

There are many advantages to a comprehensive quality assessment system. Not only does it cover a broad range of health conditions experienced by the population, but it is also designed to detect underutilization of needed services. In addition, because of its broad scope, it will be difficult for health care organizations to improve their quality scores by focusing their improvement efforts on only a few indicators or clinical areas.

Finally, this system can be effective for both internal and external quality reviews. Sufficient clinical detail exists in the system such that organizations will be able to use the resulting information to improve care, while the simple summary scores that the system generates will be an important tool for health care purchasers and consumers.

ORGANIZATION OF THIS DOCUMENT

The rest of this volume is organized as follows:

- *Each chapter* summarizes:
    - Results of the literature review for one condition.
    - Provides a table of the staff's recommended indicators based on that review.
    - Indicates the level of scientific evidence supporting each indicator along with the specific relevant citations.
- *Appendix A* provides the summary rating sheets for each condition.
- *Appendix B* shows the changes made to each indicator during the panel process, the reasons for those changes, and the final disposition of each indicator.

REFERENCES

Asch, S. M., E. A. Kerr, E. G. Hamilton, J. L. Reifel, E. A. McGlynn (eds.), *Quality of Care for Oncologic Conditions and HIV: A Review of the Literature and Quality Indicators,* Santa Monica, CA: RAND, MR-1281-AHRQ, 2000.

Brook, R. H., "The RAND/UCLA Appropriateness Method," *Clinical Practice Guideline Development: Methodology Perspectives,* AHCPR Pub. No. 95-0009, Rockville, MD: Public Health Service, 1994.

Kerr E. A., S. M. Asch, E. G. Hamilton, E. A. McGlynn (eds.), *Quality of Care for Cardiopulmonary Conditions: A Review of the Literature and Quality Indicators,* Santa Monica, CA: RAND, MR-1282-AHRQ, 2000.

Kravitz R. L., M. Laouri, J. P. Kahan, P. Guzy, et al., "Validity of Criteria Used for Detecting Underuse of Coronary Revascularization," *JAMA* 274(8):632-638, 1995.

Malin, J. L., S. M. Asch, E. A. Kerr, E. A. McGlynn. "Evaluating the Quality of Cancer Care: Development of Cancer Quality Indicators for a Global Quality Assessment Tool," *Cancer* 88:701-7, 2000.

McGlynn E. A., C. Damberg, E. A. Kerr, M. Schuster (eds.), *Quality of Care for Children and Adolescents: A Review of Selected Clinical Conditions and Quality Indicators,* Santa Monica, CA: RAND, MR-1283-HCFA, 2000a.

McGlynn E. A., E. A. Kerr, C. Damberg, S. M. Asch (eds.), *Quality of Care for Women: A Review of Selected Clinical Conditions and Quality Indicators,* Santa Monica, CA: RAND, MR-1284-HCFA, 2000b.

Park R. A., Fink A., Brook R. H., Chassin M. R., et al., "Physician Ratings of Appropriate Indications for Six Medical and Surgical Procedures," *AJPH* 76(7):766-772, 1986.

Schuster M. A., S. M. Asch, E. A. McGlynn, et al., "Development of a
Quality of Care Measurement System for Children and Adolescents:
Methodological Considerations and Comparisons With a System for
Adult Women," *Archives of Pediatrics and Adolescent Medicine*
151:1085-1092, 1997.

Selby J. V., B. H. Fireman, R. J. Lundstrom, et al., "Variation among
Hospitals in Coronary-Angiography Practices and Outcomes after
Myocardial Infarction in a Large Health Maintenance Organization,"
N Engl J Med 335:1888-96, 1996.

Shekelle P. G., J. P. Kahan, S. J. Bernstein, et al., "The
Reproducibility of a Method to Identify the Overuse and Underuse of
Medical Procedures," *N Engl J Med* 338:1888-1895, 1998b.

Shekelle P. G., M. R. Chassin, R. E. Park, "Assessing the Predictive
Validity of the RAND/UCLA Appropriateness Method Criteria for
Performing Carotid Endarterectomy," *Int J Technol Assess Health
Care* 14(4):707-727, 1998a.

1. ACNE[1]

Lisa Schmidt, MPH, Eve A. Kerr, MD, and Kenneth Clark, MD

The general approach to summarizing the key literature on acne was to review relevant sections of two medical text books (Vernon and Lane, 1992; Paller et al., 1992) as well as journal articles chosen from a MEDLINE search of all English language articles published between the years of 1990 and 1997 on the treatment of acne.

IMPORTANCE

Acne is the most common skin disorder seen in the United States, affecting approximately 17 million persons (Tolman, 1992). Acne can persist into mid-adulthood in some persons, and can also present initially in adulthood. Overall, acne affects approximately ten percent of the U.S. population (Glassman et al., 1993). Acne was the most common reason for visits to dermatologists over the two year period from 1989 to 1990, accounting for 16.6 percent of all visits (Nelson, 1994). Although acne is not associated with severe morbidity, mortality, or disability, it can produce psychological effects. Furthermore, in severe cases, acne can lead to physical scarring which may exacerbate the emotional effects of the disease.

SCREENING

Screening patients for acne is not recommended.

DIAGNOSIS

Common acne is a disorder of the pilosebaceous glands and is characterized by follicular occlusion and inflammation (Paller et al., 1992). Acne occurs primarily on the face, but it can occur on the back, chest, and shoulders. Four factors contribute to the development of acne: 1) the sebum excretion rate, 2) sebaceous lipid composition,

---

[1] This chapter is a revision of one written for an earlier project on quality of care for women and children (Q1). The expert panel for the current project was asked to review all of the indicators, but only rated new or revised indicators.

3) bacteriology of the pilosebaceous duct, and 4) obstruction of the pilosebaceous duct. The anaerobic bacterium *Propionibacterium acnes* appears to play an important role in the pathogenesis of acne (Paller et al., 1992). *P. acnes* is capable of releasing lipolytic enzymes that convert the triglycerides in sebum into irritating fatty acids and glycerol, which may contribute to inflammation (Paller et al., 1992).

There are six types of acne lesions: comedones, papules, pustules, nodules, cysts, and scars. Individual patients may have one or more predominant type of lesion or a mixture of many lesions (Paller et al., 1992).

With the aim of guiding treatment, Vernon and Lane (1992) and Glassman et al. (1993) recommend the following history elements in diagnosing acne (Indicator 1):

- age at onset of acne;
- location (face, back, neck, chest);
- aggravating factors (stress, seasons, cosmetics, creams);
- previous treatments;
- family history of acne; and
- medications and drug use.

The physical examination should include:

- location of acne;
- types of lesions present;
- severity of disease (numbers of each type of lesion and intensity of inflammation); and
- complications (extent and severity of hyperpigmentation and scarring).

Location, previous treatment, and potentially aggravating medications were felt to be especially important.

TREATMENT

Medical treatment of acne is determined by the extent and severity of disease, prior treatments, and therapeutic goals. Each regimen must be followed for a minimum of four to six weeks before determining whether it is effective (Vernon and Lane, 1992). Table 1.1 lists guidelines to be used in the treatment of acne.

Table 1.1

Guidelines for the Treatment of Acne

Clinical Appearance	Treatment
Comedonal Acne - no inflammatory lesions	Topical tretinoin *or* benzoyl peroxide
Mild to Moderate Inflammatory Acne - red papules, few pustules	Topical tretinoin *and* benzoyl peroxide *and/or* topical antibiotic If acne is resistant to above therapy, add oral antibiotic.
Moderate to Severe Inflammatory Acne - red papules, many pustules	Topical tretinoin; topical antibiotic *or* benzoyl peroxide; *and* oral antibiotics
Severe Nodulocystic Acne - red papules, pustules, cysts and nodules	Topical tretinoin; benzoyl peroxide *or* topical antibiotic; oral antibiotics; *and* consider isotretinoin

Source: Adapted from Weston and Lane (1991), Vernon and Lane (1992) Nguyen (1994), and Taylor (1991).

Tretinoin and Benzoyl Peroxide

Topical keratolytic therapy is recommended as the primary treatment for comedonal acne to prevent new acne lesions as well as to treat preexisting ones (Paller et al., 1992). Two classes of keratolytics, tretinoin (retin A) and benzoyl peroxide, can be used alone or in combination with each other and will control 80 to 85 percent of acne (Taylor, 1991; Weston and Lane, 1992; Nguyen, 1994). Cream preparations of both tretinoin and benzoyl peroxide should be used because they are less irritating to the skin than gel forms. Tretinoin has a propensity to severely irritate the skin if used incorrectly. To avoid irritation, a low strength (0.025 percent) cream should be applied every other night for one week and then nightly. In addition, because skin treated with tretinoin is more sensitive to sun exposure, sunscreen should be used. Tretinoin should be avoided during pregnancy because of the potential of photoisomerization to isotretinoin, a teratogen (Weston and Lane, 1992; Vernon and Lane, 1992). Improvement of acne after treatment of tretinoin can take six to 12 weeks and flare-ups of acne can occur during the first few weeks due to surfacing of the lesions onto the skin (Nguyen, 1994). Benzoyl peroxide is available over-the-counter in various strengths and applications (gels, creams, lotions, or soaps). All concentrations seem to be therapeutically equivalent (Nguyen, 1994). Mild redness and scaling of the skin may occur during the first week of use.

Topical Antibiotics

Topical antibiotics decrease the quantity of *P. acnes* in the hair follicles. However, they are less effective than oral antibiotics because of their difficulty in penetrating sebum-filled follicules (Nguyen, 1994). Topical erythromycin and clindamycin are similar in efficacy and can be used once or twice a day (Weston, and Lane, 1992; Nguyen, 1994). Some percutaneous absorption may rarely occur with clindamycin, resulting in diarrhea and colitis (Weston and Lane, 1992; Nguyen, 1994). Topical antibiotics are frequently used in combination with keratolytics and are most useful for maintenance therapy if improvement after one to two months of oral antibiotics is observed (Weston and Lane, 1992).

Oral Antibiotics

Patients with moderate to severe inflammatory acne will require oral antibiotics in addition to topical therapy (Indicator 2). Tetracycline and erythromycin are the most commonly used systemic antibiotics. Minocycline is also effective with more convenient dosing; however, its cost limits its use to those patients with severe or recalcitrant acne (Nguyen, 1994; and Glassman et al., 1993).

Isotretinoin

The oral retinoid isotretinoin has been very efficacious in nodulocystic acne resistant to standard therapeutic regimens. In appropriate regimens, isotretinoin has resulted in long-term remission of acne in approximately 60 percent of patients treated (Weston and Lane, 1992). Because of its severe teratogenicity, isotretinoin should be avoided during pregnancy (Weston and Lane, 1992). Side effects of isotretinoin include dryness and scaliness of the skin, dry lips and

32

occasionally dry eyes and nose. It can also cause decreased night vision, hypertriglyceridemia, abnormal liver function, electrolyte imbalance, and elevated platelet count. Glassman et al. (1993) recommend monthly liver function tests to monitor potential for liver toxicity (Indicator 4). Up to ten percent of patients experience mild hair loss, but the effect is reversible (Weston and Lane, 1992). Because of the seriousness of these side effects, isotretinoin should be reserved for patients with severe acne who have failed previous therapy (Indicator 3)(Glassman et al., 1993; Nguyen, 1994; Vernon and Lane, 1992; and Weston and Lane, 1992).

FOLLOW-UP

Follow-up visits for acne should be scheduled initially every four to six weeks. Ideal control is defined as no more than a few new lesions every two weeks (Weston and Lane, 1992).

REFERENCES

Glassman P, Garcia D, and Delafield J. 1993. *Outpatient Care Handbook*. Philadelphia, PA: Hanley and Belfus, Inc.

Nelson C. 10 March 1994. Office visits to dermatologists: National Ambulatory Medical Care Survey, United States, 1989-90. *Advance Data*. National Center for Health Statistics. U.S. Department of Health and Human Services, Hyattsville, MD.

Nguyen QH, Kim YA, Schwartz RA, et al. July 1994. Management of acne vulgaris. *American Family Physician* 50 (1): 89-96.

Paller AS, Abel EA, Frieden IJ. 1992. Dermatologic problems. In *Comprehensive Adolescent Health Care*. Editors: Friedman SB, Fisher M, and Schonberg SK, 584-64. St. Louis, MO: Quality Medical Publishing, Inc.

Taylor MB. June 1991. Treatment of acne vulgaris. *Postgraduate Medicine* 89 (8): 40-7.

Tolman EL. 1992. *Acne and Acneiform Dermatoses*. In: *Dermatology, 3rd Edition*. Philadelphia PA: W.B. Saunders Company.

Vernon HJ and Lane AT. 1992. Skin disorders. In *Textbook of Adolescent Medicine*. Editors: McAnarney ER, Kreipe RE, Orr DP, and Comerci GD, 272-82. Philadelphia, PA: W.B. Saunders Company.

Weston WL and Lane AT. 1991. Acne. In *Color Textbook of Pediatric Dermatology*. 15-25. St. Louis, MO: Mosby-Year Book, Inc.

RECOMMENDED QUALITY INDICATORS FOR ACNE

The following indicators apply to men and women age 18 and older who have acne. These indicators were endorsed by a prior panel and reviewed but not rated by the current panel.

Indicator	Quality of Evidence	Literature	Benefits	Comments
Diagnosis				
1. For patients presenting with a chief complaint of acne, the following history should be documented in their chart: a. location of lesions (back, face, neck, chest), b. previous treatments, and c. medications and drug use.	III	Glassman, et al., 1992; Vernon and Lane, 1992	Improve acne; decrease psychological effects of acne; decrease potential physical scarring.	An adequate history is necessary to determine any potential causes or exacerbating factors of the acne and to document severity and response to treatments.
Treatment				
2. If oral antibiotics are prescribed, papules and/or pustules must be present.	III	Vernon and Lane, 1992; Glassman et al., 1993; Weston and Lane, 1992	Improve acne; decrease psychological effects of acne; decrease potential physical scarring.	If only comedones are present, antibiotics should not be prescribed since they are not effective for comedones and have potential toxicities.
3. If isotretinoin is prescribed, there must be documentation of cysts and/or nodules.	III	Vernon and Lane, 1992; Glassman et al., 1993; Weston and Lane, 1992; Nguyen, 1994	Improve acne; decrease psychological effects of acne; decrease potential physical scarring.	Isotretinoin has potential for liver toxicity. Its use should be restricted to those with severe, recalcitrant nodulocystic acne.
Follow-up				
4. If isotretinoin is prescribed, monthly liver function tests should be performed, for three months.	III	Glassman et al., 1993	Prevent liver disease.	Isotretinoin has the potential effects on the liver such as toxicity or failure.

Quality of Evidence Codes

I	RCT
II-1	Nonrandomized controlled trials
II-2	Cohort or case analysis
II-3	Multiple time series
III	Opinions or descriptive studies

35

2. ALCOHOL DEPENDENCE[1]

Patricia Bellas, MD

We relied on four main sources to construct quality indicators for problems related to consumption of alcohol. Three of these sources are reports of federally sponsored task forces: the United States Preventive Services Task Force (USPSTF), the Institute of Medicine (IOM), and the National Institutes of Health (NIH), and the fourth main source is a review article by Fleming (1993). Where these core references cited studies to support individual indicators, we have referenced the original source. In addition to a hand search of bibliographies, a targeted MEDLINE search for additional English language review articles published from 1995 to 1997 was performed.

IMPORTANCE

Alcohol is consumed by over half of all American adults. It is estimated that up to 20 percent of patients seen in primary care settings satisfy diagnostic criteria for alcohol abuse or dependence (Allen et al., 1995). Alcohol dependence can be associated with a number of medical problems, including alcohol withdrawal syndrome, psychosis, hepatitis, cirrhosis, pancreatitis, thiamine deficiency, neuropathy, dementia, and cardiomyopathy. Table 2.1 shows the reported prevalence of alcohol abuse and dependence from large community surveys using structured interviews.

---

[1] This chapter is a revision of one written for an earlier project on quality of care for women and children (Q1). The expert panel for the current project was asked to review all of the indicators, but only rated new or revised indicators.

Table 2.1

Prevalence of Alcohol Abuse and Dependence, by Age and Gender

Age Group	Men	Women
18-29 years	17-24%	4-10%
30-44 years	11-14%	2-4%
45-64 years	6-8%	1-2%
Over 65	1-3%	<1%

Source: USPSTF, 1996.

Although approximately ten percent of all users meet criteria for dependence, many "problem drinkers" have medical and social problems that can be attributed to alcohol use without true dependence. This condition is often referred to as alcohol abuse or harmful drinking. In addition, many drinkers are at risk for future problems due to regular or binge drinking (also known as "hazardous or problem drinking"). These non-dependent heavy drinkers account for the majority of alcohol-related morbidity and mortality in the general population. Daily heavy alcohol consumption has been associated with an increase in blood pressure, risk of cirrhosis, hemorrhagic stroke, and cancers of the oropharynx, larynx, esophagus, and liver (USPSTF, 1996). Observational studies have found an increase in all-cause mortality beginning at four drinks per day in men and more than two drinks per day in women (USPSTF, 1996; Fuchs et al., 1995).

Nearly one half of the more than 100,000 annual deaths attributed to alcohol are due to injuries, including traffic fatalities, fires, drownings, homicides, and suicides. In 1992, 45 percent of traffic fatalities were related to alcohol (Madden and Cole, 1995), and nearly half of all trauma beds were occupied by patients who were injured while under the influence of alcohol (Gentilello et al., 1995). The far-reaching social consequences of problem drinking are significant. Those who abuse alcohol have a higher risk of divorce, depression, suicide, domestic violence, unemployment, and poverty. Intoxication may lead to unsafe sexual behavior and its sequelae. Children are at risk for an array of psychosocial problems related to alcohol abuse of their parents (USPSTF, 1996).

SCREENING

The purpose of screening may be two-fold: to identify both regular or binge drinkers, and those who already have experienced the consequences of excessive alcohol abuse or who are dependent on alcohol (see definition below). Early detection and intervention may reduce ongoing medical and social problems due to drinking and reduce future risks from excessive alcohol use (USPSTF, 1996). The American Psychiatric Association (APA) has identified the following components as required for definitions of alcohol *dependence*:

1. regular or binge use;

2. tolerance of psychoactive effects, and/or

3. physical dependence; and

4. a pattern of compulsive use with or without interference with social function.

The APA (1994) defines alcohol *abuse* as a social disorder distinct from dependence in that there is no tolerance or pattern of compulsive use, but only harmful social, occupational, psychological, physical, or legal consequences of repeated use. Accurately assessing patients for drinking problems may be difficult. The diagnostic standard is an in-depth, structured interview. Routine measures of biochemical markers such as gamma-glutamyl transferase are probably less sensitive and certainly less specific than clinical history in detecting dependence and abuse (Hoeksema and de Bock, 1993; USPSTF, 1996).

Many physicians are unaware of their patients' problem or hazardous alcohol use. Primary care providers should ascertain regular or binge use by asking patients about the quantity and frequency of their alcohol consumption (Indicator 1). This "regular or binge use of alcohol" is usually defined as more than two drinks per day, 11 drinks per week, or five drinks in any one day in the last month (a "drink" is generally defined in ethanol equivalents, with one ounce representing one to two drinks). In addition, all patients hospitalized for trauma, hepatitis, pancreatitis, or gastrointestinal bleeding should be screened at least once during their hospital stay (Indicator 2). Although estimates of the sensitivity of direct questioning are as much as 50 percent lower than that of self-administered questionnaires, direct questioning can serve as a screen for further evaluation (Fleming, 1993; Cyr and Wartman, 1988; NIH, 1993).

Many validated screening questionnaires for alcohol abuse and dependence have been developed that focus on consequences of drinking and perceptions of drinking behavior. The Michigan Alcoholism Screening Test (MAST) reportedly has a sensitivity between 84 and 100 percent and a specificity between 87 and 95 percent for alcohol abuse or dependence (Cyr, 1988). Because the MAST is a lengthy questionnaire, it is not appropriate as a brief screen. Several shorter versions of the MAST, such as the Short MAST (or SMAST), have been proposed, but may be less sensitive and specific (Selzer et al., 1975). The much shorter and more widely used CAGE has only four items and an estimated sensitivity and specificity for alcohol abuse or dependence of 74 to 89 percent and 79 to 95 percent, respectively. However, it is less sensitive for detecting early problem or heavy drinking (USPSTF, 1996). Limitations to the MAST and CAGE as screening instruments are their emphasis on dependence rather than on early problem drinking, and their failure to distinguish between current and lifetime problems. Sensitivity and specificity also are influenced by the "cut score" that is used to define a positive screen (e.g., using one versus two positive responses on the CAGE). Many other questionnaires are available, including the Self-Administered Alcoholism Screening Test (SAAST) (Swenson and Morse, 1975); the Alcohol Use Disorder Identification (AUDIT) (Babor and Grant, 1989); and the Health Screening Survey (HSS) (Fleming and Barry, 1991). In addition, modifications have been made to existing questionnaires for application to special populations, as with the Adolescent Drinking Index (Allen et al., 1995) for young people and the MAST-G for the elderly. These questionnaires may help the clinician better assess the likelihood of problem or binge drinking. Positive responses should be followed with a more detailed interview with the patient or family members to confirm alcohol abuse or dependence (USPSTF, 1996) (Indicator 3).

TREATMENT

Regular or binge drinkers who do not meet criteria for dependence can benefit from medical intervention (Indicator 4). There have been many clinical trials of the effect of brief office counseling on heavy or problem drinkers. Brief interventions are time-limited strategies that directly focus on reducing alcohol use in the nondependent drinker. These interventions include assessment and direct feedback, contracting and goal setting, behavioral modification techniques, and the use of written self-help materials (NIH, 1993). Treatment goals are usually controlled, moderate drinking instead of abstinence (Wilk et al., 1997). Optimal session length and number of visits have not been established. A meta-analysis by Wilk et al. (1997) reviewed 12 randomized controlled trials (RCTs) of brief counseling. Eligible subjects were heavy drinkers who consumed between 15 to 35 drinks per week. Most of the trials excluded dependent drinkers. Heavy drinkers receiving the brief intervention were almost twice as likely to moderate their drinking for six to 12 months after the intervention compared with the control group (Wilk et al., 1997). In addition, a recently published study (Fleming et al., 1997) of brief physician advice to reduce alcohol describes a significant reduction in seven day alcohol use, episodes of binge drinking, and a two-fold reduction in hospital days in intervention drinkers (men who drank more than 14 drinks a week and women who drank more than 11 drinks a week).

Treatment of alcohol dependence is usually divided into three phases:

1. detoxification;
2. treatment and rehabilitation; and
3. relapse prevention.

The IOM reviewed more than 60 controlled trials evaluating specific treatments in one or another of these three phases, including inpatient and outpatient rehabilitation, mutual help groups, supportive psychotherapy, disulfuram, benzodiazapines, and aversion therapy. Although various treatment modalities have clinical trial support when compared with no treatment at all, the IOM concluded that there was insufficient evidence to recommend any one modality over another. The

Secretary's Eighth Special Report to Congress on Alcohol and Health (NIH, 1993) came to a similar conclusion, although the authors emphasized the need to tailor the treatment to the individual patient. In particular, they noted a RCT of 200 women in which subjects assigned to a female gender versus a mixed male/female gender treatment group remained in treatment longer and had higher rates of program completion (Dahlgren and Willander, 1989). We propose simply that the medical record should indicate referral for one of the above-mentioned treatment modalities for alcohol-dependent patients (Indicator 5).

FOLLOW-UP

For alcohol-dependent patients, the core references agree that relapse prevention is the most difficult and least evaluated phase of treatment. Most of the predictors of relapse (psychosocial stressors, mood state, concomitant psychiatric diagnoses) are difficult to modify. Two randomized trials compared aftercare protocols and found no difference in relapse rates by protocol, but did find that those who did not drop out relapsed less often. The outcome could be a result of self-selection of motivated patients. Observational trials of perhaps the most widely known aftercare program, Alcoholics Anonymous (AA), have found that patients who subscribe to the "12-Step" AA philosophy relapse less often (Gilbert, 1991; Cross, 1990), but these results could also be due to patient self-selection. A trial of randomized court-mandated AA meeting attendance versus no treatment showed no long-term difference in the likelihood of relapse (Brandsma et al., 1980). Given this weak evidence, we cannot recommend a quality indicator requiring any particular aftercare program.

For nondependent drinkers, there are no clear trials evaluating follow-up separately from brief interventions. It also appears that screening for alcohol use or questioning patients regarding their intake level may have a treatment effect, leading to an overall reduction in consumption (Fleming, 1997). We will follow Fleming's recommendation that providers review all regular or binge drinkers' alcohol consumption at subsequent visits (Fleming, 1993) (Indicator 6).

REFERENCES

Allen J, Maisto S, and Connors G. 1995. Self-report screening tests for alcohol problems in primary care. *Archives of Internal Medicine* 155: 1726-1730.

Babor TF and Grant M. 1989. From clinical research to secondary prevention: International collaboration in the development of the alcohol use disorders identification test (AUDIT). *International Perspectives* 13 (4): 371-4.

Brandsma JM, Maultsby MC, and Welsh RJ. 1980. *Outpatient treatment of alcoholism: A review and comparative study*. Baltimore, MD: Univ. Part. Press.

Committee of the Institute of Medicine, Division of Mental Health and Behavioral Medicine. 1990. *Broadening the Base of Treatment for Alcohol Problems*. Washington, DC: National Academy Press.

Cross GM, CW Morgan, AJ Mooney, et al. March 1990. Alcoholism treatment: A ten-year follow-up study. *Alcoholism: Clinical and Experimental Research* 14 (2): 169-73.

Cyr MG, and SA Wartman. 1 January 1988. The effectiveness of routine screening questions in the detection of alcoholism. *Journal of the American Medical Association* 259 (1): 51-4.

Dahlgren L and A Willander. July 1989. Are special treatment facilities for female alcoholics needed? A controlled 2-year follow-up study form a specialized female unit (EWA) versus a mixed male/female treatment facility. *Alcoholism: Clinical and Experimental Research* 13 (4): 499-504.

Fleming MF. 1993. Screening and brief intervention for alcohol disorders. *Journal of Family Practice* 37 (3): 231-4.

Fleming M, et al. 1997. Brief physician advice for problem alcohol drinkers. A randomized controlled trial in community-based primary care practices. *Journal of the American Medical Association* 277 (13): 1039-45.

Fleming MF, and KL Barry. 1991. The effectiveness of alcoholism screening in an ambulatory care setting. *Journal of Studies on Alcohol* 52 (1): 33-6.

Fuchs CS, MJ Stampfer, GA Colditz, et al. 11 May 1995. Alcohol consumption and mortality among women. *New England Journal of Medicine* 322 (2): 95-9.

Gentilello L, et al. 1995. Alcohol interventions in trauma centers. *Journal of the American Medical Association* 274 (73): 1043-8.

Gilbert FS. 1991. Development of a "steps questionnaire". *Journal of Studies on Alcohol* 52 (4): 353-60.

Hoeksema HL, and GH de Bock. The value of laboratory tests for the screening and recognition of alcohol abuse in primary care patients. *Journal of Family Practice* 37 (3): 268-76.

Madden C, and Cole T. 1995. Emergency intervention to break the cycle of drunken driving and recurrent injury. *Annals of Emergency Medicine* 26: 177-179.

National Institutes of Health. September 1993. Eighth Special Report to the U.S. Congress on Alcohol and Health -- from the Secretary of Health and Human Services. *U.S. Department of Health and Human Services, Washington, D.C.*

Selzer ML, A Vinokur, and L van Rooijen. 1975. A self-administered short Michigan Alcoholism Screening Test (SMAST). *Journal of Studies on Alcohol* 36 (1): 117-26.

Swenson WM, and RM Morse. April 1975. The use of a self-administered alcoholism screening test (SAAST) in a medical center. *Mayo Clinic Proceedings* 50: 204-8.

US Preventative Services Task Force. 1996. *Guide to Clinical Preventative Services, 2nd ed.* Baltimore: Williams & Wilkins.

Wilk A, Jensen N, and Havighurst T. 1997. Meta-analysis of randomized control trials addressing brief interventions in heavy alcohol drinkers. *Journal of General Internal Medicine* 12: 274-283.

RECOMMENDED QUALITY INDICATORS FOR ALCOHOL DEPENDENCE

The following indicators apply to men and women age 18 and older. Only the indicators in bold type were rated by this panel; the remaining indicators were endorsed by a prior panel.

Indicator	Quality of Evidence	Literature	Benefits	Comments
Screening				
1. All new patients or those receiving a routine history and physical should be screened[2] for problem drinking. This assessment of pattern of alcohol use should include at least one of the following: • Quantity (e.g., drinks per day); • Binge drinking (e.g., more than 5 drinks in a day in the last month).	II-III	Fleming 1993; USPSTF, 1996; NIH, 1993.	Reduce alcohol-associated pathology.[1]	Diagnosis of alcohol dependence requires regular or binge use. Increased detection of problem drinkers may lead to counseling, detoxification, and ultimately cessation of alcohol intake. In addition, screening may in itself have an intervention effect on those problem drinkers who are not dependent and early identification of those at risk for problem drinking may alter their pattern of drinking with brief counseling intervention.
2. All patients hospitalized with the following conditions should be screened[2] for problem drinking at least once during their hospital stay. a. trauma; b. hepatitis; c. pancreatitis; d. gastrointestinal bleeding.	III	Madden & Cole, 1996; NIH, 1993; Gentilello, 1995	Reduce alcohol-associated pathology.[1]	Hospitalized patients may have a higher prevalence of problem drinking, which frequently goes undetected. There is a high prevalence of problem drinking in those who present with trauma. There is good evidence that interventions to treat both dependent and nondependent drinkers may lead to a reduction in alcohol consumption and may at least reduce hospital day utilization.
Diagnosis				
3. The record should indicate more detailed screening for dependence, tolerance of psychoactive effects, loss of control, and consequences of use with a validated screening questionnaire (examples include but are not confined to the CAGE, MAST, HSS, AUDIT, SAAST, and SMAST), if the medical record indicates the patient is a regular or binge drinker.[3]	II	Fleming, 1993; Babor & Grant, 1989; Swenson & Morse, 1975; Selzer et al, 1975; USPSTF, 1996	Reduce alcohol-associated pathology.[1]	Diagnosis of alcohol dependence requires evidence of dependence, loss of control, and negative consequences. Sensitivity and specificity of questionnaires are 49-100% and 75-95%, respectively. These questionnaires are screening tools for more severe alcohol problems and should be validated by more in-depth interview or referral. Increased detection of alcohol dependence may lead to detoxification, treatment, and cessation.

Indicator	Quality of Evidence	Literature	Benefits	Comments
Treatment				
4. Regular or binge drinkers[3] should be advised to decrease their drinking.	I	Fleming et al., 1997; Wilk et al., 1997; USPSTF, 1996; NIH, 1993	Reduce alcohol-associated pathology.[1]	There is good evidence that brief counseling can reduce alcohol consumption in problem drinkers. In addition, it may lead to reduced utilization of hospital days.
5. Patients diagnosed with alcohol dependence should be referred for further treatment to at least one of the following: • inpatient rehabilitation program; • outpatient rehabilitation program; • mutual help group (e.g., AA); • substance abuse counseling; • aversion therapy.	I	NIH, 1993	Reduce alcohol-associated pathology.[1]	Multiple clinical trials show effectiveness of various treatment modalities, though no one treatment has consistently been demonstrated to be most effective.
Follow-up				
6. Providers should reassess the alcohol intake of patients who report regular or binge drinking[3] at the next routine health visit.	III	Fleming, 1993; Fleming et al., 1997	Reduce alcohol-associated pathology.[1]	Prevention of relapse is the most difficult phase of treatment. Experts recommend frequent reassessment to evaluate success of intervention. It appears that simply querying persons regarding their alcohol intake may lead to a reduction in consumption.

Definitions and Examples

[1] Alcohol associated pathology includes: cirrhosis, pancreatitis, gastrointestinal bleeding, cardiomyopathy, assault, suicide, and motor vehicle accidents. Cirrhosis, cardiomyopathy, and pancreatitis may cause chronic decreases in health-related quality of life due to vomiting, ascites, abdominal pain, bleeding, shortness of breath and may eventually result in mortality. Gastrointestinal bleeding has a short-term mortality risk as well as a chronic impact on health-related quality of life due to anemia and other complications. Motor vehicle accidents and assaults may result in chronic disability from injuries and death. The health-related quality of life of persons other than the patient may also be affected. Liver disease and alcohol-related trauma are more common in women.

[2] Screening should consist of an assessment of alcohol use to include at least one of the following: quantity (e.g., drinks per day) and/or binge drinking (e.g., more than 5 drinks in a day in the last month).

[3] Regular or binge drinking:

a. Patient drinks more than 2 drinks each day;

b. Patient drinks more than 14 drinks per week;

c. Patient drank more than 5 drinks in a day in the last month.

Quality of Evidence Codes

I	RCT
II-1	Nonrandomized controlled trials
II-2	Cohort or case analysis
II-3	Multiple time series
III	Opinions or descriptive studies

47

3. ALLERGIC RHINITIS[1]

Eve A. Kerr, MD, MPH

We conducted a MEDLINE search of review articles on rhinitis between the years of 1990-1997 and selected articles pertaining to allergic rhinitis. We also performed a MEDLINE search of randomized controlled trials on allergic rhinitis patients between January 1990 and May 1997. Identified studies tended to use investigative therapies or compare new formulations of nasal steroids or antihistamines to previously used formulations. Since the general approach to treatment of allergic rhinitis is currently not controversial, these were not separately reviewed.

IMPORTANCE

Allergic rhinitis ranks thirteenth among the principal diagnoses rendered by physicians, based on the 1991 National Ambulatory Medical Care Survey (National Center for Health Statistics [NCHS], 1994c), accounting for over 11 million visits to the physician in that year. In fact, allergic rhinitis affects about 20 percent of the American population (Bernstein, 1993). Allergic rhinitis results in a limitation of daily activities, and time lost from school and work (Bernstein, 1993). Complications of allergic rhinitis include serous otitis media (especially in children) and bacterial sinusitis (Kaliner and Lemanske, 1992).

DIAGNOSIS

The history is the fundamental diagnostic tool in allergic rhinitis. Symptoms include sneezing, itching of the nose, eyes, palate or pharynx, nasal stuffiness, rhinorrhea and post-nasal drip (Kaliner and Lemanske, 1992). A careful history of allergen exposure may reveal exacerbating antigens (Indicator 1). In addition, one should inquire as

---

[1] This chapter is a revision of one written for an earlier project on quality of care for women and children (Q1). The expert panel for the current project was asked to review all of the indicators, but only rated new or revised indicators.

to use of medications, especially nose drops or sprays (Indicator 2).
On physical exam, pale, edematous nasal turbinates and clear secretions
are characteristic. Temperature elevation, purulent nasal discharge, or
cervical adenopathy should indicate the possibility of sinusitis,
otitis, pharyngitis, or bronchitis (Kaliner and Lemanske, 1992).

Selected skin testing with appropriate allergens is the least time-
consuming and expensive diagnostic modality when confirmation of
allergen sensitivity is necessary. Specific serum IgE determinations,
although more expensive, may also be employed. Results need to be
interpreted in the context of the patient's history. Total IgE levels
and peripheral eosinophil counts are neither sensitive nor specific.
Nasal smears for eosinophils are not specific for allergic rhinitis
(Kaliner and Lemanske, 1992).

TREATMENT

Treatment rests with allergen avoidance, use of pharmaceutical
agents and, when indicated, immunotherapy. Careful counseling regarding
allergen avoidance is the mainstay of treatment (Naclerio, 1991)
(Indicator 3). If it is unclear which allergen causes moderate to
severe symptoms, skin testing should be performed (Naclerio, 1991). In
addition, oral antihistamines (first- or second-generation H1-
antagonistic drugs) are appropriate first-line agents, and decrease
local and systemic symptoms of allergic rhinitis (Kaliner and Lemanske,
1992; Bernstein, 1993).

Antihistamines may also be used in combination with decongestants
for symptomatic relief. Topical nasal decongestants should be used for
a maximum of four days (Indicator 4). Nasal cromolyn sodium can be
useful as a single agent, but requires regular, frequent dosing for
optimal benefit (Bernstein, 1993). Topical nasal corticosteroids are
effective in treating allergic rhinitis, but have no effect on ocular
symptoms. Local burning, irritation, epistaxis and, very rarely, nasal
septal perforation, are the reported side effects. Currently, both
antihistamines and topical steroids have been advocated as first-line
agents (Kaliner and Lemanske, 1992)(Indicator 3).

Immunotherapy should be considered if symptoms are present more than a few weeks of the year and medication and avoidance measures are ineffective (Naclerio, 1991). Allergy injections are reported to reduce symptoms in more than 90 percent of patients (Bernstein, 1993). Reported toxicities, although uncommon, include hives, asthma and hypotension. The duration of treatment for optimal effect and maintenance of benefits after treatment cessation is unclear (Creticos, 1992).

REFERENCES

Bernstein, and Jonathan A. 1 May 1993. Allergic rhinitis: Helping patients lead an unrestricted life. *Postgraduate Medicine* 93 (6): 124-32.

Creticos, and Peter S. 25 November 1992. Immunotherapy with allergens. *Journal of the American Medical Association* 268 (20): 2834-9.

Kaliner, Michael, Lemanske, and Robert. 25 November 1992. Rhinitis and asthma. *Journal of the American Medical Association* 268 (20): 2807-29.

Naclerio, and Robert M. 19 September 1991. Allergic rhinitis. *New England Journal of Medicine* 325 (12): 860-9.

National Center for Health Statistics. 1994. *National Ambulatory Medical Care Survey: 1991 summary*. U.S. Department of Health and Human Services, Hyattsville, MD.

RECOMMENDED QUALITY INDICATORS FOR ALLERGIC RHINITIS

The following indicators apply to men and women age 18 and older. These indicators were endorsed by a prior panel and reviewed but not rated by the current panel.

Indicator	Quality of evidence	Literature	Benefits	Comments
Diagnosis				
1. If a diagnosis of allergic rhinitis is made, the search for a specific allergen by history should be documented in the chart (for initial history).	III	Kaliner and Lemanske, 1992, Naclerio, 1990	Decrease nasal congestion, rhinorrhea, and itching.	Allergen avoidance is the mainstay of treatment.
2. If a diagnosis of allergic rhinitis is made, history should include whether the patient uses any topical nasal decongestants.	III	Bernstein, 1993	Decrease nasal congestion, rhinorrhea, and itching.	Chronic use of topical nasal decongestants can cause rhinitis medicamentosa and may mimic allergic rhinitis.
Treatment				
3. Treatment for allergic rhinitis should include at least one of the following: • allergen avoidance counseling; • antihistamines; • nasal steroids; • nasal cromolyn.	I-III	Naclerio, 1991; Kaliner and Lemanske, 1992	Decrease nasal congestion, rhinorrhea, and itching.	These have proven efficacy in allergic rhinitis.
4. If topical nasal decongestants are prescribed for patients with allergic rhinitis, duration of treatment should be for no longer than 4 days.	II	Stanford et al., 1992; Barker, 1991	Decrease nasal congestion, rhinorrhea, and itching.	Longer treatment may cause rebound congestion.

Quality of Evidence Codes

I	RCT
II-1	Nonrandomized controlled trials
II-2	Cohort or case analysis
II-3	Multiple time series
III	Opinions or descriptive studies

53

4. BENIGN PROSTATIC HYPERPLASIA (BPH)

Steven Asch MD, MPH, and John Roland Franklin, MD

The AHCPR *Clinical Practice Guideline for Benign Prostatic Hyperplasia: Diagnosis and Treatment* (1994) was the starting point for this review. We also performed a MEDLINE literature search and hand checked bibliographies for more recent reviews.

IMPORTANCE

Prostatic hyperplasia, symptoms of prostatism, urodynamic presence of obstruction, and bladder muscle or detrusor response to obstruction interact in a symptom complex commonly referred to as benign prostatic hyperplasia (BPH). BPH obstructing the bladder neck initially causes bladder detrusor muscle hypertrophy. Eventually, the detrusor muscle decompensates, resulting in collagen deposits between the smooth muscles, poor bladder tone, and diverticula formation. Transmission of increased bladder pressures can cause upper tract injury (dilatation or hydronephrosis of ureters and renal pelvis, and renal insufficiency). Over seven percent of patients with BPH will have evidence of hydronephrosis by intravenous pyelography prior to surgery. Thirty-three percent of these patients had associated renal insufficiency (McConnell, 1994).

BPH is the most common benign tumor in the aging male population. Fifty percent of 60 year old males have been observed to have histological evidence of prostatic hyperplasia, increasing to 90 percent for men at 85 years. Half of the men with histologic evidence of hyperplasia will develop macroscopic enlargement of the prostate gland, and half of these men will develop clinical symptoms of prostatism (Isaacs, 1990). Approximately one in every four men in the United States will be treated for symptoms of prostatism by age 80 (Barry, 1997). Although the introduction of effective pharmacotherapies has decreased the frequency of transurethral prostatectomies (TURPs) (Holtgrewe, 1989; Graves, 1995), it remains one of the most commonly performed major operations. In 1993, Medicare paid for approximately 256,000 TURPs in the United States (Graves, 1995). The national annual cost of treating patients with BPH is about $4 billion (Chirikos, 1996).

SCREENING

Screening of asymptomatic men for prostatic hyperplasia is not recommended. While silent prostatism (anatomic hyperplasia and urodynamic evidence of obstruction without symptoms of prostatism) has been observed, it is rare and no treatment is usually recommended.

DIAGNOSIS

The focal point in the diagnosis of BPH is the presence of recent symptoms of prostatism. Prostatism refers to a complex of symptoms that may be either obstructive, irritative, or both. These include urinary frequency, nocturia, urgency, urge incontinence, post void dribbling, hesitancy, weak stream, incomplete emptying, double voiding, and straining to urinate. Patients may present with any combination of these symptoms and some patients delay presentation until symptoms became intolerable. As a result, many experts recommend that providers ask all men over 50 about symptoms of prostatism (Indicator 1) (Chute, 1993; Garraway, 1991; Gilman, 1994). Although no studies have evaluated the efficacy of such symptom screening practices, proponents argue that they are warranted due to the high prevalence of prostatism and the availability of low risk therapy.

If the patient has recent symptoms of prostatism, the AHCPR Guideline recommends the use of the American Urological Association Symptom Index (AUASI) to categorize the severity of the symptoms (McConnell, 1994). The AUASI consists of seven items, each with a scale of 0 to 5 points, yielding a total score range of 0 to 35. The seven item set was chosen for its high internal validity (Cronbach's alpha = 0.85) and high test-retest reliability (r = 0.93) (Barry, 1992). Scores fall into three severity groupings: mild (scores 0 to 7), moderate (8 to 19), and severe (20 to 35). This symptom index was found to discriminate well between patients with and without BPH (area under the receiver operating curve = .85). There was high correlation (r > .85) with two previous symptom scales (Madsen, 1983; Boyarsky, 1976) as well

56

with patients' global rating of urinary difficulties (r = 0.78.). In a community-based study of 2115 men with prostatism, eight percent had none of the AUASI symptoms, 58 percent had mild symptoms (AUASI 1-7) and 33 percent had moderate to severe symptoms (AUASI 8-35) (Girman, 1994). Patients with moderate to severe symptoms (determined by AUASI) reported levels of bother and interference with daily activity four to six times higher than patients with mild symptoms. Without the AUASI, a patient's global characterization of symptoms and degree of bother may be sufficient to make a diagnosis of BPH and to plan treatment (Barry, 1992). In our proposed indicator, we allow either approach to grading the severity of symptomotology (Indicator 2) (McConnell, 1994; SCIL, 1993).

Symptoms of prostatism can result from a wide variety of other conditions, and one of the provider's primary tasks during initial evaluation is to rule out such conditions. These include: urinary tract infections, urolithiasis, urethral stricture (often from previous urethral instrumentation), bladder cancer, diabetes, Parkinson's disease, and stroke. As a result, patients with symptoms of prostatism should have at least a focused medical and surgical history, with attention placed on excluding the foregoing diseases or conditions (McConnell, 1994). We propose that the medical record document the presence or absence of at least one of the following conditions at initial evaluation of prostatism: Parkinson's disease, diabetes, stroke, and history of urethral instrumentation (Indicator 3).

The AHCPR guideline recommends that the physical examination of a patient with new symptoms of prostatism include a digital rectal examination (DRE) (McConnell, 1994) (Indicator 4), although the supporting evidence is not strong. A DRE helps the provider evaluate prostatic hypertrophy and detect prostatic malignancy. While an enlarged prostate does confirm the diagnosis of BPH, the size of the prostate does not correlate with symptom severity, degree of obstruction or treatment outcome (Roehrborn, 1986; Simonsen, 1987). DRE has a low specificity (26 to 34%) and sensitivity (33%) for detecting prostate cancer.

AHCPR determined that other tests to document obstructions, including urinary flow rate, post void residual urine measurement (PVR), and pressure-flow urodynamic studies, can only be considered optional in the initial evaluation of BPH. On the other hand, some Peer Review Organizations require PVR measurement to document urinary retention before authorizing prostatectomy. PVR can be ascertained either through ultrasound or catheterization, but studies have questioned the reproducibility of either method (Birch, 1988; Bruskewitz, 1982). Observational data indicate that urodynamic studies are the best predictors of surgical outcome, while post void residual measurement is less predictive (Griffiths, 1970; Jensen, 1988c; Andersen, 1982). We have included an indicator for quantification of urinary obstruction by uroflowometry, PVR, or pressure flow studies (Indicator 5).

Urine analysis and serum creatinine measurement are recommended by AHCPR (Indicator 6). The urine analysis is important in distinguishing urinary tract infection and bladder cancer from BPH (Holtgrewe, 1962; Melchior, 1974). Serum creatinine is essential in evaluating renal insufficiency. Beyond indentifying a relatively common BPH complication, renal insufficiency is also a strong predictor of mortality in patients following surgical treatment for BPH (Meburst, 1989; McConnell, 1994).

Prostatic specific antigen (PSA) is considered an optional test by AHCPR. Combined with the DRE, PSA increases the detection of prostate cancer over DRE alone. However, PSA was not recommended because there is: (1) significant overlap in PSA values between men with BPH and men with pathologically organ-confined cancer; (2) a lack of consensus concerning the optimal evaluation of minimally elevated PSA; and, (3) a lack of evidence showing that PSA testing reduces the morbidity or mortality of men with prostatic disease. Moreover, certain therapies, procedures, and complications for BPH affect PSA levels. Finasteride reduces PSA levels by approximately 50 percent, while prostatic biopsies, surgery, urethrocystoscopy and inflamatory processes (urinary tract infection, urinary retention, prostatitis) elevate PSA levels. On the other hand, DRE does not significantly elevate serum PSA levels (Chybowski, 1992). Strategies to overcome these difficulties have included assessing PSA velocity, PSA density, age adjusted PSA levels, race specific PSA levels, and the ratio of free and total PSA levels; though none have been completely successful (Carter, 1992; Benson, 1992). In the absence of further data, we do not recommend an indicator requiring PSA testing for patients suspected of having BPH.

TREATMENT

The AHCPR guideline recommends that the AUASI categories guide therapy. Patients with mild symptoms (AUASI ≤ 7) do not benefit from treatment but should be followed carefully. One recent study showed that 58 percent of patients with mild symptoms had progressed to moderate or severe symptoms after four years, and ten percent had undergone surgery (Barry, 1997). Additionally, certain prescription and non-prescription drugs taken by the patient may have anticholinergic properties that can impair bladder contractility, or may have sympathomimetic properties that can increase bladder outflow resistance. The AHCPR guideline recommends that BPH patients on such drugs be offered discontinuation (Indicator 7).

For patients with moderate disease, medical therapies for BPH include: alpha blocker therapy (terazosin, dotazosin and prazosin) to reduce prostatic tone, and finasteride therapy to gradually reduce prostatic size. An RCT comparing finasteride, finasteride and teraszosin, terazosin, and placebo found that finasteride was no better than placebo at reducing symptoms (Lepor, 1995; Lepor, 1996). Moreover, finasteride combined with terazosin did not improve symptom scores when compared to terazosin alone. Subgroup analysis suggests that the efficacy of finasteride may be confined to patients with prostate sizes greater than 50 grams. For that reason our proposed indicator states that patients with moderate disease be offered alpha 1 blockers first (Indicator 8).

Surgical treatment options include: transurethral incision of the prostate (TUIP), transurethral resection of the prostate (TURP), and open prostatectomy. The few randomized studies that have been conducted on the effect of these three options on either direct (symptom relief, complications) or indirect (PVR, urinary flow rate) outcomes show the treatments to be equivalent. However, they all have been proven superior to watchful waiting in the short term (see Table 4.1) (McConnell, 1994). In general, TUIP is appropriate for prostates less than 30 grams in size, and open prostatectomies are reserved for large prostates (greater than 60 grams). Balloon dilation has failed to prove efficacious in the long-term when compared with TURP and is not recommended. The AHCPR panel recommended surgical therapy when medical therapy has failed to reduce moderate symptoms (Indicator 10a), or when complications of urinary retention develop, such as renal failure (Indicator 9), recurrent UTIs (Indicator 10b), or bladder stones (Indicator 10c).

FOLLOW-UP

As most treatment for BPH aims to reduce symptoms, providers must reassess symptoms of prostatism in order to evaluate the effectiveness of interventions. For that reason, the AHCPR panel recommends that the providers administer the AUASI to all patients under therapy. We propose to allow more informal symptom follow-up as well (Indicator 11). If symptoms persist, primary bladder dysfunction may be the cause, and the guideline recommends urodynamic evaluation (Indicator 12) before any further intervention.

Table 4.1

Comparison of BPH Surgical Treatment Outcomes

Direct Treatment Outcomes	TUIP[1]	TURP[2]	Open Prostatectomy	Balloon Dilation	Watchful Waiting
Chance for improvement of symptoms (90% confidence interval)	78-83%	75-96%	94-99.8%	37-76%	31-55%
Degree of symptom improvement (percent reduction in symptom score)	73%	85%	79%	51%	Unknown
Morbidity/complications associated with surgical or medical treatment (90% confidence interval), about 20% or all complications assumed to be significant	2.2-33.3%	5.2-30.7%	7.0-42.7%	1.8-9.9%	1-5% complications from BPH[3] progression
Chance of dying within 30-90 days of treatment (90% confidence interval)	0.2-1.5%	0.5-3.3%	1.0-4.6%	0.7-9.8% (high-risk/elderly patients)	0.8% chance of death ≤90 days for 67 year old man
Risk of total urinary incontinence (90% confidence interval)	0.1-1.1%	0.7-1.4%	0.3-0.7%	Unknown	Incontinence associated with aging
Need for operative treatment for surgical complications in future (90% confidence interval)	1.3-2.7%	0.7-10.1%	0.6-14.1%	Unknown	0
Risk of impotence (90% confidence interval)	3.9-24.5%	3.3-34.8%	4.7-39.2%	No long-term followup available	About 2% of men age 67 and older become impotent each year
Risk of retrograde ejaculation (percent of patients)	6-55%	25-99%	36-95%	Unknown	0

61

Table 4.1 (Continued)

Direct Treatment Outcomes	TUIP[1]	TURP[2]	Open Surgery	Balloon Dilation	Watchful Waiting
Loss of work time (days)	7-21	7-21	21-28	4	1
Hospital stay (days)	1-3	3-5	5-10	1	0

Source: Adapted from McConnell, 1994, Attachment B.

[1] TUIP: Transurethral incision of the prostate

[2] TURP: Transurethral resection of the prostate

[3] BPH: Benign prostatic hyperplasia

REFERENCES

Andersen JT. 1982. Prostatism II. Detrusor hyperreflexiana and residual urine. Clinical and urodynamic aspects and the influence of surgery on the prostate. *Scandavian Journal of Urology and Nephrology* 16: 25-30.

Barry MJ, Fowler FJ Jr, Bin L, et al. 1997. The natural history of patients with binign prostatic hyperplasia as diagnosed by North American urologists. *Journal of Urology* 157: 10-15.

Birch NC, Hurst G, and Doyle PT. 1988. Serial residual volumes in men with prostatic hypertrophy. *British Journal of Urology* 62: 571-5.

Bruskewitz RC, Iversen P, and Madsen PO. 1982. Value of postvoid residual urine determination in evaluation of prostatism. *Urology* 20: 602-4.

Chirikos TN, et al. April 1996. Cost consequences of surveillance, medical management or surgery for benign prostatic hyperplasia. *Journal of Urology* 155 (4): 1311-1316.

Chute CG, Panser LA, Girman CJ, et al. The prevalence of prostatism: A population-based survey of urinary symptoms. *Journal of Urology* 150: 85-89.

Chybowski FM, Bergstralh EJ, and Oesterling JE. 1992. The effects of digital rectal examination on the serum prostate-specific concentration: results of a randomized study. *Journal of Urology* 148 (83-86):

Garraway, WM, et al. 24 August 1991. High prevalence of benign prostatic hypertrophy in the community. *Lancet* 338 (8765): 469-471.

Girman CJ, Epstein RS, Jacobsen SJ, et al. Natural history of prostatism: Impact of uninary symptoms on quality of life in 2115 ramdomly selected community men. *Urology* 44: 825-831.

Graves EJ. 1995. Detailed diagnosis and procedures, national hospital discharge survey, 1993. *Vital Health Statistics* 13 (122):

Griffiths HJ, and Castro J. 1970. An evaluation of the importance of residual urine. *British Journal of Radiology* 43: 409-13.

Jensen KM-E, Jorgensen JB, and Mogensen P. 3 1988. Urodynamics in prostatism III. Prognostics value of medium fill water cystometry. *Scandinavian Journal of Urology and Nephrology* Suppl (114): 78-83.

Lepor H. March 1995. Long-term efficacy and safety of terazosin in patients with benign prostatic hyperplasia. Terazosin Research Group. *Urology* 45 (3): 406-413.

Lepor H, et al. 22 August 1996. The efficacy of terazosin, finasteride, or both in benign prostatic hyperplasia. Veterans Affairs Cooperative Studies Benign Prostatic Hyperplasia Study Group. *New England Journal of Medicine* 335 (8): 533-539.

McConnell JD, Barry MJ, Bruskewitz RC, et al. February 1994. Benign Prostatic Hyperplasia: Diagnosis and treatment. *Clinical Practice Guidelines, Number 8. Agency for Health Care Policy and Research.* AHCPR Publication No. 94-0582. Rockville, MD; U.S. Department of Health and Human Services.

Roehrborn CG, Chinn HK, Fulgham PF, et al. 1986. The role of transabdomian ultrasound in the preoperative evaluation of patients with benign prostatic hypertrophy. *Journal of Urology* 135: 1190-3.

Simonsen O, Moller-Madsen B, Dorflinger T, et al. 1987. The significance of age on symptoms and urodynamic and cystolsecopic findings in benign prostatic hypertrophy. *Urological Research* 15: 355-8.

RECOMMENDED QUALITY INDICATORS FOR BENIGN PROSTATIC HYPERPLASIA (BPH)

The following indicators apply to men age 18 and older.

Indicator	Quality of Evidence	Literature	Benefits	Comments
Diagnosis				
1. Men age 50 and older who present for routine care should be asked at least once a year about recent symptoms of prostatism.	II	Chute, 1993; Garraway, 1991; Girman, 1994	Relieve symptoms by detecting and treating BPH.	No efficacy of BPH symptom screening has been established. However, the high prevalence of BPH and availability of low risk therapy warrants inquiry.
2. If the patient has recent symptoms of prostatism,[1] the provider should document one of the following on the same visit: • AUA symptom score; • How bothersome the patient considers the symptoms.	III	McConnell, 1994; SCIL, 1993	Relieve symptoms by detecting and treating BPH.	This index is recommended by the American Urologic Association and World Health Organization. Bothersome BPH is more likely to need treatment.
3. Patients with new recent symptoms of prostatism[1] should have the presence or absence of at least one of the following conditions documented: • Parkinson's disease; • Diabetes mellitus; • Stroke; • History of urethral instrumentation.	III	McConnell, 1994	Relieve symptoms by detecting and treating causes of prostatic symptoms other than BPH.	Urinary symptoms produced by these conditions require different therapeutic modalities. Previous TURP or urethral instrumentation may result in urethral stricture or bladder neck contraction.
4. Patients with new recent symptoms of prostatism[1] should be offered a digital rectal examination (DRE) on the same visit that the symptoms are noted, if they have not had a DRE in the past year.	III	McConnell, 1994	Relieve symptoms by detecting prostatic cancer.	Annual digital rectal examinations are recommended by the AUA and AHCPR. Trials have shown DRE detects cancer at earlier stages but does not reduce mortality.

65

Indicator	Quality of Evidence	Literature	Benefits	Comments
5. If a patient has new recent symptoms of moderate prostatism[2] the health care provider should offer at least one of the following within one month of the note of symptoms: • Uroflowometry; • Post void residual; • Pressure flow study	III	McConnell, 1994	Prevent complications of BPH.	Diminished flow rates and high post void residual can be indications for therapy to prevent obstructive complications, though supporting evidence is weak.
6. If a patient has new recent symptoms of prostatism,[1] the provider should order the following tests within one month of the note of symptoms, unless done in the past year: a. Urine analysis b. Serum creatinine	II, III II, III	Holtgrewe, 1962; Melchior, 1974; McConnell, 1994 Meburst, 1989; McConnell, 1994	Treat other causes of prostatic symptoms. Prevent complications of BPH.	Abnormal urine analyses may be an early sign of urinary infection, urolithiasis, urothelial malignancy and other urologic pathology. Patients with renal insufficiency should have a radiographic evaluation of their upper tracts. These patients are at a higher risk for postoperative complications; nevertheless, renal insufficiency is an absolute indication for treatment.
Treatment				
7. Patients diagnosed with BPH who report recent symptoms of prostatism,[2] and who are on anticholinergic or sympathomimetic medications, should be offered discontinuation of these medications within one month of the note of symptoms.	III	McConnell, 1994	Relieve symptoms.	Anticholinergics may reduce detrusor contractility, and sympathomimetics may increase bladder neck and prostatic tone, either or both may potentiate symptoms of prostatism.
8. Patients diagnosed with BPH who report recent symptoms of moderate prostatism[2] should be offered alpha 1 adrenergic therapy[1] within one month of the note of symptoms.	I, III	Lepor, 1995; Lepor, 1996; McConnell, 1994	Relieve symptoms.	RCTs demonstrate effectiveness in reducing symptoms of moderate prostatism. Long-term efficacy and effect on the natural history of BPH is still not defined.

Indicator	Quality of Evidence	Literature	Benefits	Comments
9. Patients diagnosed with BPH should be offered surgical therapy within one month of either of the following conditions being noted: a. Acute renal insufficiency with dilated upper tracts; b. Persistant renal insufficiency[5] after catheterization trial.	II, III	Meburst, 1989; McConnell, 1994	Relieve symptoms. Prevent renal failure.	TURP preferred over open prostatectomy because of fewer post operative complications.
10. Patients diagnosed with BPH should be offered surgical therapy[4] within two months of any of the following conditions being noted: a. Continued complaints of moderate symptoms of prostatism[2] after 6 months of alpha 1 adrenergic therapy,[3] b. More than one urinary tract infection in the past year, c. Bladder stones.	II, III	Meburst, 1989; McConnell, 1994	Relieve symptoms.	TURP preferred over open prostatectomy because of fewer post operative complications.
Follow-up				
11. Patients diagnosed with BPH who have received alpha 1 adrenergic[3] or surgical therapy[4] should have their symptoms reassessed 6 months after initiation of therapy.	III	McConnell, 1994	Relieve symptoms.	AUA score or patient report monitors effectiveness of therapy.
12. Patients with persistent recent symptoms of prostatism[1] 6 months after appropriate surgical therapy[4] should be offered urodynamic evaluation.	III	McConnell, 1994	Relieve symptoms by treating contributing cause.	Identification of primary bladder dysfunction could potentially spare the patient further surgical therapy.

Definitions and Examples

[1]Recent symptoms of prostatism: At least two of the following symptoms in the past six months: urinary frequency, nocturia, urgency, urge incontinence, post void dribbling, hesitancy, weak stream, incomplete emptying, double voiding, straining to urinate.
[2] Moderate prostatism: American Urologic Association Symptom Index (AUASI) score of 8 to 19, or by patient or physician description of bothersome symptoms.
[3] Alpha 1 adrenergic therapy: terazosin, doxazosin, prazosin.
[4] Surgical therapy: Transurethral or open prostatectomy.

67

[5] Renal insufficiency: Creatinine greater than 2.0.

<u>Quality of Evidence Codes</u>

I	RCT
II-1	Nonrandomized controlled trials
II-2	Cohort or case analysis
II-3	Multiple time series
III	Opinions or descriptive studies

5. CATARACTS

Paul P. Lee MD, JD, and Steven Asch MD, MPH

Several major projects in recent years provide core material in developing quality indicators for the management of adult-onset senile cataract. The Agency for Health Care Policy and Research (AHCPR) supported a Patient Outcomes Research Team assessment of cataract management, particularly the surgical options, and also supported the development of a practice guideline for the management of adult senile cataract (AHCPR, 1993; Powe et al., 1994; Schein et al., 1994; O'Day et al., 1993). The American Academy of Ophthalmology (1996) has published a guideline on the management of adult cataract, as has a consortium of other ophthalmic organizations (American College of Eye Surgeons, 1993). RAND and the Academic Medical Center Consortium (AMCC) assessed the appropriate indications for cataract surgery using the RAND/UCLA modified Delphi approach (Brook, 1994), and applied these indicators to cataract surgeries performed in the United States (Lee et al., 1993). Individual investigators and research teams have also published extensively on the outcomes and pre-operative predictors of functional improvement after cataract surgery (Mangione et al., 1994, 1995; Tielsch et al., 1995; Schein et al., 1995; Applegate et al., 1987; Bernth-Peterson, 1981). Finally, AHCPR and RAND developed a set of review criteria based on the AHCPR cataract management guideline (Laouri et al., 1995). Taken together, these projects provide a substantial foundation for developing quality indicators for the management of cataract.

A significant issue in understanding the recommended indicators in this chapter is the quality of supporting evidence (AHCPR, 1993; Powe et al., 1994; O'Day et al., 1993). It was not unusual for the sources we reviewed to agree on a given recommendation, with only Level III data (expert opinion) in support of it. At best, only Level II data (observational) have been published to date for these recommendations that have been scientifically assessed. In many cases, Level I (RCT) trials may be unnecessary or infeasible because the recommendations are so basic (e.g., to perform a complete pre-operative examination of the eye). As in other conditions, we have proposed Level III indicators when consensus exists among all sources.

Another important aspect of the indicators proposed in this chapter is how responsibility for them is separated among different health care providers. For example, while some indicators apply to all providers, eye care specialists alone are held accountable for indicators related to surgery and certain specialized examinations. Such a separation of responsibilities is intentional, as it reflects the current organization of health care services.

Finally, this document reflects the current emphasis in health technology assessment on the impact of a condition on patient functioning and on the prevention of patient morbidity or mortality. As such, and in conformance with current professional guidelines, the management of cataract is centered on ameliorating the effect of cataract on a person's ability to perform visual tasks and on enhancing health-related quality of life (HRQL). Thus, although a cataract is defined in this document as a lens opacity, management issues do not arise unless the lens opacity is associated with impairment of visual function.

IMPORTANCE

The prevalence of lens opacities believed to diminish visual acuity to 20/30 or worse increases with age. In population-based studies, nuclear cataracts, which are the most common form of cataract, rise from 5.7 percent among those aged 55 to 64 years to 30 percent among those aged 75 to 84 years (AHCPR, 1993; Kahn et al., 1977; Spreduto and Hiller, 1984). If the criterion is merely the presence of a lens opacity -- without visual impairment -- then the rate rises from 42 percent among those aged 52 to 64 to virtually 100 percent by the time they reach their 80s (AHCPR, 1993). From the perspective of health care delivery, the surgical removal of cataracts remains the single largest surgical expenditure for Medicare Part B, and cataract is one of the leading reasons for office visits in the United States, especially among those over age 65.

Given these high utilization rates, it is reassuring that the majority of studies suggest cataract surgeries are only rarely performed for inappropriate reasons (Tobacman et al., 1996). However, recent evidence shows that the utilization of cataract surgery in senior managed care plans, after adjusting for ocular risk factors and co-morbid medical conditions, is half that for comparable patients enrolled in the fee-for-service sector of Medicare (Goldzweig et al., 1997). Thus, concerns about under- as well as over-utilization need to be addressed in any quality indicator system.

From the patient's perspective, amelioration of the visual difficulties posed by cataract offers tremendous benefit not only in functioning and HRQL as measured by both general (SF-36) and vision-specific instruments, but also in terms of satisfaction (Tielsch et al., 1995; Schein et al., 1995; Steinberg et al., 1994). Several studies have shown that decrements in visual performance, including contrast sensitivity, are associated with significantly increased rates of falls and hip fractures (Felson et al., 1989; Tobis et al., 1985). At the same time, some patients with cataracts do not improve with either non-surgical or surgical treatment.

Definition of Cataract

For the purposes of this document, a cataract is defined as an acquired opacification of the lens. The mere presence of a lens opacity does not necessarily result in a functional impairment of vision (Mangione et al., 1995). Whether vision is defined by a test performed on an outpatient basis, such as Snellen visual acuity or contrast sensitivity, or by the ability to perform daily visual tasks, such as reading or watching TV, no study has found a consistent and clear relationship between the density of the opacity and the level of vision impairment. Thus, the inquiry into possible visual impairment is separate from the initial inquiry into whether a lens opacity exists.

SCREENING AND PREVENTION

Although screening to detect a lens opacity could be performed with either a trained examiner or photographic assessment, the yield of patients who have lens opacities with related visual impairment is so low that it raises concerns about relative costs and benefits. The Framingham study is particularly instructive in this regard, as only 12 percent of its subjects with lens opacities had visual acuity diminished to 20/30 or worse (AHCPR, 1993). Moreover, visual acuity itself is only modestly related to vision-related functioning (Mangione et al., 1995). Thus, we recommend a quality indicator requiring only that patients be asked by both primary care physicians and eye care providers whether they have functional decrements related to their vision, and make no recommendations for screening of asymptomatic patients for the presence of a lens opacity (Indicator 1).

New data exist on the potential role of several factors in the development of cataract, including ultraviolet radiation (B), diabetes mellitus, certain drugs, cigarette smoking, alcohol consumption, and low antioxidant status (AHCPR, 1993). However, no studies have yet documented that risk factor reduction prevents cataract development.

DIAGNOSIS

The diagnosis of cataracts requires the performance of a magnified eye examination, either by a trained examiner or through the use of a standardized photographic assessment. Once a lenticular opacity is detected, additional assessment is needed to determine if visual impairment exists. Traditionally, visual impairment has been defined by decreased Snellen visual acuity. Under current approaches, however, impairment is increasingly defined by degradation of visual performance on vision-related tasks or through effects on HRQL (Mangione et al., 1995). Establishing the existence of visual impairment is separate from diagnosing the presence of a lens opacity. Like all patients who present with visual complaints, suspected cataract patients should receive an assessment of their vision and visual task performance. We recommend a quality indicator specifying that the eye care provider should conduct a complete eye examination, including a dilated exam of the fundus (macula, optic nerve, vessels, and periphery) to determine if other concurrent ocular conditions might be related to the impaired visual functioning (Indicator 2).

Regardless of the endpoint of visual impairment used, all studies indicate that the success rates of cataract surgery can be significantly reduced by the presence of other ocular diseases, particularly diabetic retinopathy, glaucoma, and macular degeneration. This is due, in large part, to the potential for a separate, independent effect on visual functioning that cannot be improved by removal of the cataract (Lee et al., 1993; Mangione et al., 1995; Schein et al., 1995). The presence of ocular diseases such as high myopia or pseudoexfoliation syndrome is associated with higher immediate complication rates. This understanding is reflected in every current guideline for the care of patients with cataracts, either in limiting the guideline only to eyes without such conditions (AHCPR, 1993; American Academy of Opthalmology, 1996; American College of Eye Surgeons, 1993) or in explicitly using more restrictive indications for cataract removal (Lee et al., 1993). Thus, the decision to proceed with surgery should be made with full knowledge of the patient's ocular status, including a dilated fundus exam, and, if necessary, an ultrasound exam.

TREATMENT

A cataract does not require treatment unless the cataract itself is causing rare, secondary diseases such as phacomorphic glaucoma or lens-related uveitis, or if it sufficiently compromises the ability to monitor or treat other ocular diseases such as diabetic retinopathy or glaucoma (AHCPR, 1993; American Academy of Ophthalmology, 1996; Lee et al., 1993) (Indicator 4). Otherwise, treatment is indicated when the cataract is associated with some degree of visual impairment. In the past, the traditional reliance on Snellen visual acuity to measure visual impairment prompted the treatment of cataracts basically to improve Snellen visual acuity. Thus, for example, indications for cataract surgery were based on the Snellen visual acuity level that a patient could see (e.g., 20/60 or 20/80). Currently, however, the emphasis on functioning and well-being is shifting the basis for intervention to the patient's ability to perform visual tasks and activities of daily living related to vision, such as reading, driving safely, and work (AHCPR, 1993; American Academy of Opthalmology, 1996; American College of Eye Surgeons, 1993; Lee et al., 1993).

Because cataracts can cause a change in the refractive status of the eye, all current guidelines for the management of cataracts recommend that an up-to-date refraction be performed in all eyes with significant functional impairment thought to be due to the cataract. Although no study has documented the effectiveness of this medical intervention, there is universal support for an in-office assessment of refractive status to determine if non-surgical treatment can decrease the visual impairment to a degree significant for the patient (AHCPR, 1993; American Academy of Ophthalmology, 1996; American College of Eye Surgeons, 1993). Thus, we propose a quality indicator that stating that all patients undergoing cataract surgery should have had a refraction in the operative eye within four months before surgery (Indicator 3).

If the medical intervention results in insufficient improvement for the patient then surgical treatment may be warranted. Numerous case series and case-control studies have been performed using visual acuity as the indicator of improvement in visual functioning or impairment after surgical removal of the cataract (AHCPR, 1993; Powe et al., 1994; Schein et al., 1994; O'Day et al., 1993; Lee et al., 1993). A far smaller number of studies have used patient-reported vision-related task performance or visual functioning and HRQL as the indicator of visual impairment. However, these recent studies on vision-related functioning have not only confirmed these findings using vision-related task endpoints, but have also clearly identified that pre-operative visual acuity is not predictive of the surgical outcomes related to functioning and health-related quality of life (Mangione et al., 1995; Schein et al., 1995). Rather, factors such as the presence of other ocular diseases, the patient's age, and the degree of pre-operative functional impairment are the most important predictors of post-operative functional improvement. These studies clearly indicate that visual functioning can be improved by cataract surgery and that such initial impairment or subsequent improvement is only poorly related to Snellen

74

acuity. Thus, the decision to proceed with surgery must be made on the basis of functional impairment and not Snellen acuity; there is no role for a Snellen acuity cutoff (Indicator 5).

Due to current cataract extraction techniques, the posterior lens capsule may opacify after surgery. YAG (yttrium-argon-garnet laser) capsulotomy can be used to treat this problem. However, because the use of this technique is associated with an increased risk of complications such as retinal detachment (AHCPR, 1993), it should not be performed in every case of opacification of the posterior lens capsule. Rather, the indications for a YAG capsulotomy are similar to that of the initial cataract surgery: impaired visual functioning thought to be due to a media opacification (in this case, posterior lens capsule) or for specific medical reasons, such as monitoring or treatment of glaucoma or diabetes (AHCPR, 1993; American Academy of Ophthalmology, 1996; American College of Eye Surgeons, 1993) (Indicator 6).

FOLLOW-UP

No study has been conducted regarding the ideal follow-up intervals of patients with cataract. Guidelines suggest follow-up intervals ranging from every few months to one year (American Academy of Ophthalmology, 1996), both for continuing preventive care as well as for monitoring the cataract.

Data suggest that the rate of cataract progression is slow (AHCPR, 1993). One small study determined that the rate of vision loss over an average of almost three years was 1.5 lines of Snellen acuity per year, with a loss of nearly two lines per year among those who had any degree of loss (Gloor and Farrell, 1989). Unfortunately, no data exist on the natural history of vision-related functioning due to untreated cataract. Thus, we make no recommendations on the frequency of follow-up exams among those with cataracts who do not undergo cataract surgery. However, as noted in the screening section, all guidelines agree that patients should be asked about their degree of visual functioning, with specific attention given to whether impairment of visual tasks or vision-related functioning exists (AHCPR, 1993; American Academy of

Ophthalmology 1996; American College of Eye Surgeons, 1993; Lee et al., 1993)(Indicator 1).

If patients are to undergo surgery, the available guidelines agree to a large degree on which pre-operative tests should be performed, what operative issues should be considered, and what post-operative management should be arranged. However, no data have been published linking the performance of any specific pre-operative test -- other than vision-related functioning assessment -- with post-operative outcomes. Further, the small amount of existing data reveals a wide variation between optometrists, ophthalmologists, and internists in the use of preoperative tests (Bass et al., 1995, 1996; Steinberg et al., 1994).

Recent studies have shown that complication rates and outcomes after four months are comparable with either a traditional extracapsular technique or a phacoemulsification technique for cataract removal (although the intracapsular technique is associated with higher immediate complication rates) (Schein et al., 1994; Steinberg et al., 1994). No other aspect of intra-operative management has been studied in a similarly detailed fashion, other than the comparability of routes of anesthesia during surgery or specific surgical maneuvers for creating incisions or removing the lens. Thus, we make no recommendation regarding the intra-operative considerations of cataract surgery.

No study has documented the ideal intervals for follow-up after surgery, or what steps should be performed during the post-operative assessment. The only published study on post-operative care patterns demonstrates variations between different provider types, but does not examine the outcomes of care by different care patterns (Bass et al., 1996). All current guidelines agree that the operating surgeon has the responsibility for managing the post-operative care of the patient (Indicator 7). Patients should be seen within 24 to 48 hours of surgery, and have a complete anterior segment examination performed to detect any complications at that time (AHCPR, 1993; American Academy of Ophthalmology, 1996; American College of Eye Surgeons, 1993) (Indicator 8). Similarly, regular follow-up exams are recommended, as is a dilated fundus examination within 90 post-operative days. However, recent data from a RAND/AHCPR-sponsored project indicates that this last

76

recommendation is rarely carried out in the community setting unless a patient complains of symptoms (Laouri et al., 1995). Thus, we make no recommendation regarding the advisability of a dilated fundus exam within the 90 day postoperative period. Finally, patients should be asked if the functional difficulty that spurred surgery improved within 90 days (Indicator 9).

REFERENCES

American Academy of Ophthalmology. 1996. *Preferred Practice Pattern: Cataract in the Otherwise Healthy Adult Eye.* American Academy of Ophthlamology, San Francisco.

American College of Eye Surgeons. 1993. *Guidelines for Cataract Practice.*

Applegate W, Miller ST, Elam JT, et al. 1987. Impact of cataract surgery with lens implantation on vision and physical function in elderly patients. *Journal of the American Medical Association* 256: 1064-66.

Bass EB, Sharkey PD, Luthra R, et al. 1996. Postoperative management of cataract surgery patients by ophthalmologists and optometrists. *Archives of Ophthalmology* 114: 1121-27.

Bass EB, Steinberg EP, Luthra R, Schein OD, Tielsch JM, and Javitt JC. 1995. Do ophthalmologists, anesthesiologists, and internists agree about preoperative testing in healthy patients undergoing cataract surgery? *Archives of Ophthalmology* 113: 1248-56.

Bass EB, Steinberg EP, Luthra R, et al. 1995. Variation in ophthalmic testing prior to cataract surgery: results of a national survey of optometrists. Cataract Patient Outcome Research Team. *Archives of Ophthalmology* 113: 27-31.

Bernth-Petersen P. 1981. Visual functioning in cataract patients: methods of measuring and results. *Acta Ophtahlmol (Copenhagen)* 59: 50-56.

Brook RH. May 1994. The RAND/UCLA appropriateness method. In: McCormick KA, Moore SR, and Siegel RA. *Clinical Practice Guideline Development: Methodology Perspectives.* AHCPR Pub. No. 95-0009 (Rockville, MD): 59-70.

Cataract Management Guideline Panel. February 1993. *Cataract in Adults: Management of Functional Impairment. Clinical Practice Guideline, Number 4.* US Department of Health and Human Services, Public Health Service, Agency for Health Care Policy and Research, Rockville, MD.

Felson D, Anderson JJ, Hannon MT, et al. 1989. Impaired vision and hip fracture. The Framingham Study. *Journal of the American Geriatric Society* 37: 494-500.

Gloor P and Farrell TA. 1989. The natural course of visual acuity in patients with senile cataracts. *Investigative Ophthamology and Visual Science* 30 (Supp): 500.

Goldzweig CL, Mittman BS, Carter GM, et al. 11 June 1997. Variations in cataract extraction rates in prepaid and fee-for-service settings. *Journal of the American Medical Association* 277 (22): 1765-1768.

Kahn HA, Leibowitz HM, Ganley JP, et al. 1977. The Framingham Eye Study: I. Outline and major prevalence findings. *American Journal of Epidemiology* 106 (1): 17-32.

Laouri M, Mittman BS, Lee PP, Mangione CM, et al. 1995. Developing quality and utilization review criteria for management of cataract in adults: Phase II final report. RAND, Santa Monica CA: PM-404-AHCPR.

Lee PP, Kamberg CJ, Hilborne LH, et al. 1993. *Cataract Surgery: a literature review and ratings of appropriateness and cruciality.* RAND, Santa Monica CA.

Mangione CM, Lee PP, and Hays R. 1995. Measurement of visual functioning and health-related quality of life in eye disease and cataract surgery. In: *Quality of Life and Pharacoeconomics in Clinical Trials*, 2nd ed. New York, NY: Raven Press.

Mangione CM, Orav EJ, Lawrence MG, et al. 1995. Prediction of visual function after cataract surgery: a prospectively validated model. *Archives of Ophthalmology* 113: 1305-11.

O'Day DM, Steinberg EP, and Dickersin K. 1993. Systematic literature review for clinical practice guideline development. *Transactions of the American Ophthalmological Society* 91: 421-36.

Powe NR, Schein OD, Gieser SC, et al. 1994. Synthesis of the literature on visual acuity and complications following cataract extraction with introacular lens implantation. Cataract Patient Outcome Research Team. *Archives of Ophthalmology* 112: 239-52.

Powe NR, Tielsch JM, Schein OD, et al. 1994. Rigor of research methods in studies of the effectiveness and safety of cataract extraction with intraocular lens implantation. Cataract Patient Outcome Research Team. *Archives of Ophthalmology* 112: 228-38.

Schein OD, Steinberg EP, Cassard SD, et al. 1995. Predictors of outcome in patients who underwent cataract surgery. *Ophthalmology* 102: 817-23.

Schein OD, Steinberg EP, Javitt JC, et al. 1994. Variation in cataract surgery practice and clinical outcomes. *Ophthlamology* 101: 1142-52.

Sperduto RD, and Hiller R. 1984. The prevalence of nuclear, cortical, and posterior subcapsular lens opacities in a gneral population sample. *Opthlamology* 91: 815-18.

Steinberg EP, Bass EB, Luthra R, et al. 1994. Variation in ophthalmic testing before cataract surgery: results of a national survey of ophthlamologists. *Archives of Ophthalmology* 112: 896-602.

Steinberg EP, Tielsch JM, Schein OD, et al. 1994. National study of cataract surgery outcomes: variation in 4-month postoperative outcomes as reflected in multiple outcome measures. *Ophthalmology* 101: 1131-40.

Tielsch JM, Steinberg EP, Cassard SD, et al. 1995. Preoperative functional expectations and postoperative outcomes among patients undergoing first-eye cataract surgery. *Archives of Ophthlamology* 113: 1312-18.

Tobacman JK, Lee PP, Zimmerman B, et al. 1996. Assessment of appropriateness of cataract surgery in ten academic medical centers in 1990. *Ophthalmology* 103: 207-15.

Tobis JJ, Reinsch S, et al. 1985. Visual perception dominance of fallers among community-dwelling older adults. *Journal of the American Geriatric Society* 33: 330-33.

RECOMMENDED QUALITY INDICATORS FOR CATARACTS

The following indicators apply to men and women age 18 and older (except where otherwise specified).

Indicator	Quality of Evidence	Literature	Benefits	Comments
Screening				
1. Patients aged 55 and older presenting for non-urgent care should be asked annually if they are having difficulty with visual function.[1]	III	Cataract Management Guideline Panel 1993; AAO, 1996; SGO, 1992; Laouri, et al., 1995	Improve visual functioning.	Determines those who might benefit from an eye evaluation and possible cataract management.
Diagnosis				
2. Patients who report difficulty with visual function[1] should be offered a complete eye exam by an optometrist or ophthalmologist. This examination should be performed at least annually and should include all of the following: • visual acuity measurement • intraocular pressure measurement; • pupil exam; • motility exam; • slit lamp exam; • dilated fundus exam.[2]	II	Cataract Management Guideline Panel 1993; AAO, 1996; SGO, 1992; Lee, 1993; Laouri, et al., 1995	Improves visual functioning.	Determines if the visual difficulty is related to the cataract. Detects the presence of other diseases that may be treated to reduce the risk of blindness (e.g., diabetes).
3. Patients should be offered refraction in the operative eye within 4 months before surgery unless a prior refraction made no improvement in otherwise stable vision in the past two years.	III	Cataract Management Guideline Panel 1993; AAO, 1996; SGO, 1992; Lee, 1993; Laouri, et al., 1995	Improves visual functioning.	Determines if a non-surgical intervention may be successful in delaying the need for surgery.

	Indicator	Quality of Evidence	Literature	Benefits	Comments
Treatment					
4.	Patients with cataracts should be offered surgery if any of the following situations are present: a. phacomorphic glaucoma; b. phacolytic glaucoma; c. lens-related uveitis; d. disrupted anterior lens capsule in otherwise phakic eye; e. cataract prevents adequate monitoring or treatment of glaucoma or diabetes.	III	Cataract Management Guideline Panel 1993; AAO, 1996; SGO, 1992; Lee, 1993	Prevent progression of disease.	
5.	In the absence of a medical indication for cataract surgery,[3] the ophthalmologist should offer cataract surgery only when both of the following conditions are met: • the patient's visual functioning is impaired;[1] • there is either a normal fundus exam[2] or a statement that the surgeon believes the patient's visual function would improve after the surgery.	II	Cataract Management Guideline Panel 1993; AAO, 1996; SGO, 1992; Lee, 1993; Mangione, 1995; Mangione, 1994; Tielsch, 1995; Schein, 1995; Bernth-Petersen, 1981; Laouri, et al., 1995	Improve visual function.	Snellen acuity cutoffs do not predict improvement, functional assessments do.
6.	YAG capsulotomy should not be offered unless one condition from each of the following categories is met: • presence of opacity or impairment of the patient's visual function[1]; • there is either a normal fundus exam[2] or a statement that the surgeon believes the patient's visual function would improve after the surgery.	III	Cataract Management Guideline Panel 1993; AAO, 1996; SGO, 1992	Avoid surgical complications.	

82

Follow-up

Indicator	Quality of Evidence	Literature	Benefits	Comments
7. Within 90 days of surgery, the surgeon should do at least one of the following: • examine the patient; • refer the patient for further care; • document inability to contact patient.	III	Cataract Management Guideline Panel 1993; AAO, 1996; SGO, 1992	Improve visual functioning.	Provides continuity of care. Evaluates functional improvement. Detects complications of surgery.
8. Within 48 hours of surgery, an optometrist or ophthalmologist should offer patients who have undergone cataract extraction a complete anterior segment eye examination, including all of the following: • visual acuity measurement; • intraocular pressure measurement; • slit lamp exam.	II	Cataract Management Guideline Panel 1993; AAO, 1996; SGO, 1992	Improve visual functioning.	Detects potential intraocular infections or bleeding complications of surgery.
9. Patients who have undergone cataract extraction should have their visual functioning[1] assessed within 90 days of surgery.	II	Cataract Management Guideline Panel 1993; AAO, 1996; SGO, 1992; Laouri, 1995	Improve visual functioning.	Evaluates improvement after surgery.

83

Definitions and Examples

1 Difficulties with or impairment of visual function include problems with glare, recreational activities, reading, driving, employment, IADLSs, ADLs, mobility.

2 Dilated fundus exam must include documentation of the: optic nerve, macula, vasculature, and retinal periphery.

3 Medical indications for cataract surgery:
a. phacomorphic glaucoma;
b. phacolytic glaucoma;
c. lens-related uveitis;
d. disrupted anterior lens capsule in otherwise phakic eye;
e. cataract prevents adequate monitoring or treatment of glaucoma or diabetes.

Quality of Evidence Codes

I	RCT
II-1	Nonrandomized controlled trials
II-2	Cohort or case analysis
II-3	Multiple time series

84

6. CHOLELITHIASIS

Deidre Gifford, M.D.

Background information for this review was obtained by performing a MEDLINE search for English language review articles on the topic of cholelithiasis for the years 1990 to 1997. A focused search on the topic of diagnosis of cholelithiasis was also carried out. In addition, the summary of the NIH consensus conference on gallstones and laparoscopic cholecystectomy (1993) was reviewed. This document, along with the American College of Physicians' "Guidelines for the Treatment of Gallstones" and the accompanying background paper (Ransohoff, 1993) form the primary sources of information used in developing this chapter.

IMPORTANCE

Gallstone disease is common. Approximately 10 to 15 percent of the adult population in the United States has gallstones, and about one million new cases are diagnosed annually (NIH, 1993). By the age of 75, an estimated 35 percent of women and 20 percent of men have developed gallstones (ACP, 1993). Gallstones are more common in women, and are associated with parity (number of pregnancies), obesity, rapid weight loss, age and ethnicity (NIH, 1993). As a result of gallstones, approximately 600,000 cholecystectomies are performed annually in the US. The annual overall cost associated with this condition has been estimated at more than five billion dollars (NIH, 1993).

Most cases of gallstones remain asymptomatic. The most common symptom associated with gallstones is biliary pain. Complications from gallstones include acute cholecystitis, gallstone pancreatitis, common bile duct obstruction, ascending cholangitis, gallstone ileus or (rarely) gallbladder cancer. Death from gallstones is uncommon, accounting for approximately 5,000 deaths per year in the US. These deaths are usually in the elderly and caused by biliary complications and the associated treatment (Ransohoff, 1993).

SCREENING

No specific recommendations regarding screening for gallstones in asymptomatic individuals were identified from the literature search.

DIAGNOSIS

Gallstones are generally diagnosed by ultrasound, or less commonly by oral cholecystography or plain x-ray. In an asymptomatic individual, they may be discovered incidentally at the time of laparotomy for another condition, or at the time of imaging for another indication. Ultrasound is a non-invasive, sensitive and specific method of diagnosing gallstones (ACP, 1988). Because the treatment of gallstones is guided by the presence or absence of symptoms (see below), the determination of whether an individual's symptoms are related to the gallstones, or the gallstones are an incidental finding in someone with non-biliary symptoms, is an important element of diagnosis. However, we did not find any diagnostic algorithms or decision rules which allow the clinician to accurately differentiate biliary from non-biliary symptoms in the person with gallstones.

TREATMENT

Treatment for gallstones can include expectant management, non-surgical therapy to "dissolve" the stones while leaving the gallbladder intact, and cholecystectomy via laparoscopy or laparotomy. Non-surgical therapy includes oral bile acids, direct instillation of contact solvents into the gallbladder, and extracorporeal shock wave lithotripsy (ESWL) plus oral bile acid therapy. None of these methods is currently widely used in the US (Ransohoff, 1993). Oral bile acid therapy effectively dissolves stones in individuals with small stones made up primarily of cholesterol. However, therapy takes up to two years to complete, and gallstones recur in approximately 50 percent of patients (Schoenfield, 1993). Direct instillation of contact solvent into the gallbladder is an experimental therapy, and involves repeated instillations by an interventional radiologist. ESWL uses acoustic shock waves to break up the gallstones into small pieces, which are further dissolved and passed with the use of oral bile acid therapy. This therapy is primarily effective in individuals with a solitary gallstone less then 2 cm in diameter, or approximately 12 percent of patients having surgery for gallstones (Ransohoff, 1993). Ninety percent of patients with a single stone treated with ESWL and oral bile acids will have complete dissolution of stones after one year. Thirty percent of those treated will have a recurrence of pain, but gallstone complications following lithotripsy are rare.

Surgical treatment of gallstones has traditionally been carried out via laparotomy. This operation is considered safe and effective, and the standard against which newer therapies should be measured (NIH, 1993). Mortality rates from open cholecystectomy are generally low, but vary depending on the age of the patient and whether or not the surgery is carried out for prophylaxis or in the presence of a biliary tract complication. Mortality rates for women are approximately half of those for men. Mortality rates for prophylactic open cholecystectomy (following pain or in those without symptoms) range from 0.05 percent for a 30 year old woman to 6.1 percent for an 80 year old man. For open cholecystectomy following a biliary complication, the range increases to 0.2 to 24.6 percent (Ransohoff, 1993). There are no good estimates of morbidity following open cholecystectomy; however, common bile duct injury is the most serious complication, and occurs in approximately 0.1 to 0.2 percent of cases (Ransohoff, 1993).

In the last decade, laparoscopic cholecystectomy has become increasingly popular. This method uses four small incisions in the abdominal wall, and is generally associated with less pain and quicker recovery of function for patients. Estimates of mortality from large studies are not yet available, but mortality appears to be low. Common bile duct injury may be more common with laparoscopic cholecystectomy than with open cholecystectomy (Ransohoff, 1993).

Ransohoff et al. (1993) developed a model which describes the trade-offs of treatment versus expectant management of gallstones, depending on the likelihood of a patient developing complications in the future and of mortality from those complications. For this study, the authors reviewed the literature and summarized the probabilities of recurring symptoms, complications, and death for patients with asymptomatic and symptomatic gallstones.

Individuals who have a complication of gallstone disease (including acute cholecystitis, acute pancreatitis, common bile duct stones, cholangitis, or gallstone ileus) have a 30 percent chance of developing another complication within three months if not treated with cholecystectomy. Prompt cholecystectomy following one of these complications is effective in preventing recurrent complications. Early surgery is avoided if the patient's condition contraindicates surgery (Ransohoff 1993, NIH 1993) (Indicator 1).

Among individuals with asymptomatic gallstones, the rate of development of any symptom or complication is approximately one to four percent per year (Ransohoff, 1993; NIH, 1993). In addition to the low incidence of pain or complications, natural history studies show that the majority of those who do develop a problem will present initially with pain. Those who do develop a complication will almost always have a preceding episode of biliary pain (NIH, 1993), making intervention at the time of the initial symptom as low risk as a cholecystectomy done in an asymptomatic individual. The modeling study demonstrated small gains or minimal loss of life expectancy (depending on methodology) when expectant management is used for individuals with asymptomatic gallstones. Both the NIH and the American College of Physicians guideline recommend that expectant management be used for individuals with asymptomatic gallstones (ACP, 1993; NIH, 1993) (Indicator 2).

Patients with symptomatic gallstones are at increased risk for developing complications of gallstone disease. Pain recurs in approximately 40 percent of individuals per year, although 30 percent will have no further episodes of pain over a ten year period. The rate of biliary complications is one to two percent per year in persons with symptomatic gallstones. The modeling study demonstrated significant loss of life expectancy for individuals with symptomatic gallstones treated with expectant management, as compared to cholecystectomy (from 63 days loss of life expectancy for a 30 year old man to 104 days for a 50 year old woman). Given this result, cholecystectomy for individuals with symptomatic gallstones is warranted, although patients may opt for expectant management if they choose to incur the risk of recurrent pain or biliary complication (Ransohoff, 1993). The NIH consensus states that "..most symptomatic patients should be treated" (Indicator 3).

FOLLOW-UP

No specific recommendations regarding follow-up of individuals with asymptomatic gallstones were identified from the literature search. Gallstones do not generally resolve spontaneously once they appear, and the number of gallstones per se does not change the management from non-surgical to surgical in the absence of symptoms. Therefore, repeated imaging of the gallbladder in the absence of symptoms does not appear to be warranted.

REFERENCES

American College of Physicians. 1993. Guidelines for the Treatment of Gallstones. *Archives of Internal Medicine* 119 (7): 620-622.

American College of Physicians and Health and Policy Committee. 1988. How to study the gallbladder. *Archives of Internal Medicine* 109: 752-754.

NIH Consensus Conference. 1993. Gallstones and Laparoscopic Cholecystectomy. *Journal of the American Medical Association* 269 (8): 1018-1024.

Ransohoff DF and Gracie WA. 1993. Treatment of gallstones. *Archives of Internal Medicine* 119 (7): 606-619.

Schoenfield LJ and Marks JW. April 1993. Oral and Contact Dissolution of Gallstones. *American Journal of Surgery* 165: 427-430.

RECOMMENDED QUALITY INDICATORS FOR CHOLELITHIASIS

The following indicators apply to men and women age 18 and older.

	Indicator	Quality of Evidence	Literature	Benefits	Comments
Treatment					
1.	Patients who are diagnosed with a complication of gallstones[1] should receive a cholecystectomy within one month of the complication, unless the medical record states that they are not a surgical candidate.	II-2[2], III	NIH, 1993; Ransohoff, 1993	Avoid morbidity and mortality from complications of gallstones.	"Prompt" cholecystectomy is generally recommended after a complication. The one month time period is arbitrary. Laparoscopic or open cholecystectomy may be used.
2.	If a patient undergoes cholecystectomy for gallstones, one of the following should be documented within the 6 months prior to surgery: • biliary pain; • complications from gallstone.[1]	II-2[2]	Ransohoff, 1993; NIH, 1993	Avoid morbidity and mortality from unnecessary cholecystectomy.	This indicator applies to both laparoscopic or open cholecyst-ectomy. The six month time period is arbitrary.
3.	Patients who are diagnosed with biliary pain[3] should be offered cholecystectomy within 6 months of the symptoms, unless the medical record states that they are not a surgical candidate.	II-2[2]	Ransohoff, 1993; NIH, 1993	Avoid morbidity and mortality from complications of gallstones.	Patient may choose not to accept therapy. The 6 month time period is arbitrary.

Definitions and Examples

[1] Complications from gallstones include: acute chclecystitis, acute gallstone pancreatitis, gallstone ileus, cholangitis and common bile duct obstruction.
[2] Refers to those cohort studies used to develop probabilities for the Ransohoff modeling study (1993).
[3] A patient is considered to have biliary pain if the medical record indicates a diagnosis of "biliary pain," or if the medical record indicates "probable biliary pain" and a diagnostic study confirms the presence of gallstones within two months of the notation of pain.

Quality of Evidence Codes

I	RCT
II-1	Nonrandomized controlled trials
II-2	Cohort or case analysis
II-3	Multiple time series
III	Opinions or descriptive studies

91

7. DEMENTIA

Alison Moore, MD

Eight practice guidelines and six reviews provided the background material in developing quality indicators for dementia (Canadian Task Force on the Periodic Health Examination [CTFPHE], 1979; National Institutes of Health Consensus Development Conference [NIH], 1987; Organizing Committee, Canadian Consensus Conference on the Assessment of Dementia [CCCAD], 1991; American Academy of Family Physicians [AAFP], 1994; Quality Standards Subcommittee of the American Academy of Neurology [ANN], 1994; Agency for Health Care Policy and Research [AHCPR], 1996; U.S. Preventive Services Task Force [USPSTF], 1996; U.S. Department of Veterans Affairs and the University Health System Consortium [USDVAUHSC], 1996; Corey-Bloom et al., 1995; Siu, 1991; Cummings, 1995; Cummings and Benson, 1992; Winograd and Jarvik, 1986; Schneider and Tariot, 1994). We also performed MEDLINE searches of the medical literature from 1990 to 1996 to supplement these references.

IMPORTANCE

Dementia is the most common type of cognitive impairment seen in ambulatory and nursing home settings. It is characterized by an acquired, persistent impairment of intellectual function that includes significant losses in at least three of the following five areas: cognition, memory, language, visuospatial skills, and personality (Cummings and Benson, 1992). Most diagnostic criteria require that the patient have a memory impairment (USDVAUHSC, 1996). This impairment in intellectual abilities interferes with the person's usual occupational and social functioning (AHCPR, 1996). While the prevalence of dementia among the U.S. adult population is five percent among persons aged 65 years, this prevalence doubles approximately every five years thereafter (Jorm et al., 1987). The prevalence of dementia also varies by health delivery setting, with higher rates among patients who are hospitalized or in long term care facilities.

Despite its high prevalence among older persons, dementia often goes unrecognized or misdiagnosed in its early stages. Clinicians fail to detect an estimated 21 to 72 percent of patients with dementia (Pinholt et al., 1987; Roca et al., 1984; World Health Organization, 1986; German et al., 1987; Callahan et al., 1995). Many health care professionals, as well as patients and family members, mistakenly view the early symptoms of dementia as inevitable consequences of aging (AHCPR, 1996).

Because demented persons are subject to impairments and disabilities in all domains of daily function (Winograd and Jarvik, 1986), care of the demented patient imposes an enormous psychosocial and economic burden on family and other caretakers. The annual cost of treating dementia has been estimated to be $113 billion (National Foundation for Brain Research, 1992).

Prevalence estimates of different causes of dementia vary widely by the population sampled and diagnostic criteria used. Most causes are irreversible. Alzheimer's disease accounts for about 50 percent of cases of dementia in North America (Cummings and Benson, 1992), with an additional ten to 20 percent attributed to vascular dementia (Heyman et al., 1991; Skoog et al., 1993; Aronson et al., 1991). Alcohol-related dementia, dementia due to Parkinson's disease, and normal-pressure hydrocephalus are other important causes of dementia (Larson et al., 1986). However, between 10 and 15 percent of dementia syndromes may be potentially reversible. The most common causes of "reversible" dementia are depression, use of certain drugs affecting mentation, and hypothyroidism (Larson et al., 1986; Clarfield, 1988).

SCREENING

Several task forces and expert panels have reviewed screening procedures for dementia and have, in general, not recommended routine screening (CTFPHE, 1979; NIH, 1987; CCCAD, 1991; AAFP, 1994; AAN, 1994; AHCPR, 1996; USPSTF, 1996; USDVAUHSC, 1996).

DIAGNOSIS

Detecting dementia before patients are severely impaired is important for several reasons: reversible causes of dementia may be identified and treated; treatments to slow the progression of Alzheimer's disease may be considered; measures can be taken to reduce the morbidity associated with dementia; and patients and their family members can anticipate and prepare for problems that will arise as the dementia progresses (USPSTF, 1996).

History

All the guidelines advise that persons suspected of having cognitive impairment should have a comprehensive history performed (CTFPHE, 1979; NIH, 1987; CCCAD, 1991; AAFP, 1994; AAN, 1994; AHCPR, 1996; USPSTF, 1996; USDVAUHSC, 1996). First, it is important to determine if the person's cognitive abilities have declined from a previous level and if the decline is interfering with the patient's usual activities (Indicator 1a and 1b). Providers should elicit information about symptoms that may indicate dementia including: a) difficulty learning and retaining new information; b) problems handling complex tasks (e.g., balancing a checkbook or preparing a meal); c) problems with reasoning (e.g., knowing what to do if the bathroom flooded); d) deficits in spatial ability and orientation (e.g., having trouble driving or navigating in familiar places); e) language difficulties (e.g., difficulty with word finding); and f) behavior changes (e.g., increased levels of suspiciousness or passivity).

In every case, an assessment should also look for delirium and depression and other treatable causes of cognitive impairment (Indicator 1e and 1f). In particular, the clinician should review both the prescription and non-prescription medications the patient may be taking as this may contribute to delirium and mimic dementia (Thompson, 1983; Larson et al., 1986; Clarfield, 1988) (Indicator 1c). Evidence of substance abuse (e.g., alcohol abuse or benzodiazepine abuse) should also be sought (Indicator 1d). In a study of the diagnostic evaluation of dementia among 200 elderly outpatients, drug toxicity was responsible for approximately ten percent of cognitive impairment, while depression was the cause in eight percent (Larson, 1986). Clarfield (1988) critically reviewed the diagnosis of dementia and found that 13 percent of 2,889 subjects were found to have potentially reversible causes of cognitive impairment. Of the 1,051 patients for whom follow-up information was reported, eight percent had dementia that reversed partially and three percent completely. Depression was the etiologic factor of the apparent dementia in 26 percent of these cases, and drugs in 28 percent. Of note, dementia cannot be diagnosed if the changes are only present during a delirium or can be attributable to another mental disorder such as major depression or schizophrenia. Generally, reliable informant reports (e.g., family members, friends, neighbors, caregivers or employees) will be necessary to obtain complete information on the patient's cognitive changes.

To establish the etiology of dementia symptoms, it is particularly important in the history to establish the chronicity of symptoms (date of onset, abrupt versus gradual) and the nature of progression (stepwise versus continuous decline, worsening versus fluctuating or improving) (AHCPR, 1996; USDVAUHSC, 1996) (Indicator 2). Asking these questions may help determine if the symptoms are due to multiple strokes (often a stepwise pattern of decline) versus Alzheimer's disease (usually a progressive decline), and whether a delirium (abrupt onset, fluctuating course, and short duration) or depression is present (abrupt onset and short duration).

If the clinician notes that the patient has any symptoms suggestive of cognitive impairment, the eight guidelines recommend a brief neurological and mental status examination to assess the etiology of the impairment (Indicator 3). A physical examination can be useful to detect co-morbid medical conditions that may be exacerbating or causing the cognitive impairment, and to detect evidence of personal neglect (e.g., malnutrition, urinary incontinence).

Brief mental status tests can be used to: 1) develop a multidimensional clinical picture; 2) provide a baseline for monitoring the course of cognitive impairment over time; 3) reassess mental status in persons who have delirium or depression on initial evaluation; and, 4) document multiple cognitive impairments as required for the diagnosis of dementia (AHCPR, 1996). In a review of studies of diagnostic testing for dementia (Siu, 1991), four very brief screens had good predictive values for cognitive impairment: recall of three items (Folstein et al., 1975), the clock drawing test (Wolf-Klein et al., 1989), forward digit span (Kokmen, 1987), and the serial sevens test (Folstein et al., 1975). Normal results on these tests markedly reduce the probability of dementia, while abnormal results increase the odds of dementia (Siu, 1991; Klein et al., 1985; Wolf-Klein et al., 1989).

A longer and commonly used instrument to screen for cognitive impairment is the Folstein Mini-Mental State Examination (Folstein et al., 1975). It is most useful in screening for moderate impairment in cognitive function and has good reliability and construct validity (Tombaugh et al., 1992). Interpretation of this score must include assessment of possible confounding factors that may affect the patient's performance, such as level of consciousness, formal education, and English language comprehension.

Persons suspected of having cognitive impairment should also be asked about their ability to perform their daily activities. Instrumental Activities of Daily Living (IADLs) include tasks that one needs to perform to live independently. These include such functions as taking medications, using the telephone, housekeeping, and transportation. When IADLs were administered to a group of community-dwelling persons over age 65, subjects who reported difficulty using the telephone, using public transportation, taking medications, or handling finances were 12 times more likely to be diagnosed with dementia (Barberger-Gateau et al., 1992).

Laboratory Evaluation

There is much overlap in the experts' recommendations regarding further laboratory evaluation of persons having abnormal mental status tests, depending upon the suspected etiology. The CCCAD recommends a complete blood count (CBC), thyroid function tests and serum electrolytes, calcium and glucose. The AAN, the USDVAUHSC, and the NIH Consensus Panel on Dementia recommend the addition of BUN/creatinine, liver function tests, serum vitamin B_{12} level, and syphilis serology. The AAN and the USDVAUHSC also recommend the following tests when clinical suspicion warrants them: sedimentation rate (to detect inflammatory disorders), serum folate (to detect folate deficiency in a person with megaloblastic anemia), HIV test (in persons with risk factors for HIV), chest x-ray (to detect severe lung disease that might

97

cause hypoxemia and secondary cognitive impairment or lung cancer with possible brain metastases), urinalysis (to detect urinary tract infection), 24 hour urine collection for heavy metals (to detect heavy metal toxicity), and toxicology screen (in persons suspected of substance abuse). These laboratory tests will detect anemia, hyper- or hypoparathyroidism, diabetes, renal failure, liver disease, thyroid disorders, vitamin B_{12} deficiency and syphilitic infection that may be causing or contributing to the patient's dementia.

Some observational data support the utility of selected laboratory tests in the evaluation of dementia. A study assessing the utility of standard blood tests in the evaluation of dementia (Larson et al., 1986) observed that five percent of 200 elderly outpatients with suspected dementia had metabolic abnormalities that may have caused or contributed to their cognitive impairment. These included hypothyroidism, hyponatremia, hyperparathyroidism and hypoglycemia. In Clarfield's (1988) review of dementia diagnosis studies, metabolic causes were presumed to be the etiologic factor in 16 percent of potentially reversible cases. Persons who have abnormalities on any of these tests should have longitudinal follow-up to initiate interventions and ensure that such interventions are effective.

In accordance with these data, we recommend a quality indicator stating that a CBC, thyroid function tests and chemistry panel (including electrolytes, BUN, creatinine, calcium and glucose) be obtained in all patients suspected of having dementia (Indicator 4). These tests may occasionally be useful in diagnosing dementia and are more frequently helpful in identifying and treating medical conditions that complicate dementia (Larson et al., 1986). Testing for the e4 allele (for apolipoprotein E4) does not predict which individuals will get Alzheimer's disease and it does not contribute to the routine evaluation of the patient with dementia (Civil et al., 1993).

Neuroimaging

As with blood tests, the USDVAUHSC does not recommend neuroimaging if the cause of dementia is apparent from the history, examination or laboratory studies. They recommend neuroimaging only in recent onset dementia patients with focal neurologic signs, atypical features, or

98

headaches (Indicator 5). The CCCAD also recommends cranial imaging if one or more of the following criteria are met:

a. age under 60 years;

b. use of anticoagulants or history of a bleeding disorder;

c. recent head trauma (i.e., if dementia started or worsened after head trauma in the last three to four months);

d. history of cancer, especially in sites that metastasize to the brain (e.g., lung, breast, renal cell, melanoma, GI tract);

e. unexplained neurologic symptoms (e.g., new onset of severe headache or seizures);

f. rapid (i.e., over one to two months) unexplained decline in cognition or function;

g. short duration of dementia (less than two years);

h. history of urinary incontinence and gait disorder early in the course of dementia (as may be found in normal pressure hydrocephalus);

i. any new localizing sign (e.g., heimparesis or Babinski's reflex); and,

j. gait ataxia.

The CCCAD states that, in the absence of these symptoms and signs, cognitive impairment, especially if present for at least one to two years, would not likely be reversible and referral for CT scanning probably would not be indicated. However, they argue that neuroimaging should be considered in every patient with dementia based on the clinical presentation, and may facilitate identification of clincally unsuspected treatable conditions such as tumor, subdural hematomas, hydrocephalus and strokes. They make the point, however, that unanticipated detection of these conditions is uncommon, particularly when clinical evaluations are performed by experienced examiners. A recent review of the utility of CT or MRI in diagnosis of an intracranial lesion or multi-infarct dementia concludes that routinely obtaining imaging studies on all patients is unwarranted, given the poor yield, number of false-positive results, and the sometimes poor outcome of "treatable" lesions (Siu, 1991; Dietch, 1983; Martin, 1987).

Consistent with this literature, our proposed indicators do not require routine imaging for intracranial disease or multi-infarct dementia.

Referral

The CCCAD states that most patients with dementia can be assessed adequately by their primary care physicians. However, there are several reasons to consider referral to a geriatrician, geriatric psychiatrist, neurologist, geriatric pyschologist or neuropsychologist: a) continuing uncertainty about the diagnosis after initial assessment and follow-up; b) request by the family or the patient for another opinion; c) the presence of significant depression, especially if it does not respond to treatment; d) possible industrial exposure to heavy metals; e) the need for help in patient's management (e.g. if there are behavioral problems) or support of the caregiver, who may be under stress; f) the need to involve other health professionals (e.g. occupational therapists, social workers and neuropsychologists) in the evaluation or management; and g) when research studies into diagnosis or treatment are being carried out (CCCAD, 1991; ANN, 1994; AHCPR, 1996). The CCCAD suggests that patients with dementia not be referred to these specialists if the dementia has been present for many years and there are no problems in management, if the patient is expected to die soon from a coexisting condition or if risky or costly interventions would be inappropriate.

Other Diagnostic Tests

The AAN does not recommend a lumbar puncture as a routine study in evaluation of dementia. They state: "assuming no contraindications, a lumbar puncture should be performed when any of the following are present: metastatic cancer, suspicion of CNS infection, reactive serum syphilis serology, hydrocephalus, dementia in a person under age 55, a readily progressive or unusual dementia, immunosuppression, and suspicion of CNS vasculitis (particularly in patients with connective tissue diseases)" (AAN, 1994).

The AAN also does not recommend EEG as a routine study but they state it "may assist in distinguishing depression or delirium from dementia and in evaluating for suspected encephalitis, Creutzfeld-Jacob disease, metabolic encephalopathy or seizures" (AAN, 1994).

TREATMENT

Many dementing illnesses are progressive, or remain stable after substantial irreversible impairment has occurred. Survival after the onset of dementia often spans a decade during which the patient undergoes a progressive loss of function and requires ongoing medical, family and community support. Cummings states that the management of demented persons has five major aspects: 1) treating the underlying disorder that is causing or contributing to the cognitive decline (e.g., vascular dementia, Parkinson's disease, depression); 2) treating the cognitive deficit in selected patients with Alzheimer's disease (e.g., tacrine); 3) addressing associated behavioral disturbances (e.g., depression, psychosis, agitation); 4) reducing the consequences of disability (e.g., treating infections, pressure sores, dehydration); and 5) addressing the needs of the caregiver (e.g., support groups, respite services, day care, legal and social work consultation) (Cummings, 1995).

Treatments to improve cognition in Alzheimer patients have been studied in randomized clinical trials. Drugs that increase brain levels of acetylcholine, such as tacrine and donepezil, have shown the most promise. Although several studies reported no benefit, the three largest trials suggested a significant but small benefit of tacrine in patients with mild to moderate dementia[1] over six to 30 weeks (Gauthier et al., 1990; Schneider and Tariot, 1994; Farlow et al., 1992; Davis et al., 1992; Knapp et al., 1994). In one trial, the benefit of tacrine on cognitive test results was comparable to delaying disease progression by two years for responders, with an overall average of five months (Farlow et al., 1992). Use of tacrine is limited by high cost (over $100 per month), four times a day dosing, and frequently gastrointestinal side effects. Up to 25 percent of patients taking lower doses, and two-thirds of those on high doses, stopped therapy due to nausea, vomiting,

---

[1] Defined as an average Mini-Mental State Examination score of 16 to 19.

or elevated liver enzymes (Schneider and Tariot, 1994; Farlow et al., 1992; Davis et al., 1992; Knapp et al., 1994). The potential for liver toxicity requires that aminotransferase levels be monitored weekly for the first six months.

Donepezil (Aricept, 1996) was approved by the FDA in November 1996 for the treatment of patients with mild to moderate Alzheimer's disease. This drug appears to be better tolerated and to have a better safety profile than tacrine. Use of donepezil has been associated with a delay in disease progression by six to eight months (Stern et al., 1994; Aricept, 1996; Rogers et al., 1995; Rogers et al., 1996). In contrast to tacrine, this drug has a long half-life and can be given once daily and requires no laboratory monitoring (Indicator 6).

Persons with vascular dementia should have risk factors for cerebrovascular disease (hypertension, smoking cessation, hypercholesterolemia) addressed (Meyer et al., 1986; Hachinski, 1992) (Indicators 8 and 9). However, the effect that addressing risk factors has on the progression of vascular dementia is not known.

Cummings, in his review of dementia, notes that behavioral symptoms associated with dementia often improve with non-pharmacological measures, such as avoiding situations that incite outbursts, developing patient-centered environments, and teaching behavior management strategies to family members and caregivers (Cummings, 1995) (Indicator 6). Generally, non-pharmacological approaches should be used before drugs to control behavior are initiated. When medication is used, the drug therapy should be guided by a specific diagnosis (e.g., psychotic symptoms) and choice of treatment target (e.g., improved night time sleep). As with all older patients, the starting doses should be smaller and doses should be increased more slowly than in younger adults. Clinicians and caregivers should be alert for potential side-effects of psychotropic agents, including sedation, confusion, and postural instability. Neuroleptics such as haloperidol or risperidone may also cause tremors, parkinsonism, akathisia, and tardive dyskinesia. The medication regimen should be reviewed regularly and drugs reduced or eliminated whenever possible. Long-acting sedatives should not be used in demented persons as they have been associated with an increased risk of confusion, ataxia, over sedation, and hip fracture among older persons (Thompson, 1983; Pomara, 1985; Greenblatt, 1977; Ray, 1987; Ray, 1989) (Indicator 10).

Finally, care of the caregiver is an essential part of the management of dementia (Council on Scientific Affairs, 1993). It is stressful to provide care to demented persons and family members provide most of that care. Community resources such as home care, day care, respite care, and extended residential care may ameliorate the burden of care. Participation in a support group may help and some caregivers may require formal psychotherapy (Indicator 7).

The USDVAUHSC recommends referral to psychologists and specialized geropsychologists to assist with the management of cognitive deficits and the associated emotional and behavioral problems that often develop in the course of dementia (Indicator 6). They further assert that social workers should be involved in the management of all patients with dementia as they may help in identifying community resources available for patients and families. Support for this recommendation is provided by a recent randomized controlled trial testing the effectiveness of a family intervention to delay nursing home placement of patients with Alzheimer's disease (Mittelman et al., 1996). The intervention consisted of providing caregivers in the treatment group with six sessions of individual and family counseling and requiring them to join support groups. Caregivers in the control group received the usual social services provided by the dementia clinic. The intervention succeeded in delaying the time that caregivers place patients with Alzheimer's disease in nursing homes by a median of 329 days.

FOLLOW-UP

Persons who have memory complaints or difficulty with daily functioning, but who don't meet criteria for dementia, should have mental and functional status tests repeated in 6 to 12 months (AHCPR, 1996) (Indicator 11). Among persons with dementia, periodic mental status tests may mark the course of the disease and assist in informing caregivers of expectant function. Abrupt changes in cognitive or functional status need to be evaluated for superimposed delirium secondary to infection, myocardial infarction, stroke, depression or adverse drug reaction. Issues of safety will need to be evaluated on an ongoing basis. Although there are no formal recommendations about the frequency of routine follow-up of demented persons, it is advisable that demented persons be seen or contacted at least every six months.

REFERENCES

Agency for Health Care Policy and Resarch. 1996. *Early Alzheimer's Disease: Recognition and Assessment*. USDHHS, Rockville, MD.

American Academy of Family Physicians. 1994. *Age charts for periodic health examination*. American Academy of Family Physicians, Kansas City, MO.

American Medical Association, and Council on Scientific Affairs. 1993. Physicians and family caregivers: A model for partnership. *Journal of the American Medical Association* 269: 1282-1284.

1996. *AriceptTM (Donepezil hydrochloride) Product Monograph*. Roerig Division of Pfizer, Inc., New York, New York.

Aronson MK, Ooi WL, Geva DL, et al. 1991. Dementia. Age-dependent incidence, prevalence, and mortality in the old. *Archives of Internal Medicine* 151: 989-992.

Barberger-Gateau P, Commenges D, Gagnon M, et al. 1992. Instrumental activities of daily living as a screening tool for cognitive impairment and dementia in elderly community dwellers. *Journal of the American Geriatric Society* 40: 1129-1134.

Callahan CM, Hendric HC, and Tierney WM. 1995. Documentation and evaluation of cognitive impairment in elderly primary care patients. *Archives of Internal Medicine* 122: 422-429.

Canadian Consensus Conference on the Assessment of Dementia, and Organizing Committee. 1991. Assessing dementia: The Canadian consensus. *Canadian Medical Association Journal* 144 (7): 851-853.

Canadian Task Force on the Period Health Examination. 1979. The periodic health examination. *Canadian Medical Association Journal* 121: 1193-1254.

Civil RH, Whitehouse PJ, Lanska DJ, and Mayeux R. 1993. Degenerative dementia. In *Dementia*. ed Whitehouse PJ, 167-214. Philadelphia: Davis.

Clarfield AM. 1988. The reversible dementias: Do they reverse? *Archives of Internal Medicine* 109: 476-486.

Corey-Bloom J, Thal LJ, Galasko D, Folstein M, Drachman D, Raskind M, and Lanska DJ. 1995. Diagnosis and evaluation of dementia. *Neurology* 45: 211-218.

Cummings JL. 1995. Dementia: The failing brain. *Lancet* 345: 1481-1484.

Cummings JL, and Benson DF. 1992. Dementia: A Clinical Approach. 2nd Edition. Stoneham MA: Butterworth-Heinemann.

Davis KL, Thal LJ, Gamzu ER, et al. 1992. A double-blind, placebo-controlled multicenter study of tacrine for Alzheimer's disease. *New England Journal of Medicine* 327: 1253-1259.

Dementia Consensus Conference. 1987. Differential diagnosis of dementing diseases. *Journal of the American Medical Association* 258 (23): 3411-3416.

Dietch JT. 1983. Computerized tomographic scanning in cases of dementia. *Western Journal of Medicine* 138: 835-837.

Farlow M, Gracon SI, Hershey LA, et al. 1992. A controlled trial of tacrine in Alzheimer's disease. *Journal of the American Medical Association* 268: 2523-2529.

Folstein MF, Folstein SE, and McHugh PR. 1975. "Mini-Mental State": a practical method for grading the cognitive state of patients for the clinician. *Journal of Psychiatric Research* 12: 189-198.

Gauthier S, Bouchard R, Lamontagne A, et al. 1990. Tetrahydroaminoacridine-lecithin combination treatment in patients with intermediate-stage Alzheimer's disease. *New England Journal of Medicine* 322: 1272-1276.

German PS, Shapiro S, Skinner EA, et al. 1987. Detection and management of mental health problems of older patients by primary care providers. *Journal of the American Medical Association* 257: 489-493.

Hachinski V. 1992. Preventable senility: A call for action against the vascular dementias. *Lancet* 340: 645-648.

Heyman A, Fillenbaum G, et al. 1991. Estimated prevalence of dementia among elderly black and white community residents. *Archives of Neurology* 48: 594-598.

Jorm AF, Korten AE, and Henderson AS. 1987. The prevalence of dementia: A quantitative integration of the literature. *Acta Psychiatrica Scandinavia* 76: 464-470.

Klein LE, Roca RP, McArthur J, et al. 1985. Diagnosing dementia. *Journal of the American Geriatric Society* 33: 483-488.

Knapp MJ, Knopman DS, Solomon PR, et al. 1994. A 30-week randomized controlled trial of high-dose tacrine in patients with Alzheimer's disease. *Journal of the American Medical Association* 271: 985-991.

Kokmen E, Naessens JM, and Offord KP. 1987. A short test of mental status: description and preliminary results. *Mayo Clinic Proceedings* 62: 281-288.

Larson EB, Reifler BV, Sumi SM, Canfield CG, and Chinn NM. 1986. Diagnostic tests in the evaluation of dementia. *Archives of Internal Medicine* 146: 1917-1922.

Martin DC, Miller J, Kapoor W, Karpf M, and Boller F. 1987. Clinical prediction rules for computed tomographic scanning in senile dementia. *Archives of Internal Medicine* 147: 77-80.

Meyer JS, Judd BW, Tawaklna T, Rogers RL, and Mortel KF. 1986. Improved cognition after control of risk factors for multi-infarct dementia. *Journal of the American Medical Association* 256: 2203-2209.

Mittelman MS, Ferris SH, Shulman E, Steinberg G, and Levin B. 1996. A family intervention to delay nursing home placement of patients with Alzheimer disease. *Journal of the American Medical Association* 276: 1725-1731.

National Foundation for Brain Research. 1992. *The cost of disorders of the brain*. National Foundation for Brain Research, Washington, DC.

Pinholt EM, Kroenke K, Hanley JF, et al. 1987. Functional assessment of the elderly: A comparison of standard instruments with clinical judgement. *Archives of Internal Medicine* 137: 484-488.

Pomara N, Stanley B, Block R, et al. 1985. Increased sensitivity of the elderly to central depressant effects of diazepam. *Journal of Clinical Psychiatry* 45: 185-187.

Quality Standards Subcommittee of the American Academy of Neurology. 1994. Practice parameter for diagnosis and evaluation of dementia: Summary statement. *Neurology* 44: 2203-2206.

Ray WA, Griffin MR, and Downey W. 1989. Benzodiazepines of long and short elimination half-life and the risk of hip fracture. *Journal of the American Medical Association* 262: 3303-3307.

Ray WA, Griffin MR, Schaffner W, Baugh DK, and Melton LJ 3d. 1987. Psychotropic drug use and the risk of hip fracture. *New England Journal of Medicine* 316: 363-369.

Roca RP, Klein LE, Kirby SM, et al. 1984. Recognition of dementia among medical patients. *Archives of Internal Medicine* 144: 73-75.

Schneider LS, and Tariot PN. 1994. Emerging drugs for Alzheimer's disease. *Medical Clinics of North America* 78: 911-934.

Siu AL. 1991. Screening for dementia and investigating its causes. *Archives of Internal Medicine* 115: 122-132.

Skoog I, Nillson L, Palmertz B, et al. 1993. A population-based study of dementia in 85-year olds. *New England Journal of Medicine* 328: 153-158.

Stern RG, Mohs RC, Davidson, et al. 1994. A longitudinal study of Alzheimer's Disease measurement: Rate and predictors of cognitive deterioration. *American Journal of Psychiatry* 161: 390-396.

Thompson TL II, Moran MG, and Nies AS. 1983. Psychotropic drug use in the elderly. *New England Journal of Medicine* 308: 134-138, 194-199.

Tombaugh TN, and McIntyre NJ. 1992. The Mini-Mental State Examination: a comprehensive review. *Journal of the American Geriatric Society* 40: 922-935.

US Department of Veterans Affairs and the University Health System Consortium. 1996. *Dementia identification and assessment: guidelines for primary care practitioners*. Technology Assessment Program, University HealthSystem Consortium; Washington, DC: Veterans Health Administration, U.S. Department of Veterans Affairs, Oak Brook, IL.

US Preventative Services Task Force. 1996. *Guide to Clinical Preventative Services, 2nd ed.* Baltimore: Williams & Wilkins.

Winograd C, and Jarvik LF. 1986. Physician management of the demented patient. *Journal of the American Geriatric Society* 34: 295-308.

Wolf-Klein GP, Silverstone FA, Levy AP, Brod MS, and Breuer J. 1989. Screening for Alzheimer's disease by clock drawing. *Journal of the American Geriatric Society* 37: 730-734.

World Health Organization. 1986. Dementia in later life: research and action: report of a WHO scientific group on senile dementia. World Health Organization, Geneva.

RECOMMENDED QUALITY INDICATORS FOR DEMENTIA

The following indicators apply to men and women age 18 and older.

Indicator	Quality of Evidence	Literature	Benefits	Comments
Diagnosis				
1. If a patient has any symptoms of cognitive impairment,[1] all of the following information should be documented:				
a. Have the patient's cognitive abilities declined from a previous level?	III	CTFP, 1979; NIH, 1987; CCCAD, 1991; AAFP, 1994; QSSAAN, 1994; AHCPR, 1996; USPSTF, 1996; USDVAUHSC, 1996.	Ensures patient's cognitive deficits are not due to a lifelong condition such as mental retardation.	Recommended by all the consensus developers and guidelines.
b. Do the patient's symptoms of cognitive impairment interfere with daily functioning?[2]	III		Improve functional status.	Recommended by all the consensus developers and guidelines. Assists in determining the extent of the cognitive impairment.
c. Medications being taken (both prescription and non-prescription);	II-2	Larson, 1986; Clarfield, 1988	Limit toxicities of medication.	Many medications may contribute to delirium and mimic dementia. Two case series observed between 3-10% of cases of dementia were actually caused by drug toxicity.
d. The use of alcohol or other substances that may affect cognition;	II-2	Larson, 1986; Clarfield, 1988	Limit contribution of alcohol to dementia.	Alcohol and sedative-hypnotics may contribute to delirium and mimic dementia. Two case series observed alcohol and medications are major cause of reversible dementia.

109

Indicator	Quality of Evidence	Literature	Benefits	Comments
e. The presence or absence of delirium;	II-2, III	CTFP, 1979; NIH, 1987; CCCAD, 1991; AAFP, 1994; QSSAAN, 1994; AHCPR, 1996; USPSTF, 1996; U.S. Department of Veterans Affairs and the University Health System Consortium, 1996; Larson, 1986; Clarfiled,1988.	Limit symptoms of dementia by treating delerium.	Symptoms of delirium may mimic dementia. Two case series observed that delirium was responsible for 3-10% cases of diagnosed dementia.
f. The presence or absence of depression.	II-2, III		Limit symptoms of dementia by treating depression.	Two case series observed between 3-8% of cases of dementia were actually due to depression.
2. All of the following information should be documented for patients with a diagnosis of dementia: a. The chronicity of symptoms (e.g. noted one week ago vs. 2 years ago, abrupt vs. gradual); b. The nature of progression (e.g., worsening, fluctuating, stable).	III	AHCPR, 1996; USDVAUHSC, 1996	Identify potentially treatable causes of dementia.	Recommended by the AHCPR and the U.S. Department of Veterans Affairs and the University Health System Consortium. May help determine if the dementia is due to multiple strokes vs. Alzheimer's disease or whether a delirium or depression is causing symptoms.

Indicator	Quality of Evidence	Literature	Benefits	Comments
3. If a patient has any new symptoms of cognitive impairment,[1] the health care provider should offer a neurological examination (including a mental status examination).	III	CTFP, 1979; NIH, 1987; CCCAD, 1991; AAFP, 1994; QSSAAN, 1994; AHCPR, 1996; USPSTF, 1996; U.S. Department of Veterans Affairs and the University Health System Consortium, 1996	Identify potentially treatable causes of cognitive impairment. Limit danger to self and environment by diagnosing severity of impairments.	Recommended by all consensus and guideline developers. Neurological examination and mental status exam may assist in determining etiology and severity of dementia.
4. If patient has any new symptoms of cognitive impairment,[1] the following blood tests should be offered within 30 days: a. CBC (if not ordered in last month), b. Chemistry panel (electrolytes, BUN, creatinine, bicarbonate, chloride, glucose, calcium) if not ordered in last 2 weeks; c. TSH if not ordered in last 6 months.	II-2, III	CCCAD, 1991; QSSAAN, 1994; U.S. Department of Veterans Affairs and the University Health System Consortium, 1996; Larson, 1986; Clarfield, 1988	Identify potentially treatable contributors to dementia.	Frequently helpful in identifying and treating medical conditions that complicate dementia. Two case series observed that metabolic abnormalities were causing or contributing to cognitive impairment in 2-5% of demented persons. Recommended by three consensus developers.

Indicator	Quality of Evidence	Literature	Benefits	Comments
5. If a patient has any new symptoms of cognitive impairment,[1] a head CT or MRI should be offered within 30 days if one or more of the following criteria is met: a. onset of dementia in the past 2 years; b. head trauma in the past 2 years; c. onset of seizures in the past 2 years; d. gait disorder in the past 2 years; e. dementia with focal neurologic findings;[3] f. dementia and headache.	III	CCCAD, 1991; QSSAAN, 1994; U.S. Department of Veterans Affairs and the University Health System Consortium, 1996	Identify potentially treatable causes of cognitive impairment.	These are indicators of potentially treatable conditions. Recommended by three consensus developers
Treatment				
6. Patients with a diagnosis of dementia and who are having behavioral problems[4] should be offered at least one of the following interventions: • counseling the caregivers about non-pharmacological measures[5] to control symptoms; • providing pharmacological means[6] to control symptoms; • referral to specialists[7] who may assist with symptoms.	III	CCCAD, 1991; QSSAAN, 1994; U.S. Department of Veterans Affairs and the University Health System Consortium, 1996; Cummings, 1995.	Improve the health and functioning of persons with dementia.	Recommended by three of the consensus developers.
7. Caregivers of demented persons should be asked about their need for support services.	I	Council on Scientific Affairs, 1993; Mittelman, 1996; U.S. Department of Veterans Affairs and the University Health System Consortium, 1996	Improve health and functioning of persons with dementia and their caregivers.	A randomized controlled trial of an intense social intervention targeted to spouses of persons with Alzheimer's disease delayed the time they placed demented persons in nursing homes by a median of 329 days.

112

Indicator	Quality of Evidence	Literature	Benefits	Comments
8. For patients diagnosed with dementia, the presence or absence of all of the following risk factors for vascular etiology should be documented: a. hypertension; b. smoking; c. hypercholesterolemia.	III	Hachinski, 1992, Meyer, 1986	Prevent CVAs.	Amelioration of risk factors for cerebrovascular disease may prevent further strokes. It is unknown whether addressing risk factors for vascular dementia affects its progression.
9. Patients with vascular or multi-infarct dementia should be offered aspirin, unless active peptic ulcer disease or aspirin intolerance is noted.	III	Hachinski, 1992, Meyer, 1986	Prevent further CVAs.	
10. Persons with dementia should not be taking long-acting sedatives.	II-1,III	Thompson, 1983; Pomara, 1985; Greenblatt, 1977; Ray, 1987; Ray, 1989	Prevent medication toxicities. Prevent falls and fractures.	Long-acting sedatives increase risk for adverse CNS effects (i.e., delirium, ataxia) and risks for hip fracture in older persons, particularly those persons with an underlying dementia. Pomara et al. demonstrated increased CNS depressant effect of diazepam in elderly. Greenblatt et al noted that excess CNS effects of flurazepam were more common in older hospitalized patients. Ray, et al.0 found association between long acting benzodiazepines and the occurrence of hip fractures in older persons.
Follow-up				
11. Patients with symptoms of cognitive impairment who do not receive a diagnosis of dementia should have documented that the provider inquired again about those symptoms within 12 months of first presentation.	III	AHCPR, 1996	Improve quality of life for persons with dementia and their caregivers.	May permit early identification of persons with dementia and allow them to plan for future. Recom-mended by AHCPR.

Definitions and Examples

[1] Symptoms of cognitive impairment include: (a) difficulty learning and retaining new information such as forgetting appointments, (b) handling complex tasks such as balancing a checkbook or preparing a meal, (c) problems with reasoning, such as knowing what to do if the bathroom flooded , (d) deficits in spatial ability and orientation such as having trouble driving or finding his or her way around familiar places, (e) language difficulties, like difficulty with word finding, (f) behavior changes such as being more suspicious or passive than usual. "New symptoms" means onset within the past 2 years.

[2] Daily functioning includes such activities as:

113

a. Activities of Daily Living (ADLs): bathing, dressing, feeding oneself, urinary continence

b. Instrumental Activities of Daily Living (IADLs): taking medications, doing housework, taking care of finances, using the telephone, preparing meals, using transportation

c. Advanced Activities of Daily Living (AADLs): working, doing hobbies, social events, sports

[3] Focal neurologic findings include asymmetry in any of the following: deep tendon reflexes, Babinsky reflexes, motor strength, cranial nerves, and visual fields.

[4] Behavioral problems: aggression, withdrawl, paranoia, hallucinations (seeing objects that are not there, like deceased parents), or delusions (believing things that are not real, such as spouse's infidelity).

[5] Non-pharmacologic measures: (a) avoiding situations that incite behavioral problems; (b) using a calm soothing tone; (c) repeating messages frequently; (d) avoiding changes in the demented person's routine; (e) trying to structure the home environment to allow unrestricted walking or pacing.

[6] Pharmacologic means include any of the following: (a) antipsychotics, including haloperidol, fluphenazine, thioridazine, molindone, thiothixene, mellaril, respirdol; (b) antidepressants, including fluoxetine, sertraline, paroxetine, nortripytline, trazadone, desipramine, doxepin; (c) anti-anxiety drugs such as busprione, temazepam, lorazepam, oxazepam; (d) anti-seizure medications such as carbamazepine.

[7] Specialists include: psychiatrists, neurologists, psychologists, registered occupational therapists, mental health nurse practitioners, and social service providers.

Quality of Evidence Codes

I   RCT
II-1   Nonrandomized controlled trials
II-2   Cohort or case analysis
II-3   Multiple time series
III   Opinions or descriptive studies

114

8. DEPRESSION[1]

Eve A. Kerr, M.D., M.P.H. and Kenneth A. Clark, M.D., M.P.H.

We relied on the following sources to construct quality indicators for depression: the AHCPR Clinical Practice Guideline *Depression in Primary Care* (AHCPR, 1993a and 1993b), as well as selected review and journal articles. We also conducted a MEDLINE search for review articles published in English between the years 1985 and 1997.

IMPORTANCE

Major depression is a common condition, affecting more than ten percent of adults between the ages of 14 and 55 annually (Kessler, 1994). Major depressive disorder is characterized by one or more episodes of major depression without episodes of mania or hypomania. By definition, major depressive episodes last at least two weeks, and typically much longer. Up to one in eight individuals may require treatment for depression during their lifetime (AHCPR, 1993b). The common age of onset is from 20 to 40; however, depression can start at any age.

Approximately 11 million people in the United States suffered from depression in 1990; a disproportionate share (7.7 million) were women (Greenberg et al., 1993). The point prevalence for major depressive disorder in Western industrialized nations is 2.3 to 3.2 percent for men and 4.5 to 9.3 percent for women (AHCPR, 1993a). Katon and Schulberg (1992) report that among general medical outpatients, the prevalence rate for major depression is between five and nine percent, and six percent for the less severe diagnosis of dysthymia. Consistent with these findings, Feldman et al. (1987) found that the point prevalence of major depressive disorder in primary care outpatient settings ranged

---

[1] This chapter is a revision of one written for an earlier project on quality of care for women and children (Q1). The expert panel for the current project was asked to review all of the indicators, but only rated new or revised indicators.

from 4.8 to 8.6 percent. The lifetime risk for developing depression is between 20 and 25 percent for women.

Depression is associated with severe deterioration of a person's ability to function in social, occupational, and interpersonal settings (Broadhead et al., 1990; Wells et al., 1989a). Broadhead, et al. (1990) found that patients with major depressive disorder reported 11 disability days per 90-day interval compared to 2.2 disability days for the general population. Roughly one-quarter of all persons with major depressive disorder reported restricted activity or bed days in the past two weeks (Wells et al., 1988). The functioning of depressed patients is comparable with or worse than that of patients with other major chronic medical conditions, such as congestive heart failure (Hays et al., 1995).

The direct costs associated with treating major depressive disorder, combined with the indirect costs from lost productivity, account for about $16 billion per year in 1980 dollars (AHCPR, 1993a). Greenberg et al. (1993) estimate that the total costs of affective disorders are $12.4 billion for direct treatment, $7.5 billion for mortality costs due to suicide, and $23.8 billion in morbidity costs due to reduction in productivity ($11.7 billion from excess absenteeism and $12.1 billion while at work).

Sturm and Wells (1994) recently demonstrated the cost-effectiveness of treatment for depression. They found that treatment consistent with standards/guidelines lowers the average cost per quality-adjusted life-year when compared to no treatment or ineffective treatment (e.g., subtherapeutic doses of antidepressants). To achieve this gain, however, total costs of care are higher.

SCREENING

The under-diagnosis of depression seriously impedes intervention efforts. The AHCPR Depression Guidelines report that only one-third to one-half of all cases of major depressive disorders are properly recognized by primary care and non-psychiatric practitioners (AHCPR, 1993a; Wells et al., 1989b). The Medical Outcomes Study (MOS) revealed that approximately 50 percent of patients with depression were detected

116

by general medical clinicians, and among patients in prepaid health plans the rates of detection were much lower than those observed for patients in fee-for-service plans (Wells et al., 1989b).

No definitive screening method exists to detect major depression. Patient self-report questionnaires are available, but are non-specific. These questionnaires can be used to supplement the results of direct interview by a clinician (AHCPR, 1993a). Burnam et al. (1988) used an eight-item screen in the MOS; however, no standard screen currently exists for clinical work.

A clinical interview is the most effective method for detecting depression (AHCPR, 1993a) (Indicator 1). Clinicians should especially look for symptoms in patients who are at high risk. Risk factors for depression include prior episodes of depression[1], family history of depressive disorder, prior suicide attempts, female gender, postpartum period, medical comorbidity, lack of social support, stressful life events; and current alcohol or substance abuse (AHCPR, 1993a).

Laboratory testing for depression is effective only in identifying underlying physiologic reasons for depression (e.g., hypothyroidism). No laboratory screening test exists for depression *per se* and thus, laboratory tests should be tailored to the patient, when indicated, as part of a diagnostic work-up. Laboratory testing should especially be considered as part of the general evaluation if: the medical review of systems reveals signs or symptoms that are rarely encountered in depression, the patient is older, the depressive episode first occurs after the age of 40 to 45, or the depression does not respond fully to routine treatment (AHCPR, 1993a).

DIAGNOSIS

The diagnosis of depression is based primarily on DSM-IV criteria. The criteria state that at least five of the following symptoms must be present during the same period to receive a diagnosis of major depression: depressed mood, markedly diminished interest or pleasure in

---

[1] One major depressive episode is associated with a 50 percent chance of a subsequent episode; two episodes with a 70 percent chance, and three or more with a 90 percent chance of recurrent depression over a lifetime (NIMH Consensus Development Conference, 1985).

almost all activities, significant weight loss/gain, insomnia/hypersomnia, psychomotor agitation/retardation, fatigue, feelings of worthlessness (guilt), impaired concentration and recurrent thoughts of death or suicide (American Psychiatric Association, 1994). The symptoms should be present most of the day, nearly daily, for a minimum of two weeks.

Practitioners need to consider the presence of other co-morbidities prior to making a diagnosis of major depression. Other factors that may contribute to the patient's mental health and which the clinician may want to treat first include: substance abuse, medications that cause depression, general medical disorder, causal, non-mood psychiatric disorder and/or grief reaction (AHCPR, 1993a) (Indicator 2). The clinician should also consider alternative diagnoses by eliciting a proper patient history. Examples of alternative diagnoses include: bipolar disorder (if the patient manifests prior manic episodes), or dysthymic disorder (if the patient has a chronic mood disturbance [sadness] present most of the time for at least two consecutive years) (AHCPR, 1993a).

TREATMENT

Treatment is more effective if provided earlier in the depressive episode, prior to the condition becoming chronic (Bielski and Friedel, 1976; Kupfer et al., 1989)(Indicator 3). Early inquiry about the presence of suicidal ideation should be made (AHCPR, 1993a) (Indicator 4). Persons who have suicidality should be asked if they have specific plans to carry out suicide in order to take the appropriate precautionary measures (AHCPR, 1993a) (Indicator 5). Persons who have suicidality and have any of the following risk factors should be hospitalized:

- Psychosis;
- Current alcohol or drug abuse or dependency;
- Specific plans to carry out suicide (e.g., obtaining a weapon, putting affairs in order, making a suicide note) (AHCPR, 1993a) (Indicator 6).

Unless noted otherwise, the remaining recommendations for treatment are drawn from the AHCPR *Depression Guideline* (AHCPR, 1993b), which were developed for the primary care setting.

Use of Antidepressant Medications

Antidepressant medications are the first-line treatments for major depressive disorder. Medications have been shown to be effective in all forms of major depressive disorder. Antidepressant medications are highly likely to be of benefit when:

1. The depression is moderate to severe;

2. There are psychotic, melancholic, or atypical symptom features;

3. The patient requests medication;

4. Psychotherapy by a trained, competent psychotherapist is not available; and,

5. The patient has shown a prior positive response to medication; and, maintenance treatment is planned.

The choice of antidepressant is less important than use of antidepressants at appropriate dosages (Wells et al., 1994) (Indicator 7). No single antidepressant medication is clearly more effective than another and no single medication results in remission for all patients. Pharmacologic doses are recommended in the AHCPR *Depression Guideline* (1993b).

The specific choice of medication should be based on:

1. Short- and long-term side effects;

2. Prior positive/negative response to medication;

3. Concurrent, nonpsychiatric medical illnesses that may make selected medications more or less risky; and/or,

4. The concomitant use of other non-psychotropic medications that may alter the metabolism or increase the side effects of the antidepressant.

5. In general, anxiolytic agents should not be used (with possible exception of alprazolam) (Indicator 8).

Use of Psychotherapy

Maintenance medication clearly prevents recurrences, while, to date, maintenance psychotherapy does not (AHCPR, 1993a). Clinicians should consider psychotherapy alone for major depression as a first-line treatment if the episode is mild to moderate AND the patient desires psychotherapy as the first-line therapy. If psychotherapy is completely ineffective by 6 weeks of treatment or if psychotherapy does not result in nearly a fully symptomatic remission within 12 weeks, then a switch to medications is appropriate due to the clear evidence of the efficacy of treatment with medications.

Medication Plus Psychotherapy

Clinicians should consider combined treatment initially with medications and psychotherapy if:

1. The depression is chronic or characterized by poor inter-episode recovery;

2. Either treatment alone has been only partially effective;

3. The patient has a history of chronic psychosocial problems; or,

4. The patient has a history of treatment adherence difficulties.

However, there is little evidence that indicates that patients being seen in primary care practices who have major depression require initial psychotherapy in addition to medication. It is recommended that medication be added to (or substituted for) psychotherapy if:

1. There is no response to psychotherapy at 6 weeks;

2. There is only partial response at 12 weeks;

3. The patient worsens with psychotherapy; or,

4. The patient requests medications and symptoms are appropriate.

Clinicians may add psychotherapy to prescribed medications if residual symptoms are largely psychological (e.g., low self-esteem) or if the patient has difficulty with adherence.

FOLLOW-UP

Most patients with major depressive disorder respond partially to medication within two to three weeks and full symptom remission is typically seen within six to eight weeks (AHCPR, 1993a). Most patients who receive time-limited psychotherapy respond partially by five to six weeks and fully by ten to twelve weeks. Office visits or telephone contacts to manage indications should occur weekly for the first three to four weeks following initial diagnosis to ensure adherence to medication regimen, adjust dosage, and detect and manage side effects (Indicator 9). Persons who are hospitalized for depression should have follow-up with a mental health specialist or primary care doctor within two weeks of discharge (AHCPR, 1993a) (Indicator 10). Patients who respond to acute phase medication should be continued on the medication at the same dose for four to nine months after they have returned to the clinically well state (AHCPR, 1993a) (Indicator 11). The depression panel recommends that patients with severe depression be seen weekly for the first six to eight weeks (AHCPR, 1993a). Once the depression has resolved, visits every four to twelve weeks are reasonable (AHCPR, 1993a). The AHCPR Depression Guideline Panel recommended the following guidelines for evaluating patients at each subsequent visit.

Failure to Respond to Medications

If the patient shows no response to the current medication by six weeks, then the clinician should both reassess accuracy of the diagnosis and reassess adequacy of treatment. Change in diagnosis or treatment plan (e.g., change of medication, referral to mental health specialist) is indicated (AHCPR, 1993b) (Indicator 12).

If the patient exhibits a partial response by six weeks, but cognitive symptoms remain, then the clinician should:

- continue treatment;
- reassess response to treatment in six more weeks;
- increase the dose of the current medication or change the medication entirely if reevaluation reveals only a partial response (alternately, referral to a mental health specialist for addition of psychotherapy may be warranted);
- consult a psychiatrist if two attempts at acute-phase medication have failed to resolve symptoms (AHCPR, 1993b).

Continuation of Treatment

The Depression Guideline Panel recommended follow-up visits at 12-week intervals, but did not have any evidence about optimal timing. At each visit during which depression is discussed, the degree of response/remission and side effects of medication should be assessed and documented during the first year of treatment (AHCPR, 1993a) (Indicator 13).

Maintenance

Maintenance treatment is designed to prevent new episodes of depression. Patients should be considered for maintenance treatment if they have had:

1. Three or more episodes of major depressive disorder; or,
2. Two episodes of major depressive disorder and other circumstance (i.e., family history of bipolar disorder, history of recurrence within one year after previously effective medication was discontinued, family history of recurrent major depression, early onset (prior to age 20) of the first depressive episode, both episodes were severe, sudden, or life-threatening in the past three years) (AHCPR, 1993b).

REFERENCES

American Psychiatric Association. 1994. Substance-related disorders. In *Diagnostic and Statistical Manual of Mental Disorders: DSM-IV*, Fourth ed. 175-205. Washington, DC: American Psychiatric Association.

Bielski RJ, Friedel RO. December 1976. Prediction of tricyclic antidepressant response: A critical review. *Archives of General Psychiatry* 33: 1479-89.

Broadhead WE, Blazer DG, George LK, et al. 21 November 1990. Depression, disability days, and days lost from work in a prospective epidemiologic survey. *Journal of the American Medical Association* 264 (19): 2524-8.

Burnam MA, Wells KB, Leake B, Landsverk J. 1988. Development of a brief screening instrument for detecting depressive disorders. *Medical Care* 26: 775-89.

Depression Guideline Panel. April 1993. *Depression in Primary Care: Volume 1. Detection and Diagnosis. Clinical Practice Guideline, Number 5.* AHCPR Publication No. 93-0550. Rockville, MD: U.S. Department of Health and Human Services, Public Health Service, Agency for Health Care Policy and Research.

Depression Guideline Panel. April 1993. *Depression in Primary Care: Volume 2. Treatment of Major Depression. Clinical Practice Guideline, Number 5.* AHCPR Publication No. 93-0551. Rockville, MD: U.S. Department of Health and Human Services, Public Health Service, Agency for Health Care Policy and Research.

Feldman E, Mayou R, Hawton K, et al. May 1987. Psychiatric disorder in medical in-patients. *Quarterly Journal of Medicine* New Series 63 (241): 405-12.

Greenberg PE, Stiglin LE, Finkelstein SN, et al. November 1993. Depression: A neglected major illness. *Journal of Clinical Psychiatry* 54 (11): 419-24.

Hays RD, Wells KB, Sherbourne CD, et al. January 1995. Functioning and well-being outcomes of patients with depression compared with chronic general medical illness. *Archives of General Psychiatry* 52: 11-9.

Katon W, Schulberg H. 1992. Epidemiology of depression in primary care. *General Hospital Pschyiatry* 14: 237-47.

Kessler RC, McGonagle KA, Zhao S, et al. January 1994. Lifetime and 12-month prevalence of DSM-III-R psychiatric disorders in the United States. *Archives of General Psychiatry* 51: 8-19.

Kupfer DJ, Frank E, Perel JM. September 1989. The advantage of early treatment intervention in recurrent depression. *Archives of General Psychiatry* 46: 771-5.

NIMH Consensus Development Conference. April 1985. Mood disorders: Pharmacologic prevention of recurrences. *American Journal of Psychiatry* 142 (4): 469-76.

Sturm R, Wells KB. June 1994. *Can Prepaid Care for Depression Be Improved Cost-Effectively?* RAND, Santa Monica CA.

US Preventative Services Task Force. 1996. *Guide to Clinical Preventative Services, 2nd ed.* Baltimore: Williams & Wilkins.

Wells KB, Hays RD, Burnam MA, et al. 15 December 1989. Detection of depressive disorder for patients receiving prepaid or fee-for-service care: Results from the medical outcomes study. *Journal of the American Medical Association* 262 (23): 3298-3302.

Wells KB, Stewart A, Hays RD, et al. 18 August 1989. The functioning and well-being of depressed patients: results from the medical outcomes study. *Journal of the American Medical Association* 262 (7): 914-9.

Wells KB, Golding JM, Burnam MA. June 1988. Psychiatric disorder and limitations in physical functioning in a sample of the Los Angeles general population. *American Journal of Psychiatry* 145 (6): 712-7.

Wells KB, Katon W, Rogers B, et al. May 1994. Use of minor tranquilizers and antidepressant medications by depressed outpatients: Results from the medical outcomes study. *American Journal of Psychiatry* 151 (5): 694-700.

RECOMMENDED QUALITY INDICATORS FOR DEPRESSION

These indicators apply to men and women age 18 and older. These indicators were endorsed by a prior panel and reviewed but not rated by the current panel.

Indicator	Quality of Evidence	Literature	Benefits	Comments
Screening				
1. Clinicians should ask about the presence or absence of depression or depressive symptoms[1] in any person with any of the following risk factors for depression: a. history of depression b. death in family in past six months, or c. alcohol or other drug abuse.	III	USPSTF, 1996	Alleviate symptoms of depression[1].	Risk factors for depression have been relatively well-defined in cross-sectional studies.
Diagnosis				
2. If the diagnosis of depression is made, specific co-morbidities should be elicited and documented in the chart: a. presence or absence of alcohol or other drug abuse; b. medication use; and c. general medical disorder(s).	III	Depression Guideline Panel, 1993a & 1993b	Alleviate symptoms of depression. Prevent complications of substance abuse[2]	Certain co-morbidities may contribute to or cause depression. The practitioner should be aware of these co-morbidities when making a treatment plan for depression. Documentation may have occurred on previous visits.

Indicator	Quality of Evidence	Literature	Benefits	Comments
Treatment				
3. Once diagnosis of major depression has been made, treatment with anti-depressant medication and/or psychotherapy should begin within 2 weeks.	I, II-1, II-2	Depression Guideline Panel, 1993a & 1993b	Alleviate symptoms of depression.[1] Reduce disability days.	Randomized controlled trials cited in the guidelines (not individually reviewed) substantiate the usefulness of medication and psychotherapy for the treatment of depression. Antidepressant medication therapy is probably the more effective sole modality. The guidelines recommend "prompt" treatment, but no definition of prompt is given. We suggest two weeks is a reasonable time interval.
4. Presence or absence of suicidal ideation should be documented during the first or second diagnostic visit.	II-2, III	Depression Guideline Panel, 1993a & 1993b	Prevent death from suicide. Prevent morbidity from suicide attempts.	Presence of suicidality is a marker for severe depression and would argue for instituting therapy with antidepressants and against psychotherapy alone. Suicidality with psychosis, drug abuse, and/or plan of action warrants hospitalization.
5. Persons who have suicidality should be asked if they have specific plans to carry out suicide.	III	Depression Guideline Panel, 1993b	Prevent death from suicide. Prevent morbidity from suicide attempts.	If a person has a plan to carry out suicide, the risk of success increases.
6. Persons who have suicidality and have any of the following risk factors should be hospitalized: 1. psychosis 2. current alcohol or drug abuse or dependency 3. specific plans to carry out suicide (e.g., obtaining a weapon, putting affairs in order, making a suicide note).	III	Depression Guideline Panel, 1993b	Prevent death from suicide. Prevent morbidity from suicide attempts.	Presence of risk factors for successful suicide in a person who admits to suicidality warrants hospitalization.
7. Antidepressants should be prescribed at appropriate dosages.	I	Depression Guideline Panel, 1993b; Wells, 1994	Alleviate symptoms of depression. Reduce disability days.	Only appropriate doses of anti-depressants will be effective in treatment, yet subtherapeutic doses are often used. For example, a patient on 25 mg of amitryptiline at bedtime is not on a therapeutic antidepressant dose. We will exclude those with renal and hepatic dysfunction from this indicator.

126

Indicator	Quality of Evidence	Literature	Benefits	Comments
8. Anti-anxiety agents should not be prescribed as a sole agent for the treatment of depression.	I	Depression Guideline Panel, 1993b	Alleviate symptoms of depression. Reduce disability days. Avoid dependence on anti-anxiety agents.	With the possible exception of alprazolam, anti-anxiety agents have not shown to be beneficial and may be harmful. Foregoing antidepressants in favor of anxiolytics deprives patients of potential benefits of antidepressant treatment.
Follow-up				
9. Medication treatment visits or telephone contacts should occur at least once in the 2 weeks following initial diagnosis.	III	Depression Guideline Panel, 1993a & 1993b	Alleviate symptoms of depression. Reduce disability days.	Once treatment is started, the practitioner needs to document improvement. Most patients improve at least partially within 3 weeks. The guidelines advocate weekly follow-up by phone or in person for 4-6 weeks. Our indicator specifies the lower end of the recommendations.
10. Persons hospitalized for depression should have follow-up with a mental health specialist or their primary care doctor within two weeks of discharge.	III	Depression Guideline Panel, 1993b	Alleviate symptoms of depression. Reduce disability days. Prevent death from suicide. Prevent morbidity from suicide attempts.	The guidelines do not specifically address time-interval between discharge and follow-up. However, given severity of disease, more than two weeks should probably not pass before re-evaluation. If the patient is also seeing a mental health specialist, the two week interval can apply to that specialist instead of the primary care provider.
11. Patients with major depression who have medical record documentation of improvement of symptoms within 8 weeks of starting medication treatment should be continued on medication treatment for at least 2 additional months.	I	Depression Guideline Panel, 1993b	Alleviate symptoms of depression. Reduce disability days.	Only appropriate duration of anti-depressants will be effective in treatment.
12. At least one of the following should occur if there is no or inadequate response to therapy for depression at 8 weeks: • Referral to psychotherapist, if not already seeing one; • Change or increase in dose of medication, if on medication; • Addition of medication, if only using psychotherapy, or • Change in diagnosis documented in chart.	III	Depression Guideline Panel, 1993a & 1993b	Alleviate symptoms of depression. Reduce disability days.	Almost all clinical depression responds at least partially by 6 weeks. If response is incomplete, the diagnosis needs to be re-evaluated and/or treatment plan changed/augmented.

127

	Indicator	Quality of Evidence	Literature	Benefits	Comments
13.	At each visit during which depression is discussed, degree of response/remission and side effects of medication should be assessed and documented during the first year of treatment.	III	Depression Guideline Panel, 1993b	Alleviate symptoms of depression. Reduce toxicities of medication. Reduce remission.	Even effectively treated patients may relapse or develop toxicities to medications. While most persons will be off of medications after one year, the optimal time to remove medications is still not well established.

Definitions and Examples

[1] Symptoms of depression include depressed mood, diminished interest or pleasure in activities, weight loss/gain, impaired concentration, suicidality, fatigue, feelings of worthlessness and guilt, and psychomotor agitation/retardation.

[2] Medical complications of substance abuse are numerous and include: for alcohol, blackouts, seizures, delerium, liver failure; for IV drugs of any kind, local infection, endocarditis, hepatitis and HIV, death from overdose; for cocaine and amphetamines, seizures, myocardial infarction, and hypertensive crises.

Quality of Evidence Codes

I	RCT
II-1	Nonrandomized controlled trials
II-2	Cohort or case analysis
II-3	Multiple time series
III	Opinions or descriptive studies

128

9. DIABETES MELLITUS[1]

Steven Asch, MD, MPH and Kenneth Clark, MD, MPH

Several recent reviews provided the core references in developing quality indicators for diabetes (Singer et al., 1991; Bergenstal, 1993; Gerich, 1989; Nathan, 1993b; Garnick et al., 1994; ECDCDM, 1997). Where these core references cited studies to support individual indicators, we have included the original references. We also performed focused MEDLINE searches of the medical literature from 1985 through 1997 to supplement these references for particular indicators.

IMPORTANCE

Diabetes is a heterogeneous, often serious, and common chronic condition. The American Diabetes Association (ADA) estimated the number of diabetics in 1997 at 16 million. The prevalence of diabetes is 26.1 per 1,000 people of all ages, and 6.8 per 1,000 in people under the age of 44. Each day, approximately 1,700 people are diagnosed with diabetes. It is the fourth leading cause of death in the United States. Diabetes occurs more frequently among women than men, and among non-whites than whites (ADA, 1997).

The complications of diabetes include visual loss, and dysfunction of the heart, peripheral vasculature, peripheral nerves, and kidneys. Diabetes is the primary cause of blindness in the United States, and diabetics are at much higher risk of developing cataracts, glaucoma, and poor near vision. The cardiovascular effects of diabetes cause heart attacks, strokes, and, together with diabetic neuropathy, amputations (Garcia et al., 1974). About half of insulin-dependent diabetics eventually develop kidney failure (Bergenstal et al., 1993). All of these complications taken together result in much higher death rates among diabetics than the rest of the population (Palumbo et al., 1976).

---

[1] This chapter is a revision of one written for an earlier project on quality of care for women and children (Q1). The expert panel for the current project was asked to review all of the indicators, but only rated new or revised indicators.

Death rates from diabetes itself (excluding complications) increase with age, ranging from 0.2 per 100,000 for those between 15 and 19 years of age to 14.6 per 100,000 for those between 50 and 54 years. Older patients experience even higher rates (National Center for Health Statistics [NCHS], 1994a). Much of the benefit of high quality care will accrue many years after the prevention of morbidity and mortality from the above-mentioned complications.

The treatment of diabetes is resource intensive, with total annual economic costs estimated at $91.8 billion in 1992 (ADA, 1997). For 1992, diabetes accounted for one of every seven dollars spent on health care (Rubin et al., 1994), and was the eighth most common reason for a patient visiting a physician's office (NCHS, 1994b).

SCREENING

This section covers screening patients who are not yet diagnosed as diabetic. Indicators for screening diabetics for complications are covered below under Diagnosis. Both the American College of Physicians (ACP) (Singer et al., 1991, in Eddy, 1991) and the Canadian Task Force (CTF) on the Periodic Health Examination (1979) have recommended that asymptomatic patients not undergo screening for diabetes, because of the poor evidence that treatment of patients so identified would prevent complications. Although many persons have asymptomatic hyperglycemia, most complications of diabetes occur late in the course of the disease, which limits the benefits of early identification. Since the publication of the ACP and CTF recommendations, the Diabetes Control and Complication Trial (DCCT) has added evidence for the efficacy of tight control in known insulin-dependent diabetics in preventing complications (1993a). However, we have found no subsequent studies directly evaluating the efficacy of screening asymptomatic patients in reducing morbidity or mortality from diabetes (Singer, 1988; CTF, 1979). In 1997, the Expert Committee on the Diagnosis and Classification of Diabetes Mellitus recommended that testing for diabetes should be considered in all individuals 45 years of age or older and, if normal, it should be repeated at three year intervals (ECDCDM). Undiagnosed Type 2 diabetes may affect 8 million individuals. The committee

130

reasoned that such patients are at increased for risk for coronary heart disease, stroke and peripheral vascular disease, and so might benefit from early detection (ECDCDM). No other expert bodies have made similar recommendations.

DIAGNOSIS

According to the criteria of the Expert Committee on the Diagnosis and Classification of Diabetes Mellitus (ECDCDM), the initial diagnosis of diabetes depends on the measurement of a fasting blood sugar greater than 126 mg/dl or a postprandial blood sugar of greater than 200 mg/dl (ECDCDM, 1997). If a recorded blood sugar meets the above criteria, we recommend as a quality indicator that the provider be required to note the diagnosis of diabetes in the progress notes or problem list (Indicator 1).

Guidelines also recommend a complete history and physical examination, dietary evaluation, urinalysis for protein, measurement of blood creatinine, and a lipid panel at the time of initial diagnosis (ADA, 1989). We do not propose any of these as quality indicators for the initial diagnosis because of the small number of incident cases in our testing sample and the difficulty of defining the time of initial diagnosis.

The Meta-analysis Research Group on the Diagnosis of Diabetes Using Glycated Hemoglobin Levels concluded that measurement of hemoglobin A1c levels may represent a reasonable approach to the diagnosis of treatment-requiring diabetics (Peters et al., 1996). However, because there are many different methods for measuring glycosylated hemoglobins and because nationwide standardization of the test has just begun, the Expert Committee on the Diagnosis and Classification of Diabetes Mellitus does not currently recommend the hemoglobin A1c test for the diagnosis of diabetes (ECDCDM, 1997). Therefore, we do not propose its use as a diagnostic quality indicator at this time.

Instead, we have concentrated on the routine diagnostic tests that known diabetics should undergo regardless of their clinical status and stage of disease. The first of these is the measurement of glycosylated hemoglobin to monitor glycemic control. A randomized controlled trial of 240 patients found that measuring hemoglobin A1c every three months led to changes in diabetic treatment and improvement in metabolic control, indicated by a lowering of average hemoglobin A1c values (Larsen et al., 1990). The landmark DCCT followed 1,441 insulin-dependent diabetics for nine years and found that tight glycemic control and lower hemoglobin A1c values decreased rates of diabetic complications (DCCT, 1993a; see under Treatment below). Despite recommendations from a number of specialty and generalist physician societies, there is great variation in the use of this test (ADA, 1993; Bergenstal et al., 1993; Garnick et al., 1994; Goldstein et al., 1994). We propose as a quality indicator that a hemoglobin A1c test be done for all diabetics at six-month intervals, which is the longest recommended interval (Indicators 2 and 3).

Home blood glucose monitoring has been shown to aid glycemic control in diabetics taking insulin. Because moderate hyperglycemia (<180 mg/dl) may not cause glycosuria, the DCCT employed home blood glucose monitoring for its population of insulin-dependent diabetics monitoring to achieve tight control, rather than the more easily tolerated urine glucose. At least one small randomized trial (n=23) has shown home blood glucose monitoring to improve glycemic control in obese insulin-dependent diabetics. The optimal frequency of monitoring has not yet been determined, although some studies have questioned patients' ability to comply with frequent measurement (Bergenstal et al., 1993; Health and Public Policy Committee, 1983; Muchmore et al., 1994; Gordon, 1991). For patients not taking insulin, randomized trials have not shown home blood glucose to be any more effective at maintaining glycemic control than urine testing (Allen et al., 1990), and observational data have failed to find any strong relationship between home blood glucose monitoring and glycemic control (Patrick, 1994; Allen et al., 1990). Specialty societies recommend that patients on insulin be offered training and equipment for home glucose monitoring, and we propose this as another indicator of diagnostic quality (ADA, 1993) (Indicator 4).

Because of the frequency of vision, cardiovascular, and renal complications among diabetics, many of which may be asymptomatic, the

ADA (1989) has recommended the following annual screening tests: eye exam, tests of triglycerides, total cholesterol, HDL cholesterol, urinalysis, and total urinary protein excretion (Indicators 2 and 3). An annual eye and vision exam conducted by an ophthalmologist, beginning at five years after diagnosis, has also been recommended by the ACP, the ADA, and the American Academy of Ophthalmology (AAO) (ACP, ADA, and AAO, 1992) (Indicators 2 and 3). Generalists detect retinopathy at an early treatable stage much less effectively than specialists (Reenders et al., 1992). The other screening recommendations have never been evaluated in controlled trials, but the conditions that are screened -- hyperlipidemia, nephropathy, and end-stage renal disease -- are both more common in diabetics and amenable to intervention (The Carter Center, 1985). Compliance with ADA screening recommendations has been estimated to vary from 20 to 50 percent (Garnick et al., 1994; Brechner et al., 1993).

Other common treatable complications of diabetes include hypertension, cellulitis, and osteomyelitis. The ADA recommends blood pressure measurement and examination of the feet at every visit to detect these complications early in their course (Indicators 2 and 3), as well as a careful history to elicit signs and symptoms of hypoglycemia and hyperglycemia. No controlled trials have examined the efficacy of a regular history and physical examination.

TREATMENT

Recent debate concerning diabetic treatment hinges on the utility of tight glycemic control. The goals of tight control and prevention of long-term complications through aggressive treatment are supported by the DCCT (1993a). The DCCT randomized 1,441 insulin-dependent diabetics into conventional therapy or intensive therapy that included daily adjustments of insulin dosage, frequent home glucose monitoring, and nutritional advice. Under the optimal circumstances present in the DCCT trial, 44 percent of the intervention group achieved glycosolated hemoglobin values under the goal of 6.05 mg/dl percent at least once, but only five percent maintained average values in that range. The intervention group developed 76 percent less retinopathy, 57 percent less albuminuria, and 60 percent less clinical neuropathy, but this reduction in diabetic complications may come at the expense of quality of life (Nerenz et al., 1992). For example, the tight control group in DCCT experienced a two- to three-fold increase in hypoglycemic episodes. The efficiency of such methods in general practice has not received adequate evaluation. Nonetheless, the ADA recommends that all diabetics over the age of seven be offered similar aggressive therapy.

Treatment strategies are different for Type 1 diabetes (complete pancreatic deficiency of insulin) and Type 2 diabetes (abnormal secretion of insulin and resistance to insulin action). In Type 1 diabetes, emphasis is placed on avoidance of diabetic ketoacidosis and tight control of blood sugar levels through the judicious use of insulin. In Type 2 diabetes, the focus shifts to control of symptoms, usually with a combination of diet, exercise, and oral hypoglycemic agents. If these measures fail to maintain adequate control in Type 2 diabetics, then insulin therapy is warranted. We will review the evidence for quality indicators for each of these treatment modalities in turn.

Adherence to the ADA-recommended diet decreases insulin and oral hypoglycemic requirements and serum lipids (Bantle, 1988). The DCCT relied on dieticians and revealed that greater adherence to dietary instructions resulted in better control (1993b). Exercise also improves glucose tolerance and may reduce or even eliminate the need for drug therapy (Raz et al., 1994). Thus, the ADA and the American Board of Family Practice (ABFP) recommend dietary and exercise counseling at both the initial diagnosis and before starting oral hypoglycemics or insulin (ADA, 1989; Bergenstal et al., 1993). We recommend as a quality indicator evaluating the medical record for evidence that all diabetics have received dietary and exercise counseling and that Type 2 diabetics have undergone a trial of this conservative therapy prior to pharmaceutical intervention (Indicator 5 and 6).

Randomized controlled trials have shown that oral hypoglycemic agents improve glycemic control and prevent hyperglycemic coma. However, the effectiveness of these agents in preventing longer-term complications of Type 2 diabetes has been questioned, particularly in the controversial UGDP Trial of the 1970s (Gerich, 1989; Kilo et al., 1980; Knatterud, 1978). The effectiveness of oral hypoglycemic agents is under study in the UK Prospective Diabetes Study (USPDS), but results are not currently available (Turner, 1995).

The biguanide metformin is a relatively new (in the U.S.) antihyperglycemic drug used in patients with noninsulin-dependent diabetes mellitus. Its efficacy in lowering blood glucose is similar to that achieved with a sulfonylurea. Unlike sulfonylurea, it does not cause weight gain and, when used as monotherapy, does not cause hypoglycemia. It can be used either as initial therapy or as an additional drug when sulfonylurea therapy is inadequate. (Campbell et al., 1996; Bailey and Turner, 1996).

At present, we recommend evaluating the medical record to determine if oral hypoglycemic therapy has been offered to symptomatic Type 2 diabetics who have already received a trial of dietary therapy (Indicator 6).

Insulin treatment is essential for Type 1 diabetics and a treatment of last resort for Type 2 diabetics. The literature contains varied recommendations on the optimal timing and content of insulin injections (Gregerman, 1991, in Barker et al., 1991; Knatterud, 1978), and no single regimen has emerged as superior. We recommend as a quality indicator that Type 2 diabetics who have failed oral hypoglycemics be offered insulin (Indicator 7).

Although quality indicators for treatment of hypertension are covered elsewhere, the intersection of diabetes and hypertension poses special treatment challenges. Control of hypertension is perhaps the most crucial step in preventing diabetic nephropathy. In particular, ACE inhibitors and possibly calcium channel blockers have been shown to reduce hyperalbuminuria and delay the progression to diabetic nephropathy (Lederle, 1992; Anderson, 1990). Beta blockers on the other hand may block the symptoms of hypoglycemia, and thus may be contraindicated in treated diabetics (Hamilton, 1990). We propose that diabetics with hypertension and proteinuria receive ACE inhibitors or calcium channel blockers as first-line pharmacotherapy if diet has failed to control blood pressure (Indicator 8).

FOLLOW-UP

A study of internists and family practitioners using patient vignettes found wide variation in recommended follow-up intervals for diabetics (Petitti and Grumbach, 1993). The ADA (1989) guidelines recommend that regular visits be scheduled every three months for insulin-dependent diabetics and every six months for other diabetics. As a minimum standard of care for patients with diabetes, we propose as a quality indicator that diabetics should visit the provider every six months (Indicator 9).

REFERENCES

Allen BT, DeLong ER, and Feussner JR. October 1990. Impact of glucose self-monitoring on non-insulin-treated patients with type II diabetes mellitus: Randomized controlled trial comparing blood and urine testing. *Diabetes Care* 13 (10): 1044-50.

American Diabetes Association. 1993. *Direct and Indirect Costs of Diabetes in the United States in 1992*. Alexandria, VA: American Diabetes Association.

American Diabetes Association. May 1988. Position Statement. *Diabetes Care* 12 (5): 365-368.

American Diabetes Association: Clinical Practice Recommendations. 1997. Standards of medical care for patients with diabetes mellitus. *American Diabetes Association* 20 (1):

American College of Physicians, American Diabetes Association, and American Academy of Ophthalmology. 15 April 1992. Screening guidelines for diabetic retinopathy. *Archives of Internal Medicine* 116 (8): 683-5.

Anderson S. 1990. Renal effects of converting enzyme inhibitors in hypertension and diabetes. *Journal of Cardiovascular Pharmacology* 15 (Suppl. 3): S11-S15.

Bailey CJ and Turner RC. 29 February. Metformin. *New England Journal of Medicine* 334 (9): 574-9.

Bantle A. 1988. The dietary treatment of diabetes mellitus. *Medical Clinics of North America* 72 (6): 1285-99.

Bergenstal RM, Hall WE, Haugen E et al. 1993. *Diabetes Mellitus: Reference Guide*, Fourth ed.Lexington, KY: American Board of Family Practice.

Brechner RJ, Cowie CC, Howie LJ, et al. 13 October 1993. Ophthalmic examination among adults with diagnosed diabetes mellitus. *Journal of the American Medical Association* 270 (14): 1714-7.

Brechner RJ, Cowie CC, Howie LJ, et al. 13 October 1993. Ophthalmic examination among adults with diagnosed diabetes mellitus. *Journal of the American Medical Association* 270 (14): 1714-7.

Campbell RK, White JR, and Saulie BA. May 1996. Metformin: a new oral biguanide. *Clinical Therapeutics* 18 (3): 360-71.

Canadian Task Force on the Periodic Health Examination. 3 November 1979. The periodic health examination. *Canadian Medical Association Journal* 121: 1193-1254.

The Diabetes Control and Complications Trial Research Group. July 1993. Expanded role of the dietitian in the Diabetes Control and Complications Trial: Implications for clinical practice. *Journal of the American Dietetic Association* 93 (7): 758-67.

Garcia MJ, McNamara PM, Gordon T, and Kannell WB. February 1974. Morbidity and mortality in diabetes in the Framingham population: Sixteen year follow-up study. *Diabetes* 23: 105-11.

Garnick DW, Fowles J, Lawthers AG, et al. 18 February 1994. Focus on quality: Profiling physicians' practice patterns. *In Press, Journal Ambulatory Care Management.*

Gerich JE. 2 November 1989. Oral hypoglycemic agents. *New England Journal of Medicine* 321 (18): 1231-45.

Goldstein DE, Little RR, Wiedmeyer H-M, et al. 1994. Is glycohemoglobin testing useful in diabetes mellitus? Lessons from the Diabetes Control and Complications Trial. *Clinical Chemistry* 40 (8): 1637-40.

Gordon D, Semple CG, and Paterson KR. 1991. Do different frequencies of self-monitoring of blood glucose influence control in type 1 diabetic patients. *Diabetic Medicine* 8: 679-82.

Gregerman RI. 1991. Diabetes mellitus. In *Principles of Ambulatory Medicine*, Third ed. Editors L. R. Barker, J. R. Burton, and P. D. Zieve, 913-51. Baltimore, MD: Williams and Wilkins.

Hamilton BP. October 1990. Diabetes mellitus and hypertension. *American Journal of Kidney Diseases* 16 (4-Suppl.1): 20-9.

Health and Public Policy Committee, and American College of Physicians. August 1983. Selected methods for the management of diabetes mellitus. *Archives of Internal Medicine* 99 (2): 272-4.

Larsen ML, Horder M, and Mogensen EF. 11 October 1990. Effect of long-term monitoring of glycosylated hemoglobin levels in insulin-dependent diabetes mellitus. *New England Journal of Medicine* 323 (15): 1021-5.

Lederle RM. 1992. The effect of antihypertensive therapy on the course of renal failure. *Journal of Cardiovascular Pharmacology* 20 (Suppl. 6): S69-S72.

Muchmore DB, Springer J, and Miller M. 1994. Self-monitoring of blood glucose in overweight type 2 diabetic patients. *Acta Diabetologica* 31: 215-9.

Nathan DM. April 1993. Diabetes Mellitus. *Scientific American* 6: 1-25.

Nathan D. 10 June 1992. Long-Term Complications of Diabetes Mellitus. *New England Journal of Medicine* 328 (3): 1676-1685.

National Center for Health Statistics. 18 August 1994. *National Ambulatory Medical Care Survey: 1992 summary*. U.S. Department of Health and Human Services, Hyattsville, MD.

National Center for Health Statistics. 1994. *Vital statistics of the United States, 1990, vol. II: Mortality-part A*. U.S. Department of Health and Human Services, Hyattsville, MD.

Nerenz DR, Repasky DP, Whitehouse FW, et al. May 1992. Ongoing assessment of health status in patients with diabetes mellitus. *Medical Care Supplement* 30 (5, Supplement): MS112-MS123.

Palumbo PJ, Elveback LR, Chu CP, et al. July 1976. Diabetes mellitus: Incidence, prevalence, survivorship, and causes of death in Rochester, Minnesota 1945-1970. *Diabetes* 25 (7): 566-73.

Patrick AW, Gill GV, MacFarlane IA, et al. 1994. Home glucose monitoring in type 2 diabetes: Is it a waste of time? *Diabetic Medicine* 11: 62-5.

Peters A, Mayer B, Davidson MD, et al. 16 October 1996. A clinical approach for the diagnosis of diabetes mellitus. *Journal of the American Medical Association* 276 (15): 1246-1252.

Petitti DB, Grumbach K. September 1993. Variation in physicians' recommendations about revisit interval for three common conditions. *Journal of Family Practice* 37 (3): 235-40.

Raz I, Hauser E, and Bursztyn M. 10 October 1994. Moderate exercise improves glucose metabolism in uncontrolled elderly patients with non-insulin-dependent diabetes mellitus. *Israel Journal of Medical Sciences* 30 (10): 766-70.

Reenders K, De Nobel E, Van Den Hoogen H, and Van Weel C. 1992. Screening for diabetic retinopathy by general practitioners. *Scandinavian Journal of Primary Health Care* 10: 306-9.

Rubin RJ, Altman WM, and Mendelson DN. 1994. Health care expenditures for people with diabetes mellitus, 1992. *Journal of Clinical Endocrinology and Metabolism* 78 (4): 809A-F.

Singer DE, Samet JH, Coley CM, and Nathan DM. 15 October 1988. Screening for diabetes mellitus. *Archives of Internal Medicine* 109: 639-49.

Singer DE, Samet JH, Coley CM, and Nathan DM. 1991. Screening for diabetes mellitus. In *Common Screening Tests*. Editor D. M. Eddy, 154-78. Philadelphia, PA: American College of Physicians.

The Carter Center. July 1985. Closing the gap: The problem of diabetes mellitus in the United States. *Diabetes Care* 8 (4): 391-406.

The Expert Committee on the Diagnosis and Classification of Diabetes Mellitus. 1997. Report of the Expert Committee on the Diagnosis and Classification of Diabetes Mellitus. *Diabetes Care* 20 (7): 1183-1197.

Turner RC and Holman RR. 28 August 1995. Lessons from the UK prospective diabetes study. *Diabetes Research and Clinical Practice* S151-7.

Turner R, Cull C, and Holman R. 1996. United Kingdom Prospective Diabetes Study 17: a 9-Year Update of a Randomized, Controlled Trial on the Effect of Improved Metabolic Control on Complications in Non-Insulin-dependent Diabetes Mellitus. *Archives of Internal Medicine* 124 (1 (Part 2)): 136-145.

US Preventative Services Task Force. 1996. *Guide to Clinical Preventative Services, 2nd ed.* Baltimore: Williams & Wilkins.

RECOMMENDED QUALITY INDICATORS FOR DIABETES MELLITUS

These indicators apply to men and women age 18 and older. Only the indicators in bold type were rated by this panel; the remaining indicators were endorsed by a prior panel.

Indicator	Quality of Evidence	Literature	Benefits	Comments
Diagnosis				
1. Patients with fasting blood sugar >126 or postprandial blood sugar >200 should have a diagnosis of diabetes noted in progress notes or problem list.	III	ADA, 1989 ECDCDM, 1997	Prevent diabetic complications.[1]	This definition of diabetes is accepted worldwide. Blood sugar tests are often ordered as part of panels.
2. Patients with the diagnosis of Type 1 diabetes should have all of the following: a. Glycosylated hemoglobin or fructosamine every 6 months. b. Eye and visual exam (annual). c. Total serum cholesterol and HDL cholesterol tests (annual). d. Measurement of urine protein (annual). e. Examination of feet at least twice a year. f. Measurement of blood pressure at every visit.	I, III	ADA, 1989; Larsen et al., 1990; ACP, ADA, and AAO, 1992	Prevent diabetic complications.[1] Prevent retinopathy, hyperlipidemia, atherosclorotic complications, and renal disease.	Randomized controlled trial of 240 patients indicated a significant decrease in hemoglobin A$_{1c}$ among those whose hemoglobin A$_{1c}$ was monitored. Time interval is that used in most clinical trials. Eye and visual exams are shown to detect retinopathy at an earlier treatable stage. Other recommendations are based on expert opinion, though studies have shown conditions they screen for to be more common in diabetics and all are susceptible to treatment with improved outcomes resulting from earlier detection.

141

Indicator	Quality of Evidence	Literature	Benefits	Comments
3. Patients with the diagnosis of Type 2 diabetes should have all of the following: a. Glycosylated hemoglobin or fructosamine every 6 months; b. Eye and visual exam (annual); c. Total serum cholesterol and HDL cholesterol tests (annual); d. Measurement of urine protein (annual); e. Examination of feet at least twice a year; f. Measurement of blood pressure at every visit.	I, III	ADA, 1989; Larsen et al., 1990; ACP, ADA, and AAO, 1992	Prevent diabetic complications. [1] Prevent retinopathy, hyperlipidemia, atherosclerotic complications, and renal disease. Reduce morbidity from foot infections.	Randomized controlled trial of 240 patients indicated a significant decrease in hemoglobin A1c among those whose hemoglobin A1c was monitored. Time interval is that used in most clinical trials Eye and visual exam are shown to detect retinopathy at an earlier treatable stage. Other recommendations are based on expert opinion, though studies have shown conditions they screen for to be more common in diabetics and all are susceptible to treatment with improved outcomes resulting from earlier detection.
4. Types 1 and 2 patients taking insulin should monitor their glucose at home unless documented to be unable or unwilling.	III	ADA, 1993	Prevent hypo-glycemic episodes. Prevent diabetic complications. [1]	A small RCT found that home glucose monitoring increases glycemic control in insulin-dependent diabetics. Another study found no difference in control by frequency of monitoring. Recommended by the ADA.
Treatment				
5. Newly diagnosed diabetics should receive dietary and exercise counseling.	II	Raz et al., 1994; Delahanty and Halford, 1993; ADA, 1989; Bergenstal et al., 1993	Reduce diabetic complications. [1]	Adherence to ADA diet decreases insulin and oral hypoglycemic requirements and serum lipids. Exercise improves glucose tolerance and may reduce or eliminate need for drug therapy. DCCT used dietitians and found that adherence to diet improved control, and the ADA and the ABFP recommend their use. No study has found that dietary counseling reduces diabetic complications.
6. Type 2 diabetics who have failed dietary therapy should receive oral hypoglycemic therapy.	III	ADA, 1989; Gerich, 1989; Bergenstal et al., 1993	Reduce diabetic complications. [1]	Observational trials have shown oral hypoglycemics to be effective in treating hyperglycemia and improving glycemic control. No studies have shown reduction of diabetic complications. Specialty societies and review articles widely recommend their use in mild-to-moderate disease before starting insulin.

142

Indicator	Quality of Evidence	Literature	Benefits	Comments
7. Type 2 diabetics who have failed oral hypoglycemics should be offered insulin.	III	ADA, 1989; Bergenstal et al., 1993	Reduce diabetic complications.[1]	Recommended by the ADA and ABFP.
8. Hypertensive diabetics with proteinuria should be offered an ACE inhibitor or a calcium channel blocker within 3 months of the notation of proteinuria.	I	Lederle, 1992; Anderson, 1990	Reduce diabetic complications.[1]	May reduce progression to diabetic nephropathy.
Follow-up				
9. All patients with diabetes should have a follow-up visit at least every 6 months.	III	Bergenstal et al., 1993; ADA, 1989	Reduce probability of severe diabetic complications.[1]	Visits for diabetic patients in control should be every 3-6 months (per ABFP). Routine monitoring facilitates early detection and treatment of complications.

Definitions and Examples

[1]Diabetic complications include visual loss and dysfunction of the heart, peripheral vasculature, peripheral nerves, and kidneys.

Synonyms for types 1 and 2 diabetes are listed below:

Type 1 diabetes	Type 2 diabetes
IDDM - Insulin-dependent diabetes Juvenile diabetes Juvenile-onset diabetes Ketosis-prone diabetes	AODM - Adult-onset diabetes MODM - Maturity-onset diabetes NIDDM - Non-insulin dependent diabetes mellitus Nonketosis-prone diabetes

Quality of Evidence Codes

I	RCT
II-1	Nonrandomized controlled trials
II-2	Cohort or case analysis
II-3	Multiple time series
III	Opinions or descriptive studies

143

10. HORMONE REPLACEMENT THERAPY

Deidre Gifford, MD, MPH

Initial background information for this review was obtained from the 1996 U.S. Preventive Services Task Force (USPSTF) chapter on postmenopausal hormone prophylaxis and the 1992 American College of Obstetricians and Gynecologists (ACOG) Technical Bulletin on hormone replacement therapy (HRT). In addition, a MEDLINE search was performed for review articles published from 1990 to 1997 on the topic of post-menopausal HRT. Topics for quality indicators were then developed and, when necessary, clinical trials specific to the indicators were reviewed. Because the areas of screening and diagnosis are not pertinent to the topic of hormone replacement, this chapter covers treatment only.

IMPORTANCE

With the average age of menopause in the United States being 51 years, and the average life expectancy for a woman after reaching menopause being 30 years, women today can expect to live approximately one-third of their lives after menopause (USPSTF, 1996). The decline in endogenous estrogen that occurs with menopause is associated with several important causes of morbidity in women, such as osteoporosis, bone fracture, and cardiovascular disease. Cardiovascular disease is the major cause of morbidity and mortality in postmenopausal women. Nearly 50 percent will develop coronary artery disease at some time, and 30 percent will die of this disease (Grady et al., 1992). It has been estimated that a 50 year old white woman has a 15 percent lifetime probability of hip fracture, a 1.5 percent probability of dying of sequelae of hip fracture, and a 32 percent lifetime risk of a vertebral fracture (Grady et al., 1992; USPSTF, 1996). Vasomotor symptoms, or "hot flashes," occur in 50 to 85 percent of women at the time of menopause, and symptoms of urogenital atrophy occur in up to 45 percent of women over the age of 60 (USPSTF, 1996).

TREATMENT

For purposes of this review, HRT refers to the systemic use of estrogen (most commonly in an oral or transcutaneous form) with or without the use of a progestin, after cessation of ovarian function. When discussing the use of estrogen alone, the term "unopposed estrogen" will be used. Post-menopausal HRT can be used for relief of vasomotor symptoms and urogenital atrophy caused by the decreased estrogen production associated with menopause. With the recognition of other potential benefits of HRT, such as reduction in the incidence of osteoporotic fractures and cardiovascular disease, more attention has been given to the use of estrogens as a preventive therapy for post-menopausal women (Grady et al., 1992). Questions about hormone replacement therapy concern the appropriate dosages and regimens, and the risks versus the benefits of its preventive use in various sub-groups of post-menopausal women.

Benefits of Hormone Replacement Therapy

HRT is generally accepted to be highly effective for relief of both vasomotor symptoms and urogenital atrophy associated with menopause. Both estrogen alone and estrogen plus progestins produce significant relief of these symptoms (ACOG, 1992; Belchetz, 1994).

Several observational epidemiologic studies have reviewed the effect of post-menopausal estrogen use on the incidence of hip fracture, with the majority showing a decreased relative risk of fracture in "ever-users" of estrogen replacement. The overall decrease in risk has been estimated at 25 percent (Grady et al., 1992). There is also evidence from clinical trials that HRT can reduce the rate of bone loss and improve bone mineral density in postmenopausal women (USPSTF, 1996). Current use of HRT, long term use (>5 years), and use close to the time of menopause have all been associated with greater reductions in fractures. However, past estrogen use provides minimal or no protection from fracture to women over the age of 75 (USPSTF, 1996). Because the median age for hip fracture is 79 (Grady et al., 1992), long-term use of HRT would be required to obtain maximal benefit for osteoporosis.

An important area of controversy in HRT concerns the decrease in risk of coronary heart disease (CHD) in women using estrogen plus progestin HRT. Many epidemiologic studies have evaluated the relationship of HRT with CHD, most of them finding a lower risk of CHD among estrogen users (Grady et al., 1992). The relative risk of CHD in ever-users of estrogen has been estimated at 0.65 (Grady et al., 1992). This estimate is based on studies where the majority of subjects were taking unopposed estrogen. Because systemic estrogen therapy decreases LDL cholesterol and increases HDL cholesterol, the effect of HRT on CHD risk is thought to be mediated at least in part by this beneficial effect on the lipid profile. However, progestins have been shown to attenuate this beneficial effect (PEPI, 1995) raising the possibility that estrogen plus progestin HRT may not lead to as great a reduction in CHD as unopposed estrogen therapy. In addition, the non-random nature of the studies of CHD risk and HRT introduces the possibility that women at lower baseline risk of CHD were prescribed estrogen therapy, leading to an over-estimate of the beneficial effects of HRT (Hemminki and Sihvo, 1993). A more conclusive estimate of the benefits of estrogen plus progestin HRT on CHD will not be available until results of randomized trials, such as the Women's Health Study, are published.

Risks of Hormone Replacement Therapy

Use of unopposed estrogen in women with intact uteri leads to a significant increase in the risk of endometrial cancer. A meta-analysis of 37 observational studies showed that unopposed estrogen use for five to ten years was associated with a six-fold increased risk of endometrial cancer, and use for more than ten years with a nine-fold increased risk (Grady et al, 1995). The addition of either continuous or cyclic progestins to the HRT regimen eliminates this increased risk of endometrial cancer (Belchetz, 1994; The Writing Group for the PEPI Trial, 1996; USPSTF, 1996). For women who do not tolerate the addition of progestins to the HRT regimen, reduction of the frequency of progestin administration or performance of annual endometrial sampling have been proposed as alternatives. However, no studies have evaluated the safety of these regimens for women on unopposed estrogen (Indicator 1).

Many epidemiologic studies have examined the association between HRT and breast cancer, with inconsistent findings (Grady et al., 1992;

USPSTF, 1996). Several overviews have reported a relative risk of 1.2 to 1.4 in current users of HRT and in women who have used estrogen for more than ten to 15 years, but no increased risk among women who had ever used HRT (USPSTF, 1996). The Nurses Health Study, a prospective cohort study, showed a 50 percent increased incidence of breast cancer in current long-term (>5 years) users of HRT compared with women who had never taken HRT (Colditz et al., 1995). No clear association between short-term HRT use and breast cancer has been documented (Grady et al., 1992). The inconsistent findings in at least 40 observational studies and six meta-analyses (USPSTF, 1996) suggest that any potential association between HRT -- especially short-term HRT -- and breast cancer is small, but the possibility of an increased risk of breast cancer with long-term use cannot be excluded.

Summary

Post menopausal HRT has well-documented beneficial effects on the vasomotor symptoms and urogenital atrophy associated with menopause. In addition, long-term use of HRT reduces the risk of fractures associated with osteoporosis and probably reduces the risk of CHD. Unopposed estrogens in women with intact uteri leads to a significant increase in endometrial cancer. A possible association exists between long-term use of HRT and breast cancer incidence.

Women with significant symptoms of menopause may find the improvement in quality of life conferred by HRT outweighs any possible risk. In asymptomatic women, it appears that the benefits of HRT are substantial, but the individual patient's preferences and feelings toward risk need to be considered (Indicator 2).

REFERENCES

American College of Obstetricians and Gynecologists. April 1992. Hormone Replacement Therapy. *ACOG Technical Bulletin* 166.

Belchetz P. 1994. Hormonal Treatment of Postmenopausal Women. *New England Journal of Medicine* 330 (15): 1062-71.

Colditz GA, Hankinson SE, Hunter DJ, et al. 1995. The use of estrogens and progestins and the risk of breast cancer in postmenopausal women. *New England Journal of Medicine* 332: 1589-93.

Ettinger B, and Grady D. 1994. Maximizing the benefit of estrogen therapy for prevention of osteoporosis. *Menopause* 1: 19-24.

Grady D, Gebretsadik T, Kerlikowske K, et al. 1995. Hormone replacement therapy and endometrial cancer risk: a meta-analysis. *Obstetrics and Gynecology* 85: 304-13.

Grady D, Rubin S, et al. 1992. Hormone Therapy To Prevent Disease and Prolong Life in Postmenopausal Women. *Archives of Internal Medicine* 117 (12): 1016-1037.

Hemminki E, and Sihvo S. December 1993. A Review of Postmenopausal Hormone Therapy Recommendations: Potential For Selection Bias. *Obstetrics and Gynecology* 82 (6): 1021-28.

US Preventive Services Task Force. 1996. Guide to Clinical Preventive Services, 2nd ed. Baltimore, MD: Williams and Wilkins.

Writing Group for the PEPI Trial. 1996. Effects of hormone replacement therapy on endometrial histology in postmenopausal woman. The postmenopausal estrogen/progestin interventions (PEPI) trial. *Journal of the American Medical Association* 275 (5): 370-5.

RECOMMENDED QUALITY INDICATORS FOR HORMONE REPLACEMENT THERAPY

The following criteria apply to women age 18 and older.

Indicator	Quality of Evidence	Literature	Benefits	Comments
1. Women with intact uteri should not use unopposed estrogen unless both of the following are true: • The patient has been tried on cyclic or continuous estrogen plus progestin regimen; • Endometrial sampling is performed yearly.	I II	Writing Group for PEPI Trial, 1996; Grady et al, 1995	Reduce risk of iatrogenic endometrial cancer.	The minimum frequency of endometrial sampling necessary has not been established.
2. Women with a new diagnosis of menopause[1] should receive counseling about the risks and benefits of HRT.	II III	USPSTF, 1996.	Reduce morbidity and mortality from cardiovascular disease and osteoporosis. Relieve symptoms of menopause.	While the benefits of using HRT have been established, the benefits of counseling have not.

Definitions and Examples

[1] Women in whom menses have ceased, either naturally or due to surgical removal of the uterus and ovaries, and in whom no other reason for amenorrhea is documented.

Quality of Evidence Codes

I	RCT
II-1	Nonrandomized controlled trials
II-2	Cohort or case analysis
II-3	Multiple time series
III	Opinions or descriptive studies

150

11. HEADACHE[1]

**Pablo Lapuerta, MD, Steven Asch, MD, MPH,
and Kenneth Clark, MD, MPH**

We identified articles on the evaluation and management of headache by conducting a MEDLINE search of English language articles between 1990 and 1997 (keywords: headache, diagnosis, treatment) and by reviewing two textbooks on primary care (Pruitt, 1995, in Goroll et al., 1995; Bleeker and Meyd, 1991, in Barker et al., 1991). Of the relevant articles that were retrieved, nine were review articles and five were observational studies. Several of these articles addressed the selection of diagnostic tests and the principles of pharmacological management, with a focus on tension headache and migraine. We did not find controlled trials that analyzed elements of an appropriate history or physical examination, and for these topics expert opinion was the primary source of information.

IMPORTANCE

Headache accounts for 18 million outpatient visits per year. Approximately 73 percent of adults in the United States report having experienced a headache within the past year. Headaches lead to 638 million work days lost per year, costing employers between $5.6 and $7.2 billion annually (Kumar and Cooney, 1995).

SCREENING

Screening for headaches is not recommended because the problem is symptomatic.

DIAGNOSIS

The International Headache Society (IHS) has developed a thorough and comprehensive etiologic classification system for headaches

---

[1] This chapter is a revision of one written for an earlier project on quality of care for women and children (Q1). The expert panel for the current project was asked to review all of the indicators, but only rated new or revised indicators.

(Dalessio, 1994). Common categories include tension, migraine, cluster, noncephalic infection (e.g., influenza), head trauma, intracranial vascular disorders (e.g., hemorrhage), intracranial nonvascular disorders (e.g., meningitis, neoplasm), substance withdrawal, and neuralgias. Much of the initial diagnostic work-up for headaches focuses on distinguishing benign etiologies such as tension headaches from the more serious causes such as meningitis, hemorrhage, or neoplasm. Once that distinction is made, clinicians should distinguish among the more common benign etiologies in order to prescribe the most efficacious treatment (Pruitt, 1995, in Goroll et al., 1995).

All sources recommend a detailed history as the first step in making these distinctions. Essential elements include: a temporal profile (chronology, onset, frequency); associated symptoms (nausea, aura, lacrimation, fever); location (unilateral, bilateral, frontal, temporal); severity; family history; and, aggravating and alleviating factors (Dalessio, 1994; Bleeker and Meyd, 1991, in Barker et al., 1991) (Indicator 1). There is some disagreement about the essential elements of the neurologic examination, although most sources recommend at least an evaluation of the cranial nerves, a fundoscopic examination to rule out papilledema, and examination of reflexes (Dalessio, 1994; Larson et al., 1980; Frishberg, 1994) (Indicator 2).

One of the most difficult decisions in the diagnosis of new onset headache is the indication for computerized tomography (CT) and magnetic resonance imaging (MRI) of the head for possible structural lesions such as arteriovascular malformations, subdural hematomas, and tumors. Several observational studies suggest that a head CT scan is a low-yield evaluation tool in patients with normal neurological examinations (Larson et al., 1980; Masters et al., 1987; Becker et al., 1988; Nelson et al., 1992; Becker et al., 1993; Frishberg, 1994); however, severe headaches in such patients may indicate subarachnoid hemorrhage, and constant headaches may indicate intracranial tumors. As a consequence, the National Institutes of Health (NIH) Consensus Panel issued guidelines on the use of CT that recommended imaging only when the patient has an abnormal neurological examination or a severe or constant headache (NIH, 1981)(Indicator 3). Others have expressed reservations that using severity alone as a criterion for head imaging may lead to extensive overuse (Pruitt, 1995, in Goroll et al., 1995; Becker et al., 1988). A summary statement issued in 1993 by the American Academy of Neurology (AAN) reviewed 17 case series to define the yield of CT or MRI scanning in headache patients. In 897 migraine patients, they found only four abnormalities, none of which were clinically unsuspected. Of the 1,825 patients with headaches and normal neurologic examinations, 2.4 percent had intracranial pathology. Based on these data, the AAN recommended against scanning suspected migraine patients, but concluded there was insufficient evidence to recommend for or against scanning other headache patients with normal neurologic examinations.

Head trauma is a strong indication for imaging. In a study of 3,658 head trauma patients, the Skull X-Ray Referral Criteria Panel identified focal neurologic signs, decreasing level of consciousness, and penetrating skull injury as indications for CT scanning (Masters et al., 1987). In a separate study of 374 blunt trauma patients, there were seven abnormal head CT results in patients without abnormal neurological findings, but the best initial treatment for these cases was observation alone (Nelson et al., 1992).

Although there is still some debate on the proper indications for CT or MRI in headache patients, there is little controversy surrounding the use of skull radiographs in such patients. Clinical trials have shown skull radiographs to be poor predictors of adverse outcomes in patients with head trauma or in others presenting for evaluation of headache (Masters et al., 1987)(Indicator 4).

TREATMENT

Our quality indicators address the two most common etiologies for headaches: migraine and tension headaches. The treatment of migraine headache depends on the frequency and severity of symptoms. Placebo-controlled trials support the use of aspirin, acetaminophen, and nonsteroidal anti-inflammatory medications in mild cases (Kumar and Cooney, 1995). For more severe pain, clinicians often rely on ergot preparations, antiemetics, opioids, and sumatriptan. Ketorolac, a nonsteroidal agent, has been shown to be effective in treating moderate to severe headaches (Kumar and Cooney, 1995). Although clinical trials have found intravenous dihydroergotamine to be effective in reducing both pain and emergency room use, three clinical trials failed to find any effect of oral ergotamines on migraine pain (Kumar and Cooney, 1995). Metoclopramide and chlorpromazine also have clinical trial support in the treatment of acute migraine headaches (Kumar and Cooney, 1995). The newest agent in the migraine pharmacopoeia is sumatriptan, a 5-hydroxytryptamine 1D agonist, available in both injectable and oral form in the U.S. Sumatriptan reduced the pain and associated symptoms of migraine headaches in 70 to 90 percent of subjects in several clinical trials (Kumar and Cooney, 1995) (Indicator 6). However, sumatriptan should not be used concurrently with ergotamine due to an interactive vasoconstrictive effect (Raskin, 1994; Kumar and Cooney, 1995) (Indicator 9). For the same reason, both sumatriptan and ergotamine preparations should be avoided in patients with uncontrolled hypertension, angina, or atypical chest pain (Indicator 11).

A consensus exists that prophylactic treatment is indicated if a patient has more than two migraine headaches per month. This concept has been endorsed by the International Headache Society. Controlled clinical trials support the use of beta blockers, valproic acid, calcium channel blockers, tricyclic antidepressants, naproxen, aspirin, cyproheptadine, and valproate (Indicator 8). No clinical trials have compared these agents with one another in preventing migraines (Raskin, 1993; Sheftell, 1993; Raskin, 1994; Rapoport, 1994; Kumar and Cooney, 1995).

Treatment options for tension headaches include aspirin, acetaminophen, and nonsteroidal anti-inflammatory agents. Because of their small number of side effects compared to other treatment agents, these medications should be tried first in patients with acute mild migraine or tension headaches (Indicator 5). At least one clinical trial found prophylaxis with tricyclic antidepressants to be beneficial. Tricyclic antidepressants have been effective in reducing the frequency and severity of headache attacks in some patients (Kumar and Cooney, 1995)(Indicator 7). Tension headache and migraine have been considered to be part of a continuum of the same process and, as a result, clear distinctions between appropriate treatments for the two diagnoses are not always present. Although clinical trials support the effectiveness of oral opioid agonists and barbiturates in these two conditions, most sources recommend against initial therapy with these agents due to the risk of dependence (Markley, 1994) (Indicator 10). Butorphonal nasal spray has been encouraged as an outpatient opioid agent because it is less addictive and has been shown to reduce emergency room visits for severe migraine headache (Markley, 1994; Kumar, 1994).

FOLLOW-UP

The need for physician visits depends on the frequency and severity of headache and cannot be precisely defined. Indeed, most people in the U.S. who experience headaches do not seek evaluation or treatment from physicians (Kumar and Cooney, 1995). Accepted guidelines for specialist referral are not present in the literature, and most cases of migraine and tension headache can be handled adequately by a primary care physician.

REFERENCES

American Academy of Neurology. 1993. Summary statement: The Utility of Neuroimaging in the Evaluation of Headache in Patients With Normal Neurological Examinations.

Becker LA, Green LA, Beaufait B, et al. 1993. Use of CT scans for the investigation of headache: A report from ASPN, Part 1. *Journal of Family Practice* 37 (2): 129-34.

Becker L, Iverson DC, Reed FM, et al. 1988. Patients with new headache in primary care: A report from ASPN. *Journal of Family Practice* 27 (1): 41-7.

Bleecker ML, and CJ Meyd. 1991. In *Principles of Ambulatory Medicine, Third ed.* Headaches and facial pain. Barker LR, JR Burton, and PD Zieve, ed. 1082-96. Williams and Wilkins.

Dalessio DJ. May 1994. Diagnosing the severe headache. *Neurology* 44 (Suppl. 3): S6-S12.

Frishberg BM. July 1994. The utility of neuroimaging in the evaluation of headache in patients with normal neurologic examinations. *Neurology* 44: 1191-7.

Kumar KL. June 1994. Recent advances in the acute management of migraine and cluster headaches. *Journal of General Internal Medicine* 9: 339-48.

Kumar KL and Cooney TG. Headaches. *Medical Clinics of North America* 79 (2): 261-86.

Larson EB, Omenn GS, and Lewis H. 25 January 1980. Diagnostic evaluation of headache: Impact of computerized tomography and cost-effectiveness. *Journal of the American Medical Association* 243 (4): 359-62.

Markley HG. Chronic headache: Appropriate use of opiate analgesics. *Neurology* 44 (Suppl. 3): S18-S24.

Masters SJ, McClean JS, Arcarese, et al. 8 Jan 1987. Skull x-ray examinations after head trauma: Recommendations by a multidisciplinary panel and validation study. *New England Journal of Medicine* 2: 84-91.

National Institutes of Health. 4 November. Computed tomographic scanning of the brain. NIH consensus statement (online) 4(2): 1-7.

Nelson JB, Bresticker MA, and Nahrwold DL. November 1992. Computed tomography in the initial evaluation of patients with blunt trauma. *The Journal of Trauma* 33 (5): 722-7.

Pruitt AA. 1995. Approach to the patient with headache. *Primary Care Medicine: Office Evaluation and Management of the Adult Patient.* 3rd ed. 821-9. Philadelphia, PA: J.B. Lippincott Company.

Rapoport AM. Recurrent migraine: Cost-effective care. *Neurology* 44 (Suppl. 3): S25-S28.

Raskin NH. 1993. Acute and prophylactic treatment of migraine: Practical approaches and pharmacologic rationale. *Neurology* 43 (Suppl. 3): S39-S42.

Raskin NH. 1994. Headache. *Western Journal of Medicine* 161 (3): 299-302.

Sheftell FD. August 1993. Pharmacologic therapy, nondrug therapy, and counseling are keys to effective migraine management. *Archives of Family Medicine* 2: 874-9.

RECOMMENDED QUALITY INDICATORS FOR HEADACHE

The following apply to men and women age 18 and older who have headaches. These indicators were endorsed by a prior panel and reviewed but not rated by the current panel.

Indicator	Quality of Evidence	Literature	Benefits	Comments
Diagnosis				
1. Patients with new onset headache should be asked about all of the following: 1. location of the pain; 2. associated symptoms; 3. temporal profile; 4. severity; 5. family history; and 6. aggravating or alleviating factors.	III	Dalessio, 1994; Larson et al, 1980; Frishberg, 1994	Decrease symptoms of sinusitis and prevent potential complications of mastoiditis, and periosteal and epidural abscess. Decrease neurologic symptoms from migraines. Reduce tension headache symptoms and side effects of unwarranted therapy. Preserve neurologic function.	Location can distinguish sinus, tension, and cluster headaches. Associated symptoms can distinguish migraine and cluster headaches. Temporal profile can distinguish tumors, cluster, and tension headaches. Severity can distinguish hemorrhage. Family history can distinguish migraine. Accurate diagnosis of sinusitis can prompt antibiotic or decongestant treatment. Accurate diagnosis of migraine, cluster, and tension headaches can prompt appropriate treatment (see below). Accurate diagnosis of tumors can prompt lifesaving radiation or surgery.
2. Patients with new onset headache should have an examination evaluating all of the following: 1. cranial nerves; 2. fundi; 3. deep tendon reflexes; and 4. blood pressure.	III	Dalessio, 1994; Larson et al, 1980; Frishberg, 1994	Preserve neurologic function.	Abnormal neurologic examination is an indication for CT or MRI scanning. Increased detection of tumors, cerebrovascular accidents, and intracranial hemorrhage can lead to lifesaving radiation or surgery.
3. CT or MRI scanning is indicated in patients with new onset headache and any of the following circumstances: 4. abnormal neurological examination; or 5. severe headache.	III	NIH Consensus Statement, 1981	Preserve neurologic function.	Recommendations of NIH Consensus Panel on Computed Tomographic Scanning of the Brain.

Indicator	Quality of Evidence	Literature	Benefits	Comments
4. Skull x-rays should not be part of an evaluation for headache.	II	Masters et al, 1987	Avoid side effects (e.g., radiation) of skull x-ray. Avoid delays in CT or MRI scanning where indicated.	Four observational trials found a combined incidence of pathology of 0.7% in patients who would not otherwise receive a CT or MRI scan.
Treatment				
5. Patients with acute mild migraine or tension headache should have tried aspirin, tylenol, or other nonsteroidal anti-inflammatory agents before being offered any other medication.	I	Kumar and Cooney, 1995	Reduce migraine symptoms[1] with fewest side effects[2] from other potential agents.	More effective than placebo in reducing headaches, nausea and photophobia, but no effect on vomiting.
6. For patients with acute moderate or severe migraine headache, one of the following should have been tried before any other agent is offered: • ketorolac; • sumatriptan; • dihydroergotamine; • ergotamine; • chlorpromazine; or • metoclopramide.	I	Kumar and Cooney, 1995; Raskin, 1993; Raskin, 1994; Sheftell, 1993; Rapoport, 1994	Reduce migraine symptoms.	All listed agents have clinical trial support, but none have been compared against one another. Clinical trials did not find an effect for oral ergot preparations alone, though they have not been evaluated in their usual combination with caffeine or barbiturates.
7. Recurrent moderate or severe tension headaches should be treated with a trial of tricyclic antidepressant agents, if there are no medical contraindications to use.	I	Kumar and Cooney, 1995	Reduce rate of tension headache recurrence. Improve quality of life and functioning.	Clinical trials show reduction in pain scores.

159

Indicator	Quality of Evidence	Literature	Benefits	Comments
8. If a patient has more than 2 moderate to severe migraine headaches each month, then prophylactic treatment with one of the following agents should be offered: • beta blockers; • calcium channel blockers; • tricyclic antidepressants; • naproxen; • aspirin; • fluoxitene; • valproate; or • cyproheptadine.	I	Kumar and Cooney, 1995; Sheftell, 1993; Markley, 1994	Reduce rate of recurrent migraine symptoms.	All listed agents have clinical trial support, but none have been compared against one another.
9. Sumatriptan and ergotamine should not be concurrently administered.	III	Kumar and Cooney, 1995	Avoid adverse effects of vasoconstriction: exacerbation of chest pain in ischemic disease, hypertension, painful extremities.	Synergistic effect may cause prolonged vasoconstriction.
10. Opioid agonists and barbiturates should not be first-line therapy for migraine or tension headaches.	III	Markley, 1994; Kumar, 1994	Avoid adverse effects of opiate therapy[2].	Other less habit-forming alternative treatment should be tried first. If patient has already tried other medications at home, administration of opioid agonists is not considered first line.
11. Sumatriptan and ergotamine should not be given in patients with a history of: uncontrolled hypertension, atypical chest pain, or ischemic heart disease or angina.	II	Kumar and Cooney, 1995; Raskin, 1994	Avoid adverse effects of vasoconstriction (see above).	Both drugs cause vasoconstriction.

160

<u>Definitions and Examples</u>

[1] Migraine symptoms include: headache, nausea, photophobia, vomiting, phonophobia, scotomota, and other focal neurologic symptoms.

[2] Side effects of migraine therapeutic agents include:

    Ergotamines: vasoconstriction, exacerbation of coronary artery disease, nausea, abdominal pain, and somnolence;

    Opiates: dependence, somnolence, and withdrawal;

    Phenothiazines: dystonic reactions, anticholinergic reactions, and insomnia.

<u>Quality of Evidence Codes</u>

I	RCT
II-1	Nonrandomized controlled trials
II-2	Cohort or case analysis
II-3	Multiple time series
III	Opinions or descriptive studies

12. HIP FRACTURE

Alison Moore, MD

Several recent reviews identified through a focused literature search provided the core references in developing quality indicators for the evaluation and management of hip fracture (Zuckerman et al., 1996; Rubin, 1995). Where these core references cited studies to support individual indicators, we have included the original references.

IMPORTANCE

There are over 250,000 hip fractures in the United States each year, with 90 percent occurring in patients over the age of 50 (Cummings et al., 1990). With the aging of the population, the annual number of hip fractures is projected to double by the year 2040 (Cummings et al., 1990; Cummings et al., 1985). A hip fracture generally occurs in the proximal femur. Such injuries are divided by anatomical area into the following three categories: 1) Femoral neck fractures, which are located in the area distal to the femoral head but proximal to the greater and lesser trochanters; 2) Intertrochanteric fractures, which occur in the metaphyseal region between the greater and lesser trochanters; and 3) Subtrochanteric fractures, which occur just below the lesser trochanter (Zuckerman et al., 1996). Femoral neck and intertrochanteric fractures account for over 90 percent of hip fractures, occurring in approximately equal proportions (Gallagher et al., 1980; Alffram, 1964).

The estimated incidence of hip fracture in the United States is 80 per million population (Cummings et al., 1985; Gallagher et al., 1980). The incidence increases with age, doubling for each decade after 50 years, and is two to three times higher in women than in men (Gallagher et al., 1980; Hedlund and Lindgren, 1987). Other risk factors for hip fracture include a maternal history of hip fracture (Cummings et al., 1995), physical inactivity (Paganini-Hill et al., 1991), excessive consumption of alcohol and caffeine (Hernandez-Avila et al., 1991), low body weight (Farmer et al., 1989), tall stature (Nevitt and Cummings, 1993), previous hip fracture (Finsen and Benum, 1986), use of certain psychotropic medications (Ray et al., 1989), residence in institutions (Niemann and Mankin, 1968), visual impairment (Cummings et al., 1995), and dementia (Gates et al., 1986). Osteoporosis is an important contributing factor because it decreases the skeleton's resistance to injury. Approximately 90 percent of hip fractures in the elderly result from a simple fall (Baker and Harvey, 1985).

The health of older adults deteriorates after hip fracture, and efforts to reduce the incidence of hip fracture could lower subsequent mortality, morbidity, and health services use (Wolinsky et al., 1997).

SCREENING

There are no recommendations for quality indicators related to screening because it is a symptomatic condition.

DIAGNOSIS

Clinical Features

A common presentation of hip fracture is that of an elderly person who falls and then experiences hip pain or pain referred to the knee with concomitant difficulty standing or walking. On physical examination, the individual may experience groin or hip pain to palpation on the side of the fracture, and the affected leg may be externally rotated and shortened.

Radiography

Persons suspected of having a hip fracture should have radiographs with an anteroposterior view of the pelvis and a true lateral view of the hip (Zuckerman, 1996) (Indicator 1). Additionally, if no fracture in seen on radiograph among persons who report hip pain with difficulty standing or walking after a fall, an anteroposterior view obtained with the hip internally rotated 15 to 20 degrees will provide an optimal image of the femoral neck and may reveal a fracture not evident on the standard anteroposterior view. If this radiograph is also normal and clinical findings support the diagnosis of a hip fracture, technetium-99m bone scanning or magnetic resonance imaging (MRI) is appropriate (Rizzo et al., 1993) (Indicator 1). The bone scan is a sensitive indicator of a hip fracture unrecognized on traditional radiography, although in elderly patients the fracture may not appear until two or three days after the injury. It has been shown that MRI is as accurate as bone scanning in the assessment of occult hip fracture, and reliable results can be obtained within 24 hours after the injury (Zuckerman, 1996).

TREATMENT

The primary goal of treatment is to return the patient to his or her level of function before the fracture. For most patients with hip fracture, this goal is best accomplished with surgery followed by early mobilization. For some patients, however, surgery poses a substantially increased risk of morbidity or mortality. Specifically, a hip fracture patient with a recent or concurrent myocardial infarction has an excessively high risk of perioperative mortality because of the risk of reinfarction. This risk remains at a minimum of 15 percent until six months after myocardial infarction (Tarhan et al., 1972). Surgery should also be delayed for patients in whom anticoagulation therapy cannot be safely discontinued for 48 to 72 hours perioperatively. Non-operative management may also be preferable for non-ambulatory patients with marked dementia who experience minimal discomfort within the first few days after the injury.

Preoperative Care

A careful medical evaluation should be performed on each patient who will undergo surgical repair (Zuckerman et al., 1995). This includes a complete history and physical examination, electrocardiogram, and laboratory evaluation that includes CBC, PT, PTT, electrolytes, BUN, creatinine, glucose, liver function tests, and urinalysis (Indicator 2). This evaluation is performed to reduce risks associated with the surgical repair and anesthesia.

Timing of Surgery

In general, surgical repair should take place as soon after the injury as possible, usually within 24 to 48 hours of diagnosis. Longer intervals before surgery may increase the risk of postoperative medical complications and mortality at one year (Zuckerman et al., 1995). Medical complications include deep venous thrombosis (DVT), secondary pulmonary embolism, other pulmonary complications such as pneumonia, urinary tract infection, and skin breakdown. However, a delay in surgery may be necessary to stabilize an acute medical condition (Kenzora et al., 1984; Sexson and Lehne, 1987).

Type of Surgical Repair

The type of surgery is based on: location of the fracture, bone quality, displacement, and comminution; age, level of function before the injury, and ability to participate in a postoperative rehabilitation program; and the experience of the surgeon. Femoral neck fractures can be treated by either internal fixation with multiple screws or prosthetic replacement. Internal fixation is generally used in patients with non-displaced or minimally displaced fractures and in younger patients (<70 years) with displaced fractures. Because the incidence of nonunion and osteonecrosis is much higher with displaced fractures (30-40%) than with non-displaced fractures (<10%) (Barnes et al., 1976), prosthetic replacement is generally preferred in older patients with displaced fractures. Non-displaced fractures are usually treated by internal fixation with a sliding hip screw or similar device.

Prophylactic Perioperative Antibiotics

There exists modest support for the use of prophylactic antibiotics based on one case series and one RCT. Most studies, however, do not have the statistical power to detect clinically meaningful differences given the low rate of postoperative infection in orthopedic procedures without antibiotics. Aagaard et al. (1994) reviewed 688 patients who underwent hip fracture repair and found a significantly lower rate of deep wound infection in the group receiving prophylactic antibiotics (0.6% vs. 4.6%). Pavel et al. (1974) randomized 1,591 patients to receive prophylactic antibiotics (1 hour preoperatively and intraoperatively) or placebo. Patients receiving prophylactic antibiotics had a postoperative infection rate of 2.8 percent as compared with 5.0 percent in the placebo group (p = 0.03). Three additional RCTs of placebo versus antibiotics (Hjortrup et al., 1990; McQueen et al., 1990; Boyd et al., 1973) and one case series (Gerber et al., 1993) failed to find a significant benefit of prophylactic antibiotics. However, in all three studies, deep wound infection rates were consistently low at about five percent. Assuming a reduction in risk of 40 percent (based on the data of Pavel, et al., 1974), sample sizes of over 525 patients would be required to detect a significant difference between groups. The largest sample size in the three trials was 502 patients.

We found no studies addressing the timing of antibiotic administration. However, in a large case series of 2,847 elective surgeries, wound infection rates were found to be lowest when antibiotics were administered within two hours before surgery (Classen et al., 1992).

In summary, there is evidence from one RCT supporting the use of prophylactic antibiotics in hip fracture patients. Antibiotics appear to reduce the risk of deep wound infections from a baseline of five percent to approximately three percent. Antibiotics should be administered within two hours before surgery (Indicator 3). Our proposed indicator allows for administration at any time on the day of surgery due to difficulties to allow for documentation variability.

The duration of antibiotic treatment after surgery is quite variable and generally reflects the individual physician's preference rather than scientific data. Most physicians continue to administer broad-spectrum antibiotics for 48 hours after surgery, even though there are no data indicating that a 48 hour regimen is more effective than a 24 hour regimen. Cephalosporins are used most commonly, except in patients with a known allergy to these agents.

Postoperative Management

Early Mobilization

One of the most important aspects of postoperative management is early mobilization to prevent the complications associated with prolonged recumbency. One randomized trial evaluated early mobilization (usually within 24 hours of surgery) as part of a program that also included early discharge from the hospital and a comprehensive rehabilitation program during and after hospitalization (Cameron et al., 1994). Although this trial of 252 patients found no differences in physical independence of patients at four months, it showed that early mobilization could reduce health care costs. Based on these limited data, we recommend as a quality indicator that rehabilitation should begin the first day after surgery, with the patient moving from the bed to a chair and progressing as soon as possible to standing and walking (Koval et al., 1995) (Indicator 4).

Prophylactic Thromboembolics

The prevention of thromboembolic complications is critical after a hip fracture. In addition to early mobilization in order to prevent venous stasis (Koval et al., 1994), patients should receive prophylactic thromboembolic medication (Indicator 5). The regimens differ, but all have some degree of efficacy (Feldman et al., 1993; Gerhart et al., 1991). Six randomized trials (Collins et al., 1988; Antiplatelet Trialists' Collaboration, 1994; Powers et al., 1989; Berqvist et al., 1979; Clagett and Reisch, 1988; Leyvraz et al., 1991) support the use of low-dose heparin (5000 units q8 to 12 hours) with an overall reduction in risk of developing DVT of 64 percent, based on data pooled across the trials (overall reduction from 49 percent in placebo to 28 percent in heparin groups) (Collins et al., 1988). Low-dose heparin appears to increase the risk of major bleeding episodes by about 30 percent as compared with patients receiving placebo, but the absolute difference is small (overall rates 3.5 percent in heparin groups as compared with 2.9 percent in placebo) (Collins et al., 1988). The use of aspirin as a prophylactic agent has been examined in a meta-analysis of ten traumatic orthopedic trials (Antiplatelet Trialists' Collaboration, 1994). Aspirin was found to reduce the risk of DVT by 31 percent and reduce the risk of pulmonary embolism by 60 percent. When data from all surgical, orthopedic, and high-risk medical patients were analyzed together, the absolute excess of major bleeding episodes due to aspirin was three per 10,000 patients.

Powers et al. (1989) compared low-dose warfarin (i.e., warfarin started immediately after surgery with INR of 2.0 to 2.7) to aspirin and placebo and found DVT prevalence rates of 20 percent in the warfarin group, 41 percent in the aspirin group, and 46 percent in the placebo group (p=.005). Berqvist et al. (1979) have reported that dextran 70 has equal or greater efficacy when compared with low-dose heparin.

Additional data on the effectiveness of other prophylactic agents are available only from general surgical trials and trials examining total hip replacement. In a meta-analysis of general surgical trials (Clagett and Reisch, 1988), dextran was found to lower the incidence of DVT from 24.2 to 15.6 percent. Pooled data from five trials found the incidence of DVT in the dextran groups to be twice that of the heparin group. This meta-analysis also revealed some efficacy of pneumatic compression stockings. Heparin has been compared to low-molecular-weight heparin in one RCT of patients undergoing total hip replacement (Leyvraz et al., 1991). Patients receiving low-molecular-weight heparin were significantly less likely to develop proximal vein thrombosis as compared with the unfractionated heparin group (2.9% vs. 13.1%). The duration of enoxaparin therapy in hip replacement has also been examined. Four studies suggest an incidence of DVT after discharge as high as 24 percent that can be significantly reduced by one month of enoxaparin therapy.

In summary, there is strong evidence supporting the use of low-dose heparin as prophylaxis for DVT starting on admission to the hospital (Indicator 5). Aspirin also appears to have some benefit, but to a lesser extent, and may be considered in patients at high risk for hemorrhagic complications. One study supports the use of low-dose warfarin. There are insufficient data at this time to support the use of enoxaparin or other prophylactic agents.

Pressure Ulcer Prevention and Management

Pressure ulcers are a significant cause of morbidity in patents with hip fracture, with an incidence of 66 percent. For the prevention of pressure ulcers in high-risk patients, guidelines of the Agency for Health Care Policy and Research (AHCPR) support the efficacy of identifying high-risk individuals with a validated risk assessment tool (e.g., Norton and Braden scales). The optimal frequency for reassessing high-risk patients is not known.

With regard to clinical interventions designed to prevent or manage pressure ulcers once they have occurred, the evidence is less strong. Fair research-based evidence cited in the AHCPR guideline supports repositioning and turning every two hours if consistent with overall

169

patient goals. Data from six controlled trials and one RCT support placing at-risk individuals on a pressure-reducing device (foam, static air, alternating air, gel, or water mattress) (Indicator 6).

The remainder of data regarding the prevention and management of pressure ulcers are drawn from expert opinion and consensus panels. Recommendations include avoiding skin exposure to moisture due to incontinence, perspiration, or wound drainage; avoiding positioning on bony prominences, specifically the greater trochanter; minimizing friction and shear forces; improving nutrition; and utilizing trapeze devices to assist in transfers or bed changes. Due to the difficulty of identifying patients who are at risk for pressure ulcers from the medical record, we are not recommending any quality indicators related to these interventions.

Urinary Tract Management

Urinary retention is commonly observed in postoperative hip fracture patients. Successful strategies to reduce voiding problems might lead to decreased morbidity. We identified two RCTs examining urinary bladder management in patients undergoing orthopedic surgery (Skelly et al., 1992; Michelson et al., 1988). One study examined patients with a recently sustained hip fracture and the other examined patients undergoing hip or knee replacement. Both studies randomized patients to immediate removal of the urinary catheter postoperatively or to removal of the urinary catheter in the morning after surgery (Michelson et al., 1988) or 48 hours after surgery (Skelly et al., 1992). The findings of these studies were inconsistent; one found that immediate removal of the catheter was associated with lower rates of retention (Skelly et al., 1992) and the other found lower rates of retention with delayed removal of the catheter (Michelson et al., 1988). In both studies there were no significant differences in the incidence of urinary tract infections. Thus, we do not recommend a quality indicator in this area.

Prevention and Management of Delirium

Delirium occurs in an estimated 30 to 50 percent of patients with hip fracture (Michelson et al., 1988). The occurrence of delirium in hospitalized patients has been shown to increase length of stay and the

risk of complications, mortality, and institutionalization.
Furthermore, the majority of patients who develop delirium have at least
some persistent symptoms as much as six months later (Levkoff et al.,
1992). In patients with hip fracture, delirium is also likely to
interfere with rehabilitation activities. Eight cohort studies have
examined the risk factors for developing delirium, but only one
specifically focused on patients with hip fracture (Gustafson et al.,
1988) and many studies lack statistical power. Nevertheless, the
assembled studies indicate a number of recurring modifiable risk factors
for developing delirium, including electrolyte and metabolic laboratory
abnormalities, use of medications with psychoactive properties, and
infection. Three studies that have systematically examined etiologies
have also been very small and lack adequate statistical power. These
findings, however, all indicate a number of common etiologies that
include fluid and electrolyte abnormalities, infection, drug toxicity,
metabolic disorders, and low perfusion.

Based on these data, we recommend as a quality indicator that
patients undergoing surgery for hip fracture have electrolytes, BUN,
glucose, CBC, urinalysis, history of alcohol use, and medication history
documented preoperatively (Indicator 2).

FOLLOW-UP

Reducing Risk Factors for Hip Fracture

Data from four case-control studies and four prospective studies
indicate that lower body weight, cigarette smoking, caffeine intake, use
of long-acting sedatives, and physical inactivity have been identified
as risk factors for hip fracture (Cooper et al., 1988; Cummings et al.,
1995; Farmer et al., 1989; Grisso et al., 1991; Kiel et al., 1990; Meyer
et al., 1993; Paganini-Hill et al., 1981; Paganini-Hill et al., 1991).
Cummings et al. (1995) prospectively studied the potential risk factors
in 9,516 white women who were 65 years of age or older. Over a four-
year period, 192 women had a first hip fracture not due to motor vehicle
accidents. In multivariate age-adjusted analyses, modifiable risk
factors included treatment with long-acting benzodiazepines or
anticonvulsant drugs, high caffeine intake, weight loss, physical

171

inactivity, impaired visual function, and low calcaneal bone density. The relative risk of having a hip fracture for each of these risk factors ranged from 1.2 to 2.0. Women with multiple risk factors had an especially high risk of hip fracture. In contrast, walking for exercise was associated with a reduced relative risk for hip fracture of 0.7.

A randomized controlled trial of low-dose nasal calcitonin was conducted among 287 women within six to 36 months of menopause. These women were randomly allocated to three years of treatment with either 500 mg per day (5 days a week) of calcium or the same amount of calcium plus 50 IU of nasal salmon calcitonin per day (5 days a week). Persons treated with salmon calcitonin and calcium had improvements in lumbar spine bone mineral density as compared with patients receiving calcium alone (Reginster et al., 1994).

The efficacy and safety of calcitriol in the treatment of postmenopausal osteoporosis was evaluated in a three year prospective randomized trial of 622 women who had one or more vertebral compression fractures. Women received treatment with calcitriol at 0.25 micrograms twice a day or supplemental calcium at one gram per day or elemental calcium daily for three years. Those in the calcitriol group had a significant reduction in the rate of non-vertebral fractures during the second and third years of treatment, as compared with women who received calcium (9.3 vs. 25 fractures per 100 patient-years in the second year, 9.9 vs. 31.5 fracture per 100 patient-years in the third year) (Tilyard et al., 1992).

To determine if vitamin D and calcium reduce the risk of hip fractures among elderly women, Chapuy et al. (1992) studied the effects of supplemental vitamin D and calcium on the frequency of hip fractures and other non-vertebral fractures in 3,270 ambulatory women (mean age, 84 years). Women were randomized to receive 1.2 grams of elemental calcium and 800 IU of vitamin D or a placebo for 18 months. Women who had received vitamin D and calcium had 43 percent fewer hip fractures and 32 percent fewer non-vertebral fractures.

The efficacy of alendronate was tested in a randomized controlled two year study of 188 postmenopausal women aged 42 to 75 years with low bone mineral density of the lumbar spine (Chestnut et al., 1995). Women who were taking alendronate daily had a five percent increase in hip bone mineral density. The Fracture Intervention Trial aimed to investigate the effect of alendronate on the risk of fractures in postmenopausal women with low bone mass. In this study, 2,027 women were randomly assigned placebo or alendronate (5 mg daily for 24 months, followed by 10 mg daily for 12 months). The women were followed for 36 months. The relative risk for hip fracture for alendronate vs. placebo was 0.49 (confidence interval 0.23-0.99).

Based on these data, we recommend including in a quality indicator for follow-up, that providers assess and address relevant modifiable risk factors for hip fracture including cessation of long-acting benzodiazepines or anticonvulsant drugs when possible, improving visual function when possible, and advising patients to reduce caffeine intake and increase physical activity (Indicator 7). Among patients with low bone mineral density, physicians should also offer patients treatments including estrogen, calcium, vitamin D, calcitonin, and alendronate.

REFERENCES

Aagaard H, Noer HH, and Torholm C. 1995. Antibiotic prophylaxis in Danish orthopedic alloplastic surgery. *Ugeskrift for Laeger* 157 (17): 2439-2442.

Alffram P. 1964. An epidemiological study of cervical and trochanteric fractures of the femur in an urban population. *Acta Orthopedica Scandinavia Supplmental* 65: 1-109.

Baker SP, and Harvey AH. 1985. Falls in the elderly. *Clinical Geriatric Medicine* 1: 501-512.

Barnes R, Brown JT, Garden RS, and Nicoll EA. 1976. Subcapital fractures of the femur: A prospective review. *Journal of Bone and Joint Surgery (British Edition)* 58: 2-24.

Boyd RJ, Burke JF, and Colton T. 1973. A double-blind clinical trial of prophylactic antibiotics in hip fractures. *Journal of Bone and Joint Surgery (American Edition)* 55 (6): 1251-1258.

Cameron ID, Lyle DM, and Quine S. 1994. Cost effectiveness of accelerated rehabilitation after proximal femoral fracture. *Journal of Clinical Epidemiology* 47 (11): 1307-1313.

Clagett GP, and Reisch JS. 1988. Prevention of venous thromboembolism in general surgical patients. Results of meta-analysis. *Annals of Surgery* 208 (2): 227-240.

Classen DC, Evans RS, Pestotnik SL, et al. 1992. The timing of prophylactic administration of antibiotics and the risk of surgical-wound infection. *New England Journal of Medicine* 326 (5): 281-286.

Collins R, Scrimgeour A, Yusuf S, and Peto R. 1988. Reduction in fatal pulmonary embolism and venous thrombosis by perioperative administration of subcutaneous heparin. Overview of results of randomized trials in general, orthopedic, and urologic surgery. *New England Journal of Medicine* 318 (18): 1162-1173.

Cooper C, Barker DJP, and Wickham C. 1988. Physical activity muscle strength and calcium intake in fracture of the proximal femur in Britain. *British Medical Journal* 297: 1443-1446.

Cummings SR, Kelsey JL, Nevitt MC, and O'Dowd KJ. 1985. Epidemiology of osteoporosis and osteoporotic fractures. *Epidemiological Review* 7: 178-208.

Cummings SR, Nevitt MC, Browner WS, et al. 1995. Risk factors for hip fracture in white women. *New England Journal of Medicine* 332: 767-773.

Cummings SR, Rubin SM, and Black D. 1990. The future of hip fractures in the United States: Numbers, costs, and potential effects of postmenopausal estrogen. *Clinical Orthopaedics and Related Research* 252: 163-166.

Davis FM, Woolner DF, Frampton C, et al. 1987. Prospective, multi-center trial of mortality following general or spinal anaesthesia for hip fracture surgery in the elderly. *British Journal of Anaestheology* 59: 1080-1088.

Ettinger B, Genant HK, and Cann CE. 1985. Long-term estrogen replacement therapy prevents bone loss and fractures. *Archives of Internal Medicine* 102: 319-324.

Farmer ME, Harris T, Madams NJ, et al. 1989. Anthropometric indicators and hip fracture: The NHANES I epidemiologic follow-up study. *Journal of the American Geriatric Society* 37: 9-16.

Feldman DS, Zuckerman JD, Walters I, and Sakales SR. 1993. Clinical efficacy of aspirin and dextran for thromboprophylaxis in geriatric hip fracture patients. *Journal of Orthopedic Trauma* 7: 1-5.

Felson DT, Zhang Y, Hannan MT, et al. 1993. The effect of postmenopausal estrogen therapy on bone density in elderly women. *New England Journal of Medicine* 329: 1141-1146.

Finsen V, and Benum P. 1986. The second hip fracture: An epidemiologic study. *Acta Orthopedica Scandanavia* 57: 431-433.

Gallagher JC, Melton LJ, Riggs BL, and Bergstrath E. 1980. Epidemiology of fractures of the proximal femur in Rochester, Minnesota. *Clinical Orthopaedics and Related Research* 150: 163-171.

Gates B, Fairbairn A, and Craxford AD. 1986. Broken necks of the femur in a psychogeriatric hospital. *Inquiry* 17: 383-386.

Gerber C, Strehle J, and Ganz R. 1993. The treatment of fractures of the femoral neck. *Clinical Orthopaedics and Related Research* 292: 77-86.

Gerhart TN, Yett HS, Robertson LK, Lee MA, Smith M, and Salzman EW. 1991. Lower-molecular-weight heparinoid compared with warfarin for prophylaxis of deep-vein thrombosis in patients who are operated on for fracture of the hip: A prospective, randomized trial. *Journal of Bone and Joint Surgery (American Edition)* 73: 494-502.

Grady D, Rubin SM, Petitti DB, et al. 1992. Hormone therapy to prevent disease and prolong life in postmenopausal women. *Archives of Internal Medicine* 117: 1016-1037.

Grisso JA, Kelsey JL, Strom BL, et al. 1991. Risk factors for falls as a cause of hip fracture in women. *New England Journal of Medicine* 324: 1326-1331.

Gustafson Y, Berggren D, Brannstrom B, et al. 1988. Acute confusional states in elderly patients treated for femoral neck fracture. *Journal of the American Geriatric Society* 36 (6): 525-530.

Hammond CB, Jelovsek FR, Lee KL, Creasman WT, and Parker RT. 1979. Effects of long-term estrogen replacement therapy. *American Journal of Obstetrics and Gynecology* 133: 525-536.

Hedlund R, and Lindgren U. 1987. Trauma type, age, and gender as determinants of hip fracture. *Journal of Orthopedic Research* 5: 242-246.

Hernandez-Avila M, Colditz GA, Stampfer MJ, et al. 1991. Caffeine, moderate alcohol intake, and risk of fractures of the hip and forearm in middle-aged women. *American Journal of Clinical Nutrition* 54: 157-163.

Hjortrup A, Sorensen C, Mejdahl S, et al. 1990. Antibiotic prophylaxis in surgery for hip fractures. *Acta Orthopedica Scandinavia* 61 (2): 152-153.

Hutchinson TA, Polansky SM, and Feinstein AR. 1979. Post-menopausal estrogens protect against fractures of hip and distal radius. *Lancet* 705-709.

Johnson RE, and Specht EE. 1981. The risk of hip fracture in postmenopausal females with and without estrogen drug exposure. *American Journal of Public Health* 71: 138-144.

Kenzora JE, McCarthy RE, Lowell JD, and Sledge CB. 1984. Hip fracture mortality: Relation to age, treatment, preoperative illness, time of surgery, and complications. *Clinical Orthopaedics and Related Research* 186: 45-56.

Kiel DP, Felson DT, Hannan MT, et al. 1990. Caffeine and the risk of hip fracture: The Framingham Study. *American Journal of Epidemiology* 132: 675-684.

Kiel DP, Felson DT, Anderson JJ, et al. 1987. Hip fracture and the use of estrogens in postmenopausal women. *New England Journal of Medicine* 317: 1169-1174.

Koval KJ, Skovron ML, Aharonoff GB, Meadows SE, and Zuckerman JD. 1995. Ambulatory ability after hip fracture: A prospective study in geriatric patients. *Clinical Orthopaedics and Related Research* 310: 150-159.

Koval KJ, and Zuckerman JD. 1994. Hip fractures. I. Overview and evaluation and treatment of femoral neck fractures. *Journal of the American Academy of Orthopedic Surgery* 2: 141-149.

Levkoff SE, Evans DA, Liptzin B, et al. 1992. Delirium. The occurrence and persistence of symptoms among elderly hospitalized patients. *Archives of Internal Medicine* 152 (2): 334-340.

Leyvraz PF, Bachmann F, Hoek J, et al. 1991. Prevention of deep vein thrombosis after hip replacement: Randomized comparison between unfractionated heparin and low molecular weight heparin. *British Medical Journal* 303 (6802): 543-548.

McQueen MM, LittleJohn MA, Miles RS, and Hughes SP. 1990. Antibiotic prophylaxis in proximal femoral fracture. *Injury* 21 (2): 104-106.

Meyer HE, Tverdal A, and Falch JA. 1993. Risk factors for hip fracture in middle-aged Norwegian women and men. *American Journal of Epidemiology* 137: 1203-1211.

Michelson JD, Lotke PA, and Steinberg ME. 1988. Urinary-bladder management after total joint-replacement surgery. *New England Journal of Medicine* 319 (6): 321-326.

Naessen T, Persson I, Adami HO, Bergstrom R, and Bergkvist L. 1990. Hormone replacement therapy and the risk for first hip fracture. *Archives of Internal Medicine* 113: 95-103.

Nevitt MC, and Cummings SR. 1993. Type of fall and risk of hip and wrist fractures: The study of osteoporotic fractures. *Journal of the American Geriatric Society* 41: 1226-1234.

Niemann KM, and Mankin HJ. 1968. Fractures about the hip in an institutionalized patient population. II. Survival and ability to walk again. *Journal of Bone and Joint Surgery (American Edition)* 50: 1327-1340.

Paganini-Hill A, Chao A, Ross RK, and Henderson BE. 1991. Exercise and other factors in the prevention of hip fracture: The Leisure World study. *Epidemiology* 2: 16-25.

Paganini-Hill A, Ross RK, Gerkins VR, Henderson BE, Arthur M, and Mack TM. 1981. Menopausal estrogen therapy and hip fractures. *Archives of Internal Medicine* 95: 28-31.

Pavel A, Smith RL, Ballard A, and Larsen IJ. 1974. Prophylactic antibiotics in clean orthopaedic surgery. *Journal of Bone and Joint Surgery (American Edition)* 56 (4): 777-782.

Powers PJ, Gent M, Jay RM, et al. 1989. A randomized trial of less intense postoperative warfarin or aspirin therapy in the prevention of venous thromboembolism after surgery for fractured hip. *Archives of Internal Medicine* 149 (4): 771-774.

Ray WA, Griffin MR, and Downey W. 1989. Benzodiazepines of long and short elimination half-life and the risk of hip fracture. *Journal of the American Medical Association* 262: 3303-3307.

Riis J, Lomholt B, Haxholdt O, et al. 1983. Immediate and long-term mental recovery from general versus epidural anaesthesia in elderly patients. *Acta Anaesthesiologica Scandanavia* 27: 44-49.

Rizzo PF, Gould ES, Lyden JP, and Asnis SE. 1993. Diagnosis of occult fractures about the hip: Magnetic resonance imaging compared with bone-scanning. *Journal of Bone and Joint Surgery (American Edition)* 75: 395-401.

Sexson SB, and Lehne JT. 1987. Factors affecting hip fracture mortality. *J Orthop Trauma* 1: 298-305.

Skelly JM, Guyatt GH, Kalbfleisch R, Singer J, and Winter L. 1992. Management of urinary retention after surgical repair of hip fracture. *Canadian Medical Association Journal* 146 (7): 1185-1189.

Tarhan S, Moffitt EA, Taylor WF, and Giuliani ER. 1972. Myocardial infarction after general anesthesia. *Journal of the American Medical Association* 22: 1451-1454.

Valentin N, Lomholt B, Jensen JS, Heigaard N, and Kreiner S. 1986. Spinal or general anaesthesia for surgery of the fractured hip? A prospective study of mortality in 578 patients. *British Journal of Anaesthesia* 58: 284-291.

Weiss NS, Ure CL, Ballard JH, Williams AR, and Daling JR. 1980. Decreased risk of fractures for the hip and lower forearm with postmenopausal use of estrogen. *New England Journal of Medicine* 303: 1195-1198.

Zuckerman JD, Skovron ML, Koval KJ, Aharonoff G, and Frankel VH. 1995. Postoperative complications and mortality associated with operative delay in older patients who have a fracture of the hip. *Journal of Bone and Joint Surgery (American Edition)* 77: 1551-1556.

RECOMMENDED QUALITY INDICATORS FOR HIP FRACTURE

The following apply to men and women age 18 and older.

Indicator	Quality of Evidence	Literature	Benefits	Comments
Diagnosis				
1. Patients with symptoms or signs of hip fracture[1] should be offered one of the following imaging studies of the affected hip within 1 day: • a radiograph; • a technetium-99m bone scan; • an MRI.	III	Zuckerman et al., 1996	Improve functional status by accurate diagnosis and management of hip fracture.	Recommended by all the consensus developers and articles reviewing this topic.
2. Patients who have had surgical repair of a hip fracture should have been offered a complete medical evaluation preoperatively, including all of the following: a. medical history;[2] b. physical examination;[3] c. laboratory evaluation;[4] d. electrocardiogram.	III	Zuckerman et al., 1996	Decrease morbidity and mortality.	Allows for improved identification and management of persons at increased risk for complications from surgery or anesthesia.
Treatment				
3. Patients who have had surgical repair of a hip fracture should have received antibiotics prophylactically on the same day that surgery was performed.	I III	Aagaard et al., 1995; Pavel et al., 1994	Reduce incidence of deep wound infections after surgical repair of hip fracture.	A case series of 688 patients and a randomized trial of 1591 patients found reduced rates of deep wound infections among patients who received prophylactic antibiotics (0.6% and 2.8%, respectively) compared with patients not receiving them (4.6% and 5.0%, respectively).
4. Patients who have a surgically repaired hip fracture should begin rehabilitation on post-operative day one.	I	Cameron et al., 1994	Improve functional status.	A randomized controlled trial of early mobilization after hip fracture surgery found an associated reduction in health care costs.

179

	Indicator	Quality of Evidence	Literature	Benefits	Comments
5.	Persons with hip fractures should be given prophylactic thromboembolics[5] on admission to the hospital.	I	Antiplatelet Trialists' Collaboration, 1994; Berqvist et al., 1979; Clagett and Reisch, 1988; Collins et al., 1988; Feldman et al., 1993; Gerhart et al., 1991; Koval et al., 1994; Leyvraz et al., 1991; Powers et al., 1989	Reduce incidence of deep venous thrombosis.	Lower rates of deep venous thrombosis have been found in several randomized trials using various prophylactic thromboembolics, including low-dose heparin, aspirin, and low-dose warfarin.
6.	Patients hospitalized with hip fracture who are at risk for developing pressure sores[6] should have both of the following done while hospitalized: a. Be repositioned every 2 hours; b. Be provided a pressure-reducing mattress.[7]	III	Panel on the Prediction and Prevention of Pressure Ulcers in Adults, 1992	Prevent pressure sores from developing or worsening.	

180

Indicator	Quality of Evidence	Literature	Benefits	Comments
Follow-Up				
7. Patients who have had a hip fracture should have documented within 2 months (before or after) the presence or absence of modifiable risk factors[8] for subsequent hip fracture.	I II III	Cauley et al., 1995; Chapuy et al., 1992; Chestnut et al., 1995; Cummings et al., 1995; Ettinger et al., 1985; Felson et al., 1993; Grady et al., 1992; Hammond et al., 1979; Hutchinson et al., 1979; Johnson and Specht, 1981; Kiel et al., 1987; Naessen et al., 1990; NIH, 1994; Paganini-Hill et al., 1981; Paganini-Hill et al., 1991; Reginster et al., 1994; Tilyard et al., 1992; Weiss et al, 1989	Prevent future hip fractures by addressing modifiable risk factors.	Many studies support risk reduction and drug interventions to increase bone mass.

Definitions and Examples

[1] Symptoms of hip fracture include those associated with a fall within the prior 7 days and/or at least one of the following: sudden onset of unilateral pain with walking, unilateral pain with movement, or an inability to stand. Signs of hip fracture include any of the following: pain in the affected hip with palpation and movement, and external rotation and shortening of the affected leg.

[2] Medical history refers to documentation of any medical problems or medications currently being taken.

[3] Physical examination refers to documentation of a heart, lung, abdominal, or neurologic examination.

[4] Laboratory evaluation of patients having surgical repair of hip fracture includes any one of the following: hemoglobin, hematocrit, platelet count, protime, prothrombin time, electrolytes, BUN, creatinine, glucose, urinalysis.

[5] Prophylactic thromboembolics include any one of the following: low-dose heparin (5000 units subcutaneously q8-12 hours), aspirin (325 mg daily), low-dose warfarin (to achieve an INR of 2.0-2.7, starting immediately after surgery).

[6] Patients are at risk for developing pressure sores if they have any of the following risk factors: malnutrition, unable to walk prior to the hip fracture, urinary incontinence, or a prior history of pressure sores.

181

[7] Pressure-reducing mattresses include those made of foam, air, gel, or water.

[8] Modifiable risk factors may include the following: use of long-acting sedatives or anti-convulsants, impaired vision, high caffeine intake (>3 cups/day), inactivity, smoking, and osteoporosis. Discussion of modifiable risk factors may result in the following: discontinuation of long-acting sedatives or anti-convulsants, referral to an eye specialist, reduction of caffeine intake, increasing physical activity, smoking cessation, and use of medications shown to increase bone mass (e.g., estrogen, calcium, calcitonin, calcitriol, vitamin D, and alendronate).

Quality of Evidence Codes

I   Randomized controlled trials
II-1   Nonrandomized controlled trials
II-2   Cohort or case analysis
II-3   Multiple time series
III   Opinions or descriptive

182

13. HYSTERECTOMY

Deidre Gifford, M.D.

Background information for this chapter was obtained from a MEDLINE search of review articles on the subject of hysterectomy for the years 1990 to 1997. Focused literature searches were also carried out on the topics of leiomyomata and abnormal uterine bleeding, two common indications for hysterectomy. The reviews entitled "Hysterectomy: Indications, Effectiveness and Risks" (Bernstein et al., 1995), and "Treatment of Common Non-Cancerous Uterine Conditions: Issues for Research" (AHCPR, 1995) were also used in the development of this chapter.

IMPORTANCE

Hysterectomy is the second most common major surgical procedure performed in the United States, following cesarean delivery. In 1995, an estimated 590,000 hysterectomies were performed, the majority of which were for non-cancerous indications (Wilcox, 1994). Most women who undergo hysterectomy are between the ages of 35 and 54, with the highest rate (11.8 hysterectomies per 1,000 women per year) for women aged 35 to 44 (AHCPR, 1995). By the age of 60, over one-third of U.S. women will have had a hysterectomy (Pokras, 1993).

Operative mortality related to hysterectomy has been reported at four to 36 deaths per 10,000 women (Bernstein et al., 1995). One large study of 53,000 women in the U.S. found a death rate of 19 per 10,000 hysterectomies performed (Kjerulff, 1993). Other short-term complications occurring after hysterectomy include bleeding, re-operation, damage to other internal structures and postoperative infection. Data predating the emergence of HIV/AIDS suggested that between 2 and 13 percent of patients undergoing hysterectomy received a blood transfusion. Current rates of transfusion with hysterectomy are unknown. Re-operation occurs in less than one percent of hysterectomies. The risk of bladder injury is approximately one percent. Infection is the most common form of post-operative morbidity, occurring in the bladder, the vaginal cuff or the abdominal wound. Febrile morbidity occurs in approximately one quarter of women when no prophylactic antibiotics are used, however this rate is reduced substantially with the use of prophylactic antibiotics (Bernstein et al., 1995).

Recent attention has focused on the variation in rates of hysterectomy. Rates vary between the U.S. and other developed countries (from 28 to 70 per 10,000 women), between regions within the U.S. (from 32 to 58 per 10,000), and within small geographic areas (from 24 to 81 per 10,000) (Bernstein, 1995). This variation has led to questions about the appropriate rate of hysterectomy, and the appropriate indications for performing the procedure.

TREATMENT

The majority of non-obstetrically related, non-cancer related hysterectomies are done for the indications of uterine bleeding, leiomyomata (fibroids), endometriosis, pelvic prolapse/urinary dysfunction, and chronic pelvic pain (AHCPR, 1995). In 1994, the Agency for Health Care Policy and Research (AHCPR) held a conference to review the current state of knowledge on the effectiveness of hysterectomy for these conditions and concluded that the literature on the whole was weak and incomplete. Few randomized trials comparing hysterectomy to other treatment modalities have been carried out. In addition, there is little data available on the effectiveness of hysterectomy in treating the symptoms which prompt the procedure to be performed. However, because of its importance as a common procedure affecting thousands of women per year, we have chosen to review what is known about hysterectomy. For the development of quality indicators, we have chosen to focus on two of the more common indications for hysterectomy: uterine fibroids and abnormal uterine bleeding.

Leiomyomata uteri (uterine fibroids)

Uterine fibroids, which are benign proliferations of smooth muscle cells and fibrous connective tissue, are the most common neoplasms of the female pelvis. They occur in as many as 25 percent of women of reproductive age (ACOG, 1994). Fibroids can be single or multiple, and can range in size from 1 mm to 20 cm in diameter. Although the majority of uterine fibroids are asymptomatic, these tumors are the most common indication for hysterectomy, accounting for 30 percent of all procedures (ACOG, 1994).

The most common symptom associated with fibroids is abnormal uterine bleeding. This may be in the form of inter-menstrual bleeding, heavy menstrual bleeding (menorrhagia) or both. The reason for irregular and/or heavy bleeding in the presence of myomata is unclear. Fibroids also commonly cause pelvic pressure and/or urinary complaints, depending on their size and location relative to other pelvic organs. Large fibroids can cause hydronephrosis related to ureteral compression, but the clinical significance of this finding is not known (ACOG, 1994). Infertility and recurrent spontaneous abortion have been related to fibroids anecdotally, but no controlled data exist demonstrating a clear role of fibroids in either condition.

Treatment of fibroids is dependent on their size and the extent of symptoms which they cause. Asymptomatic fibroids can be managed with observation alone; symptomatic fibroids can be treated with hysterectomy or myomectomy (removal of the myoma while leaving the uterus intact). The Maine Women's Health study followed a cohort of women with fibroids who were treated with observation alone for one year. These women had relatively mild symptoms at the beginning of the study, but no significant change in symptoms or quality of life were noted over the year of observation, suggesting that observation is a reasonable alternative in women with minimally symptomatic fibroids (Carlson, 1994). There is no medical therapy available for the permanent treatment of uterine fibroids. GnRH analogs, which induce an artificial menopause by causing a hypoestrogenic state, can cause fibroids to shrink by an average of 50 percent within three months. However the fibroids return to their pre-treatment size within 12 weeks of cessation of therapy. Long term GnRH analog treatment is currently not practical since prolonged treatment leads to bone loss and menopausal symptoms which are not well-tolerated (ACOG, 1994).

Traditionally, when the uterus reached a size equivalent to a twelve weeks gestation, hysterectomy was felt to be necessary. The rationale for this indication was that an enlarged uterus could make physical examination of the ovaries difficult, and obscure a developing ovarian cancer. In addition, there was a concern that surgery would become more difficult and morbid if the uterus was allowed to enlarge further. Neither of these rationale is supported by data, and lately the dictum of removing the asymptomatic enlarged uterus has been questioned (Carlson, 1993). In its current quality criteria for hysterectomy for leiomyomata, the American College of Obstetricians and Gynecologists (ACOG) requires that if hysterectomy is to be performed, either the uterus is large enough to be palpable abdominally and is of concern to the patient, or the patient has symptoms of excessive bleeding, pelvic discomfort or bladder pressure with urinary frequency (Indicator 1). The ACOG also states that a desire to maintain fertility and an asymptomatic leiomyomata less than twelve weeks size are contraindications to hysterectomy for fibroids (ACOG, 1994).

In summary, according to the consensus of the ACOG, it is appropriate to perform a hysterectomy for fibroids that are symptomatic in a woman who has completed her childbearing. In women with asymptomatic fibroids, watchful waiting (i.e., periodic follow-up with physical examination without other interventions) is felt to be appropriate therapy since asymptomatic fibroids cause virtually no morbidity if they remain stable in size. For women who have not completed childbearing but have symptomatic fibroids, myomectomy is an alternative therapy (ACOG, 1994).

Abnormal Uterine Bleeding (pre- and peri-menopausal)

Abnormal bleeding (i.e., bleeding which differs from the normal menstrual cycle in quantity or duration) is a common symptom among reproductive aged and peri-menopausal women. This symptom may account for as many as 20 percent of hysterectomies (Carlson 1993). Abnormal bleeding may have a number of underlying etiologies, including anovulation, uterine fibroids, cervical or endometrial polyps, endometrial hyperplasia, malignancy, infection, pregnancy or coagulopathy. Treatment of abnormal bleeding depends on the underlying cause. Bleeding that is not due to any of the definable causes listed above is often referred to as dysfunctional uterine bleeding (DUB).

In the pre- and peri-menopausal woman, medical therapy for DUB includes hormonal agents such as combination oral contraceptives or progestins, non-steroidal anti-inflammatory drugs, and GnRH analogues. Each of these classes of drugs has been tested among women with unexplained bleeding and found to be effective in decreasing menstrual blood loss in certain cases. For example, oral contraceptives can reduce blood loss by an average of 53 percent (Bernstein, 1995). Medical therapy generally works only while being administered, however, and women return to their pre-treatment state soon after the cessation of treatment. The Maine Women's Health Study followed a cohort of 400 women with abnormal bleeding, pelvic pain and fibroids who were treated with hysterectomy or non-surgical management. After one year of follow up, non-surgical management of abnormal bleeding was associated with significant reductions in days of bleeding and pain. Women treated non-surgically also showed a significant increase in mean scores for the General Health Index and the Activity Index, two measures of health-related quality of life. However, a substantial number of patients still experienced high symptom levels after one year of treatment (Carlson, 1994).

When medical therapy fails, surgical interventions include dilation and curettage, endometrial ablation and hysterectomy. Endometrial ablation is a procedure which uses electrocautery or laser to resect or ablate the endometrial lining. This procedure has been effective in eliminating symptoms in 70 to 90 percent of cases (Carlson, 1993), although a significant number of women will require re-operation due to continued bleeding. Currently, a multi-center randomized trial is underway in the U.S. comparing the effectiveness of endometrial ablation to hysterectomy for the treatment of abnormal uterine bleeding. At this point, available studies do not allow for the identification of which women are most appropriate for endometrial ablation versus hysterectomy, for the treatment of abnormal bleeding.

Because medical therapy is successful in controlling symptoms in a number of women with abnormal bleeding, and because it is not possible to identify in advance which patients will not be effectively treated by medical therapy, a trial of medical management is indicated in all women with abnormal bleeding of unknown etiology (or DUB) prior to hysterectomy (ACOG, 1989). Medical management can consist of hormonal therapy in the form of estrogens, progestins or combinations, or non-steroidal anti-inflammatory drugs (Indicator 2). Medical management may be impractical if the bleeding is sufficient to cause hemodynamic instability requiring immediate intervention.

Post-Menopausal Bleeding

Bleeding which occurs after menopause (generally defined as 12 months of amenorrhea due to cessation of ovarian function) can be a presenting symptom of cancer of the endometrium. However, most women with post-menopausal bleeding do not have an underlying malignancy. One recent population-based study in Sweden showed that only ten percent of women with post-menopausal bleeding had an underlying malignant or pre-malignant lesion, with the remainder having atrophy (50%), benign endometrium (14%), insufficient tissue for diagnosis (14%) or other benign conditions (Gredmark, 1995). This study is consistent with other studies describing histologic findings in women with post-menopausal bleeding (Feldman, 1993).

Because post-menopausal bleeding may represent endometrial cancer, further evaluation of any post-menopausal bleeding is indicated (Indicator 4). However, only a small percentage of women with this symptom will have a diagnosis which requires hysterectomy (i.e., endometrial cancer or a premalignant endometrial lesion). In the majority of women, once cancer has been excluded, either hormone replacement therapy or observation alone can be used as the initial management. Therefore, prior to undertaking hysterectomy for post-menopausal bleeding, biopsy of the endometrium should be performed. (Indicator 3).

Office endometrial biopsy is a simple method for accurately determining the status of the endometrium in women with post-menopausal bleeding. This method is as accurate as diagnostic dilatation and curettage (ACOG, 1991) and has the advantage of not requiring general anesthesia or the use of an operating room. Occasionally office biopsy is not possible in women with post-menopausal bleeding due to stenosis of the cervix or other anatomic considerations. In these cases, dilatation and curettage may be necessary to sample the endometrium.

Several recent studies have examined the use of transvaginal ultrasonography for the diagnosis of post-menopausal bleeding. These studies suggest that finding a thin endometrium (less than 3-5 mm) on transvaginal ultrasound excludes the possibility of underlying pathology in most cases (Dijkhuizen, 1996), and that this procedure might be used as a way of deciding which women with post-menopausal bleeding need a biopsy. However, there is as yet no published evidence to suggest that transvaginal sonography is either better accepted by women or more cost-effective than performing an office biopsy on all women with this symptom. In addition, there is no generally accepted cut-off point for endometrial thickness below which biopsy of the woman with post-menopausal bleeding can be avoided. It may be reasonable to use transvaginal sonography as an alternative to dilatation and curettage in women in whom office biopsy is unsuccessful. Further research is needed before sonography alone can replace biopsy in women with post-menopausal bleeding.

REFERENCES

ACOG Technical Bulletin No 162. 1991. Carcinoma of the Endometrium. 162: 1-6.

ACOG Technical Bulletin No 134. 1989. Dysfunctional Uterine Bleeding. 134: 1-5.

ACOG Technical Bulletin No 192. 1994. Uterine Leiomyomata. 1-9.

Agency for Health Care Policy and Research (AHCPR). 1995. Treatment of Common Non-Cancerous Uterine Conditions: Issues for Research. 95-0067: 1-21.

Bernstein SJ, Fiske ME, McGlynn EA, and Gifford DS. January 1995. Hysterectomy: Indications, Effectiveness, and Risks (MR-592-AHCPR).

Carlson KJ, Miller BA, and Fowler FJ. 1994. The Maine Women's Health Study: II. Outcomes of Nonsurgical Management of Leiomyomas, Abnormal Bleeding, and Chronic Pelvic Pain. 83 (4): 566-572.

Carlson KJ, Nichols DH, and Schiff I. 1993. Indications for Hysterectomy. *New England Journal of Medicine* 328 (12): 856-860.

Dijkhuizen FPHLJ, Brolmann HAM, Potters AE, et al. 1996. The accuracy of transvaginal ultrasonography in the diagnosis of endometrial abnormalities. *Obstetrics and Gynecology* 87 (3): 345-349.

Feldman S, Berkowitz RS, and Tosteson AA. 1993. Cost-effectiveness of strategies to evaluate postmenopausal bleeding. *Obstetrics and Gynecology* 81 (6): 968-975.

Gredmark T, Dvint S, Havel G, et al. 1995. Histopathological findings in women with postmenopausal bleeding. *British Journal of Obstetrics and Gynecology* 102: 133-136.

Kjerulff K, Langenberg P, and Guzinski G. 1993. The socioeconomic correlates of hysterectomies in the United States. *American Journal of Public Health* 83: 106-108.

Pokras R, and Hufnagel VG. March 1987. Hysterectomies in the United States, 1965-1984. Vital and health statistics, series 13, no. 92. *DHHS Publication No. (PHS) 87-1753*

Wilcox LS, Koonin LM, Pokras R, et al. 1994. Hysterectomy in the United States, 1988-1990. *Obstetrics and Gynecology* 83 (4): 549-555.

RECOMMENDED QUALITY INDICATORS FOR HYSTERECTOMY

These indicators apply to women age 18 and older.

Indicator	Quality of Evidence	Literature	Benefits	Comments
1. If a woman undergoes a hysterectomy with the indication of fibroid uterus at least one of the following should be recorded in the medical record: • The uterus is palpable abdominally and the patient is concerned about the fibroids; • Excessive menstrual bleeding; • Anemia; • Pelvic discomfort; or • Bladder pressure with urinary frequency.	III	ACOG, 1994	Avoid morbidity and mortality from unnecessary hysterectomy	No definitions are specified for the terms *concern, excessive* or *discomfort*. Any notation in the record will be accepted.
2. If a pre- or peri-menopausal[1] woman undergoes a hysterectomy with the indication of abnormal uterine bleeding, then the medical record should indicate that at least one month of medical therapy[2] was given in the six months prior to the hysterectomy without relief of symptoms.	III	ACOG, 1989	Avoid morbidity and mortality from unnecessary hysterectomy.	This indicator does not apply to women in whom another cause of the bleeding is noted, such as fibroids, polyps or coagulopathy.
3. Women who have a hysterectomy for post-menopausal bleeding[3] should have had a biopsy of the endometrium[4] within six months prior to the procedure.	III	ACOG, 1991	Avoid morbidity and mortality from unnecessary hysterectomy.	Hysterectomy can be avoided in the majority of women with post-menopausal bleeding who do not have a uterine malignancy.
4. Women with post-menopausal bleeding[3] should be offered an office endometrial biopsy[5] within one month of presentation.	III	ACOG, 1991	Reduce mortality from endometrial cancer by detection and treatment.	Although office biopsy may not be successful in all women, an attempted biopsy or a refusal of the patient should be documented in the record. The one-month time period is arbitrary.

Definitions and Examples

[1]Pre- or peri-menopausal: A women in whom the last menstrual period was less than 12 months ago.
[2]Medical therapy: Can include non-steroidal anti-inflammatory drugs, estrogens, progestins or estrogen/progestin combinations.

[3] Post-menopausal bleeding: Any amount of vaginal bleeding which occurs in a woman not on hormone replacement therapy and whose last menstrual period was 12 or more months ago. Unexpected vaginal bleeding in a women on hormone replacement therapy.

[4] Biopsy of the endometrium: Any pathology report documenting endometrial histology (even if insufficient for diagnosis), or documentation of a failed attempt at office biopsy and dilatation and curettage.

[5] Office endometrial biopsy: Office biopsy includes all methods of endometrial sampling (suction, curettage, Pipelle) not performed in an operating room, but excludes D&C.

Quality of Evidence Codes

I	RCT
II-1	Nonrandomized controlled trials
II-2	Cohort or case analysis
II-3	Multiple time series
III	Opinions or descriptive studies

192

14. INGUINAL HERNIA

Douglas S. Bell, M.D.

Inguinal hernia is a common problem in men that has significant associated costs and that occasionally causes death. Quality indicators for inguinal hernia are based on literature found through MEDLINE searches covering articles in English, published from 1990 to the present. Although 55 randomized controlled trials were identified, all such trials compared different surgical techniques or methods of peri-operative management. There seems to be very little data on the most important medical question: When to operate on a patient with an inguinal hernia.

IMPORTANCE

The prevalence of groin hernia is estimated to be three to four percent in the population (Wantz, 1997; Hay et al., 1995) with the lifetime incidence for males estimated at five to ten percent (Kittur & Smith, 1991). Women have 4 to 17 percent the risk of men (Wantz, 1997; Kittur & Smith, 1991). It is estimated that 700,000 herniorrhaphies are performed yearly in the U.S. (Rutkow & Robbins, 1993). Medicare allowable charges (including surgeon, anesthesia, and facility) for outpatient herniorrhaphy at a Boston teaching hospital are currently about $1,200.00 (Wantz, 1997). Since 96 percent of herniorrhaphies at one institution were performed on an outpatient basis (Wantz, 1997), national expenditures for inguinal herniorrhaphy can be estimated at least $840 million, not counting complications or lost work due to pain.

Hernias are termed *reducible* if their contents can be pushed back into the abdominal cavity. They are termed *incarcerated* if they cannot be pushed back (Kittur & Smith, 1991). An incarcerated hernia may entrap bowel and cause bowel obstruction, or it may become *strangulated* if the contents of the hernia sac become ischemic. Both of these conditions carry a relatively high mortality and warrant emergency surgery.

SCREENING

Most groin hernias progress through an asymptomatic stage when the defect may be detectable by a physician but the patient is unaware of it (Wantz, 1997). The natural history of groin hernia is of gradual enlargement until repaired. Femoral hernias are typically smaller than inguinal hernias, are more often asymptomatic, and present with strangulation more frequently (5-20% vs. 1.3-3% for inguinal hernias) (Wantz, 1997). Femoral hernias make up more than 30 percent of groin hernias in women, but only three percent of groin hernias overall (Schumpelick, Treutner, & Arlt, 1994). Little is written about the role of screening for asymptomatic hernias, but one author (a surgeon) recommends that a standing hernia check should be part of every periodic physical exam (Wantz, 1997). He does not specify whether women should be included in this recommendation. Since no evidence exists that early intervention for asymptomatic hernias produces a health benefit, screening cannot be recommended as a quality indicator at this time.

DIAGNOSIS

Hernias generally present as an insidiously growing groin mass, but there is occasionally a history of an inciting stress with the painful appearance of the mass. Strangulated hernias are invariably painful, and are often accompanied by symptoms of bowel obstruction (nausea and vomiting). Since the risk of strangulation is greatest in the first months and years after the patient's first awareness of a hernia (Gallegos, Dawson, Jarvis, & Hobsley, 1991), the time since the patient's first awareness of a hernia should be recorded in the chart when the provider initially documents a hernia's presence (Indicator 1).

Hernias are usually visible to the examiner's naked eye, but in men the examiner may check the inguinal ring by invaginating the skin of the scrotum with an examining finger. About 30 percent of inguinal hernias in men are of the *direct* type, which arise more medially than the *indirect* type (Schumpelick et al., 1994). Because direct inguinal hernias tend to have a wider base, their risk of strangulation may be up to ten times lower (Schumpelick et al., 1994). Even experienced surgeons, however, can distinguish direct from indirect hernias on physical exam in only 70 percent of cases (Schumpelick et al., 1994). Patients should be examined standing for groin hernias, since the hernia sac is likely to reduce when the patient is supine (Wantz, 1997). Details of exam technique are unlikely to be recorded in the chart, so quality indicators cannot be recommended based on the physical examination.

The accuracy of ultrasound in differentiating direct from indirect hernias was 73 percent in one study. It is thought to add little to a surgeon's examination (Schumpelick et al., 1994). CT and MRI may be used to diagnose hernias but they should not be necessary (Wantz, 1997). No quality indicators for testing are recommended.

TREATMENT

Treatment for incarcerated hernia is clearly emergency surgery. Mortality increases sharply if surgery is delayed, due either to delayed patient presentation or to misdiagnosis. In one case series, patients presenting for surgery within 24 hours of the onset of strangulation symptoms had a 1.4 percent mortality. Those presenting within 24 to 47 hours of symptom onset had a 10 percent mortality, and those presenting after 48 or more hours had a 21 percent mortality rate. More than half of patients presented at 24 hours or more; given this sharp rise in mortality with delayed surgery, quality care for patients with strangulation should include moving them urgently to surgery (Williams and Hale, 1966). Patients diagnosed with a strangulated or incarcerated inguinal hernia should have emergency groin exploration within 24 hours of presentation (Williams & Hale, 1966; Andrews, 1981) (Indicator 2).

Elective herniorrhaphy for non-incarcerated hernia is a much more difficult topic. The expert opinion among surgeon authors is that the high mortality of emergency surgery warrants elective herniorrhaphy for all patients with a hernia large enough that they are aware of it, unless they are terminally ill (Wantz, 1997; Schumpelick et al., 1994; Gallegos et al., 1991; Nehme, 1983; Tingwald & Cooperman, 1982). Although it may be safer to defer surgery for direct than indirect hernias, this distinction cannot be made reliably on exam, as noted above. Trusses are an alternative management option used more frequently in Britain than in the U.S. or in other parts of Europe (Cheek, Williams, & Farndon, 1995). They are thought by many surgeons to cause tissue atrophy, increasing the risk of hernia recurrence after repair, but there is no convincing data for or against this hypothesis (Cheek et al., 1995). Femoral trusses should probably never be used, since they are more likely to precipitate strangulation (Cheek et al., 1995), and they compress the femoral vessels (Wantz, 1997). Surgeons generally agree that trusses should only be used as a temporizing measure, if they are used at all (Wantz, 1997; Cheek et al., 1995).

The opposite conclusion about trusses, however, is offered by a decision analysis of elective herniorrhaphy versus truss in elderly patients, shown in Figure 14.1 (Neuhauser, 1977). A 65 year old patient was taken as the base-case and given the 1972 age-specific life expectancy of 13.3 years. Mortality from elective and emergency herniorrhaphy was estimated from 1971 Medicare hospital discharge data. The risk of strangulation was estimated to be 0.29 percent per year, based on an unpublished population-based study done in Cali, Columbia, where elective herniorrhaphy is essentially unavailable. This risk was extrapolated over the average 13.3 years of remaining life by assuming a constant hazard: $1 - (1 - .0029)^{13.3} = 0.038$. Strangulation was assumed to occur on average halfway through the 13-year time period. Hernia recurrence after elective operation was also modeled, but it contributed negligibly to mortality so it is excluded from Figure 14.1. Under these assumptions, elective herniorrhaphy in a 65 year old results in a reduction in life expectancy of .036 years (13 days). One sensitivity analysis showed that even assuming a "perfect surgeon" with no mortality from elective surgery, the life-year benefit was only 0.00922 years. The marginal cost of elective surgery over the truss strategy was estimated to be $1,110, resulting in a cost-effectiveness ratio for this "perfect surgeon" of $120,471 per life-year saved. The author concluded that elective inguinal herniorrhaphy can only be justified by quality of life benefits (e.g., by improved self-image, decreased discomfort), and not by survival benefits.

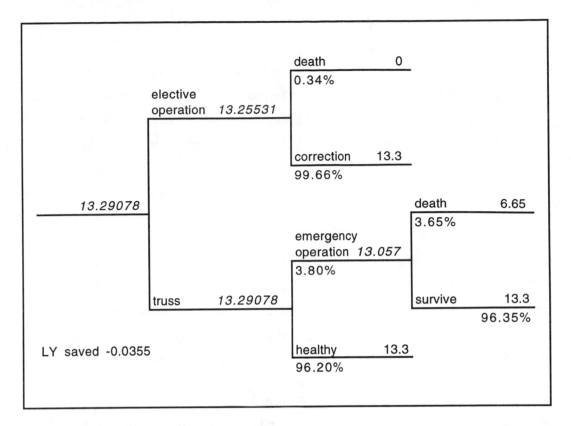

* Utilities are expressed as life-years (not quality-adjusted). Values in italics are calculated utilities for branch points.
Source: Newhauser, 1977

Figure 14.1 - Decision Analysis for Elective Herniorrhaphy in a 65 Year Old

Since the time of Neuhauser's analysis, however, male life expectancy at age 65 has increased to 15.4 years (National Center for Health Statistics, 1996) and mortality from elective herniorrhaphy has almost certainly declined. The true values for other parameters remain more uncertain. Table 14.1 compares Neuhauser's estimates with those from several other studies. The first two studies extracted data from the charts of elderly patients who had presented for elective or emergency herniorrhaphy. The studies by Hay and Liem provide prospective mortality rates from recent randomized controlled trials of alternative techniques for elective herniorrhaphy. Finally, Wantz quotes a modern mortality rate for elective herniorrhaphy based on the experience of the Shouldice Hospital in Toronto, where there have been 29 peri-operative deaths in 215,000 elective herniorrhaphies performed since 1945. Note, however, that these lower mortality rates occurred in populations that included a lower proportion of elderly persons.

Mortality from emergency surgery in other studies has also been significantly higher than the estimate used by Neuhauser.

Gallegos et al. (1991) used Kaplan-Meier survival analysis to model the risk of strangulation over time. Data were obtained by extracting from charts the duration that a hernia had been present prior to either strangulation or elective herniorrhaphy. They found that the risk of strangulation in the first three months after the onset of a hernia (2.8%) represents a significant part of the five year risk of strangulation (8.6%). The median time to strangulation was two years. This study provides the first evidence for the belief that newer hernias pose a higher risk of strangulation, presumably because they have a smaller orifice. It also calls into question Neuhauser's assumption that the strangulation hazard remains constant over time.

Table 14.1

Summary of mortality estimates for elective and emergency herniorrhaphy, and estimates of risk of strangulation.

Study	n	Mean age	Mortality from Elective Surgery	Mortality from Emergency Surgery	Risk of Strangulation (% per year)
Neuhauser (1977)	--	65	0.34%	3.65%	0.29%/yr.
Tingwald et al. (1982)	62	77	0	18%	--
Nehme (1983)	1496	78	1.3%	16%	--
Andrews (1981)	167	68	--	13.6%	--
Gallegos et al. (1991)	439	59	--	--	8.6%/5 yr.
Hay et al. (1995)	1578	54	0.25 %	--	--
Liem et al. (1997)	998	55	0	--	--
Wantz (1997)	215,000	--	0.013%	--	--

Figure 14.2 shows an updated version of Neuhauser's decision analysis created for this review, assumes a 65 year old man presenting with a new inguinal hernia. It is presented as supportive evidence for a quality indicator specifying the desirability of offering elective herniorrhaphy in patients with new (less than two years) hernias (Indicator 3). Base-case assumptions include: a potential survival benefit of 12.6 years (a discount rate of three percent was applied to the 15.4 year male life-expectancy at age 65); mortality from elective surgery of 0.16 percent (data from the 2 prospective trials of herniorrhaphy were pooled); a total risk of strangulation of 8.6 percent (the 5-year risk from Gallegos et al.); and a median time to strangulation of two years after hernia onset (also from Gallegos et al.). To give the benefit of doubt to the truss strategy, the mortality from emergency surgery is left at 3.65 percent.

The resulting model estimates that elective herniorrhaphy provides a small survival benefit in the 65 year old. Dividing this benefit into the $1,200 Medicare-allowable charge for outpatient herniorrhaphy (Wantz, 1997) produces a cost-effectiveness ratio of $92,000 per life-year, as shown in Figure 14.2. Subtracting conservative cost estimates for the truss strategy of $50 for the truss and $10,000 for emergency surgery, the cost-effectiveness improves to $26,100. By comparison, coronary artery bypass graft surgery (CABG) is estimated to have a cost-effectiveness over medical management of $5,600 for patients with left main disease, $12,000 for patients with 3 vessel disease, and $75,000 for patients with two-vessel disease (Tengs et al., 1995).

The above model is fairly sensitive to changes in the parameter estimates. Changing just the mortality of elective herniorrhaphy to that of the Shouldice hospital (Wantz, 1997) improves the cost-effectiveness ratio to $10,800. Changing just the mortality of emergency herniorrhaphy to 13 percent (Gallegos et al., 1991) improves the cost-effectiveness ratio to $3,480. Reducing the strangulation risk worsens cost-effectiveness such that at a seven percent total risk the ratio is $71,400. At a 5.2 percent strangulation risk elective surgery loses its survival benefit for a 65 year old man. Reducing the subject's age to 55 (the average age in the prospective herniorrhaphy trials) increases his discounted life expectancy to 16.8 years, which improves cost-effectiveness in the base-case to $17,400. At this age, elective surgery loses its survival benefit at a strangulation risk of five percent. Elective herniorrhaphy would be *cost-saving* if its total costs are less than the costs of emergency surgery (discounted for their occurrence in the future) multiplied by the risk of strangulation. In the base-case, elective herniorrhaphy becomes cost-saving if the discounted cost of emergency surgery exceeds $14,000.

This analysis does not use more modern methods of modeling outcomes over time (Sonnenberg & Beck, 1993). It does not model the expected changes in mortality with age. changes in strangulation risk over time (after onset of the hernia), nor changes in quality of life after herniorrhaphy. More complicated analysis is beyond the scope of the current module. The current decision analysis, however, is at least helpful for integrating the available data and for understanding the small expected benefits in relation to the relatively low costs of herniorrhaphy.

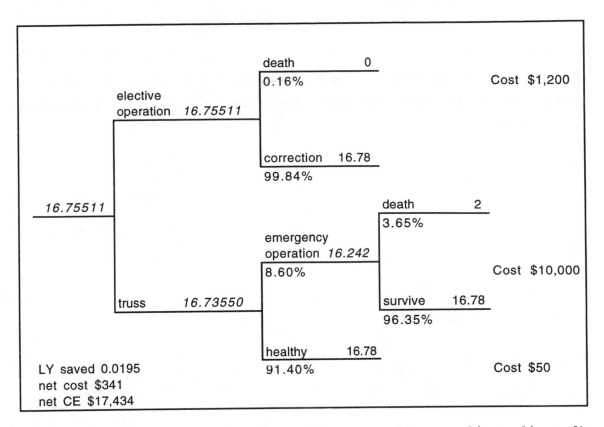

* Utilities are expressed as life-years (not quality-adjusted).
Values in italics are calculated utilities for branch points.
    Source: Newhauser, 1977

Figure 14.2 - Decision analysis for elective herniorrhaphy based on Newhauser but using newer estimates of mortality and strangulation risk. Assumes a 65 year old man with a new inguinal hernia.*

Current evidence therefore does not support a definitive answer on the benefit of elective herniorrhaphy. If, however, the study by Gallegos, et al. (Gallegos et al., 1991) is correct, patients with a reasonable life-expectancy probably do have at least a small survival benefit if their hernia is repaired in the first few years after its appearance. A conservative quality indicator might therefore be: patients younger than 65 with an inguinal hernia that has appeared within the last two years should be offered elective herniorrhaphy (Indicator 3). This quality indicator would rely on documentation of an inguinal hernia in the assessment section of a visit note. Although transient, insignificant hernias may be picked up by a screening examination alone, this would occur only rarely; therefore, an exception for these is not recommended.

FOLLOW-UP

We did not identify any data or expert opinion to support quality indicators for follow-up intervals for patients with inguinal hernias.

REFERENCES

Andrews NJ. 1981. Presentation and outcome of strangulated external hernia in a district general hospital. *British Journal of Surgery* 68 (5): 329-32.

Cheek CM, Williams MH, and Farndon JR. 1995. Trusses in the management of hernia today. *British Journal of Surgery* 82 (12): 1611-3.

Gallegos NC, Dawson J, Jarvis M, and Hobsley M. 1991. Risk of strangulation in groin hernias. *British Journal of Surgery* 78 (10): 1171-3.

Hay JM, Boudet MJ, Fingerhut A, and et al. 1995. Should ice inguinal hernia repair in the male adult?: the gold standard. A multicenter controlled trial in 1578 patients. *Annals of Surgery* 222 (6): 719-27.

Kittur DS & Smith GW. 1991. Abdominal Hernias. Principles of Ambulatory Medicine. LR Barker JR Burton & PD Zieve, ed. Baltimore MD: Williams & Wilkins.

National Center for Health Statistics. 1996. Vital statistics of the United States 1992. Vol II, Sec 6 Life Tables. Washington DC: Public Health Service.

Nehme AE. 1983. Groin hernias in elderly patients: Management and prognosis. *American Journal of Surgery* 146 (2): 257-60.

Neuhauser D. 1977. Elective inguinal herniorrhaphy versus truss in the elderly: Costs Risks and Benefits of Surgery. JP Bunker BA Barnes & F Mosteller, New York: Oxford University Press.

Rutkow IM & Robbins AW. 1993. Demographic classificatory and socioeconomic aspects of hernia repair in the United States. *Surgical Clinics of North America* 73 (3): 413-26.

Schumpelick V, Treutner KH, and Arlt G. 1994. Inguinal hernia repair in adults. *Lancet* 344 (8919): 375-9.

Sonnenberg FA & Beck JR. 1993. Markov models in medical decision making: a practical guide. *Medical Decision Making* 13 (4): 322-38.

Tengs TO, Adams ME, Pliskin JS, and et al. 1995. Five-hundred life-saving interventions and their cost-effectiveness. *Risk Analysis* 15 (3): 369-90.

Tingwald GR, and Cooperman M. 1982. Inguinal and femoral hernia repair in geriatric patients. *Surgery, Gynecology and Obstetrics* 154 (5): 704-6.

Wantz GE. 1997. A 65-year-old man with an inguinal hernia. *Journal of the American Medical Association* 277 (8): 663-9.

Williams JS & Hale HW. 1966. The advisability of inguinal herniorrhaphy in the elderly. *Surgery, Gynecology and Obstetrics* 122 (1): 100-4.

RECOMMENDED QUALITY INDICATORS FOR INGUINAL HERNIA

These indicators apply to men and women age 18 and older.

	Indicator	Quality of Evidence	Literature	Benefits	Comments
Diagnosis					
1.	For a patient < age 65 diagnosed with inguinal hernia, the medical record should document the time duration since the patient first noticed symptoms of hernia.	III	Gallegos et al., 1991	Improve survival by diagnosing newer hernias.	Newer hernias have a higher risk of strangulation and therefore necessitate elective herniorrhaphy.
Treatment					
2.	A patient diagnosed with a strangulated or incarcerated inguinal hernia should have emergency groin exploration within 24 hours of presentation.	III	Williams & Hale, 1966	Improve survival.	Strangulation that is present > 60 hours is associated with a 20-fold higher mortality. While we were not able to find a study that examined the optimal time to surgery, surgical sources generally state that under 12 hours is optimal. However, we stipulate 24 hours because it may be practically difficult to ascertain a 24-hour time frame from the medical record.
3.	For a patient < age 65 diagnosed with inguinal hernia appearing within the prior 2 years, the medical record should document that elective herniorrhaphy was offered.	III	Gallegos et al., 1991; Neuhauser, 1977	Improve survival.	It is conservative to use age 65 and a 2-year duration in this indicator. Benefit depends largely on strangulation risk estimated by Gallegos, et al.

Quality of Evidence Codes

I	RCT
II-1	Nonrandomized controlled trials
II-2	Cohort or case analysis
II-3	Multiple time series
III	Opinions or descriptive studies

205

15. LOW BACK PAIN (ACUTE)[1]

Elizabeth A. McGlynn, Ph.D and Kenneth A. Clark, MD, MPH

The principal reference for this review is the Clinical Practice Guideline (Number 14) of the Agency for Health Care Policy and Research (AHCPR), titled Acute Low Back Problems in Adults (Bigos et al., 1994). The 23-member multidisciplinary panel based their findings and recommendations on a systematic review and analysis of the literature, their own expertise, public testimony, peer review, and some pretesting in outpatient settings. Where this reference cited studies to support individual indicators, the original references have been included. In addition, a targeted MEDLINE search of the medical literature from 1985 through 1996 was performed to supplement these references for particular indicators.

IMPORTANCE

Although there are a number of methodological challenges in estimating the prevalence of low back pain (Loeser and Volinn, 1991), studies concur that it is the second leading cause of work absenteeism in the United States (Deyo and Bass, 1989). The lifetime prevalence of low back pain has been estimated to be 60 to 80 percent, and the one year prevalence is 15 to 20 percent (Andersson, 1991). Among the working age population, approximately half report symptoms of back pain during a one-year period (Vallfors, 1985; Sternbach, 1986). Approximately five to ten percent of low back patients experience chronic problems (Lahad et al., 1994), but these individuals account for nearly 60 percent of health care expenditures for low back pain.

There is evidence that many patients with low back pain who cannot perform their usual activities may be receiving care that is either inappropriate or suboptimal (Bigos et al., 1994). The evidence includes

---

[1] This chapter is a revision of one written for an earlier project on quality of care for women and children (Q1). The expert panel for the current project was asked to review all of the indicators, but only rated new or revised indicators.

substantial variations in the rates of hospitalization and surgery for low back problems (Deyo, 1991; Kellett et al., 1991; Volinn et al., 1992) and variations in the use of diagnostic tests (Deyo, 1991). For example, in a study conducted in Washington state, the rate of surgery for low back pain varied 15-fold among the 39 counties in the state (Volinn et al., 1992). The most likely explanation for this variation is differences in physicians' practice styles. A study of the effect of physician practice style on low back patient outcomes found that a low-intensity intervention style characterized by self-care, fewer prescription medications, and less bed rest produced long-term pain relief and functional outcomes that were similar to more intensive styles, while also being less costly and associated with higher levels of patient satisfaction (Von Korff et al., 1994). There are also patients who appear to have more disability after treatment than before, particularly those who have undergone surgery, those treated with extended bed rest, and those treated with longer-term use of high-dose opioids (Bigos et al., 1994).

The lack of consensus on appropriate treatment for low back pain suggests that there is probably considerable variation in practice patterns across the country. The recent promulgation of a clinical practice guideline by the AHCPR offers an opportunity for developing tools to monitor the use of both recommended and nonrecommended practices. This may provide a substantial incentive for decreasing the variation in care and reducing poor quality care.

In 1990, the direct medical costs of low back pain treatment were $24 billion (Lahad, 1994). The costs of work days lost plus disability payments have been estimated to be more than three times the national expenditures on medical treatment, suggesting that the total annual costs of back pain may exceed $100 billion.

The costs of different approaches to treating back pain vary considerably. One study examining the costs and outcomes of three different management styles for back pain found differences in the average one-year costs of treatment ranging from $428 for patients seen by "low-intensity" physicians to $768 for patients seen by "high-intensity" physicians (Von Korff et al., 1994). The difference between the low- and high-intensity management costs was reduced from $340 to $277 when case mix variables were taken into account. Because the lower intensity practice style produced similar outcomes, that style would certainly be judged to be more cost effective.

SCREENING AND PRIMARY PREVENTION

There is no strong evidence to suggest that primary preventive strategies for low back pain are effective. The literature evaluating the effectiveness of four prevention strategies was recently reviewed (Lahad et al., 1994). The strategies included back and aerobic exercises, education, mechanical supports, and risk factor modification. The authors did not examine worksite-specific preventive measures, although all of the prevention studies included in the review were conducted in work settings.

Exercise may offer some protection against the development of back pain. Four randomized trials of exercise interventions have been conducted (Gundewall et al., 1993; Donchin et al., 1990; Kellet et al., 1991; Linton et al., 1989). All four studies were conducted in specific worksites with relatively small study populations ranging from 66 to 142 subjects. None of the studies followed subjects for longer than 18 months. The trials were consistent in their findings that fewer lost work days occurred in the preventive intervention groups as compared with the control groups. Among epidemiological studies, seven found an association between fitness or flexibility and decreased low back pain, but four of these studies showed no protective effect of exercise (Lahad et al., 1994). The authors of the review conclude that, taken together, the studies suggest that exercise is mildly protective (Lahad et al., 1994).

General education does not contribute to preventing low back pain. Five randomized trials of educational interventions have been conducted (Daltroy et al., 1993; Walsh and Schwartz, 1990; Donchin et al., 1990; McCauley, 1990; Linton et al., 1989). As with the exercise studies, these trials also enrolled small numbers of subjects and were conducted in specific work sites. Only one of the randomized trials of educational intervention found a decrease in subsequent low back pain

(Linton et al., 1989); however, this trial also included exercise, which makes it difficult to determine the independent role of education. Among the other four trials, three had intermediate positive outcomes and all four had long-term negative outcomes. The authors conclude that there is minimal support in the literature for the use of educational strategies (Lahad et al., 1994).

The use of orthotic devices has not been shown to prevent low back pain. Two trials examining the use of lumbar corsets for the prevention of low back pain have been conducted (Reddell et al., 1992; Walsh and Schwartz, 1990). One trial had a very low compliance rate for the intervention groups: 58 percent of those assigned to wear a back belt stopped wearing it before the end of the study. Based on an intention-to-treat analysis, the intervention group had a trend toward increased frequency of back pain (Reddell et al., 1992). The other trial found that subjects assigned to an educational intervention plus lumbar corsets had a greater increase in knowledge and decrease in work days lost compared with controls (2.5-day decrease vs. 0.4-day increase). The authors of the review article conclude that, given the contradictory findings in these two trials, there is insufficient evidence to allow for a recommendation to be made regarding the use of orthotic devices for low back pain prevention (Lahad et al., 1994).

Several risk factors have been associated with increased risk of developing low back pain, including smoking, obesity, and psychological functioning. Studies have shown an association between smoking and back pain, indicating that risk is increased by 1.5 to 2.5 times compared with nonsmokers (Deyo and Bass, 1989). Similarly, an association between obesity and back pain has been observed, but no interventions have been conducted to determine the effect of weight reduction on back pain (Deyo and Bass, 1989). The psychological factors include depression, anxiety, and job stress, but no intervention studies of reducing psychological risk factors to prevent back pain have been conducted. The authors of the review article conclude that, while there are other health-related reasons to suggest the importance of interventions to modify these three risk factors, there is no evidence that demonstrates that a reduction in back pain will be the result (Lahad et al., 1994).

As reviewed in this section, there is no strong evidence supporting preventive strategies for acute low back pain. Therefore, screening patients for acute low back pain is not recommended.

DIAGNOSIS

The AHCPR's clinical practice guideline on the assessment and treatment of acute low back problems in adults (Bigos et al., 1994) indicates that the medical history is important in assessing whether the patient is suffering from a serious underlying condition such as cancer or spinal infection. The guideline recommends that the history include questions about age, history of cancer, unexplained weight loss, immunosuppression, duration of symptoms, responsiveness to previous therapy, pain that is worse at rest, history of intravenous drug use, and urinary tract or other infection. Symptoms of leg pain or problems walking due to leg pain may suggest neurological problems such as herniated disc or spinal stenosis. The elements of the suggested medical history along with estimates of the sensitivity and specificity of those elements are provided in the guideline document (Indicator 1). An algorithm is provided for the use of responses to the initial assessment. The guideline panel noted that factors such as work status, educational level, workers compensation issues, and depression may affect patients' responses to questions on the history of their symptoms, and may also influence treatment outcomes (e.g., time for return to work).

Elements of the physical examination such as inspection, palpation, observation, and specialized neuromuscular evaluation are also reviewed in the AHCPR guideline, and estimates of the sensitivity and specificity of each element in making differential diagnoses are provided (Indicator 2). The guideline concludes that for 95 percent of patients with acute low back problems, no special interventions or diagnostic tests are required within the first month of symptoms.

TREATMENT

There are a wide variety of treatments for low back pain that are currently in use. The clinical care methods reviewed by the panel were patient education about symptoms, structured patient education ("back school"), medications to control symptoms, physical treatments to control symptoms, activity modifications, bed rest, exercise, special diagnostic tests, and surgery. A summary of the panel's findings and recommendations regarding each of these treatment approaches follows.

Symptom Education

The panel recommends educating patients about expectations for recovery and recurrence, safe and effective methods of symptom control, reasonable activity modifications, methods for limiting recurrence of symptoms, the appropriate circumstances for special investigations, and the effectiveness and risks of diagnostic and treatment measures if symptoms persist. The panel indicated that such educational interventions may reduce utilization of medical care, decrease patient apprehension, and increase the speed of recovery.

Medications

The panel concluded that both acetaminophen and nonsteroidal anti-inflammatory drugs (NSAIDs) were adequate for achieving pain relief; however, acetaminophen may have fewer side effects than NSAIDs. Muscle relaxants were found to be no better than NSAIDs in relieving low back symptoms, while also having more substantial side effects -- especially drowsiness. Opioids were found to be no more effective than NSAIDs or acetaminophen in providing pain relief, with side effects including decreased reaction time, clouded judgment, drowsiness, and risk of physical dependence. A number of other medications (e.g., oral steroids, colchicine, antidepressants) were not recommended for the treatment of low back pain (Indicator 3).

Physical Treatments

Spinal manipulation for patients without radiculopathy is effective in reducing pain and may speed recovery within the first month. The evidence after one month is inconclusive. Transcutaneous electrical nerve stimulation, lumbar corsets and support belts, shoe lifts and supports, spinal traction, biofeedback, trigger point injections, ligamentous and sclerosant injections, facet joint injections, epidural injections, and acupuncture were not recommended for the treatment of acute back pain (Indicator 4). For patients with radiculopathy, epidural steroid injections were considered an option after failure of conservative treatment and as a means of avoiding surgery.

Activity Modifications

The panel recommended that patients with acute low back problems temporarily limit heavy lifting, prolonged sitting, and bending or twisting the spine. The activity limitations should take into account the age and clinical status of the patient as well as the demands of the patient's job. These modifications should be considered time-limited, which can be emphasized by setting goals for a timely return to normal activity.

Bed Rest

Prolonged bed rest (i.e., more than 4 days) was not recommended because it may increase rather than decrease debilitation (Indicator 5). The panel recommended a gradual return to normal activities and bed rest of short duration only for patients with severe initial symptoms of primary leg pain. A recently published randomized controlled trial found that continuing ordinary activities within the limits permitted by pain led to more rapid recovery than either bed rest or back-mobilizing exercises (Malmivaara et al., 1995).

Exercise

The panel recommended that the initial goal of exercise programs be to prevent debilitation due to inactivity, and then to increase activity tolerance with the goal of returning patients to their highest level of functioning. Exercise programs designed to improve general endurance (aerobic fitness) and muscular strength of the back and abdomen were considered particularly beneficial.

Special Diagnostic Tests

For patients whose symptoms persist longer than one month, in spite of the above-listed recommended treatments, additional diagnostic and treatment procedures may be considered. The tests are of two types: tests for evidence of physiologic dysfunction, and tests for evidence of anatomic dysfunction. Tests in the former category include electromyography, sensory evoked potentials, thermography, general laboratory screening tests, and bone scan. The appropriate indications for and timing of these tests are provided in the guideline document. Tests in the latter category include plain myelography, magnetic resonance imaging, computed tomography (CT), CT-myelography, discography, and CT-discography. These tests must be combined with information from the medical history, physical examination, and/or physiologic tests because the results can be difficult to interpret and many symptomatic patients may not show defects.

Surgery

Lumbar discectomy may provide faster pain relief in patients with severe and disabling leg symptoms who have failed to improve after one to two months of adequate nonsurgical treatment. However, there is little difference in long-term (4-10 years) outcomes of discectomy as compared with conservative care, and the procedure is quite expensive. Among methods of discectomy, direct methods of nerve root decompression were recommended over indirect methods. The role of patient preferences was emphasized, but only if adequate information about efficacy, risks, and expectations is presented.

Surgery for spinal stenosis was not recommended within the first three months of symptoms. Decisions about this surgery should take into account the patient's lifestyle, preferences, other medical problems, and the risks associated with surgery.

Spinal fusion was not recommended during the first three months of symptoms in the absence of fracture, dislocation, or complications of tumor or infection. Spinal fusion was recommended for consideration after decompression in patients with combined degenerative spondylolisthesis, stenosis, and radiculopathy. Patients under age 30 with significant spondylolisthesis and severe leg pain may also be considered candidates for spinal fusion.

FOLLOW-UP

There are no clear indications for routine follow-up of acute low back pain.

REFERENCES

Alcoff J, E Jones, P Rust, et al. 1982. Controlled trial of imipramine for chronic low back pain. *Journal of Family Practice* 14 (5): 841-6.

Andersson GBJ. 1991. The epidemiology of spinal disorders. In *The Adult Spine: Principles and Practice*. Editor Frymoyer JW, 107-46. New York, NY: Raven Press, Ltd.

Bigos S, Bowyer O, Braen G, et al. December 1994. *Acute Low Back Problems in Adults: Clinical Practice Guideline No. 14*. Agency for Health Care Policy and Research, U.S. Public Health Service, Department of Health and Human Services, Rockville, MD.

Coxhead CE, H Inskip, TW Meade, et al. 16 May 1981. Multicentre trial of physiotherapy in the management of sciatic symptoms. *Lancet* 8229: 1065-8.

Daltroy LH, MD Iversen, MG Larson, et al. March 1993. Teaching and social support: Effects on knowledge, attitudes, and behaviors to prevent low back injuries in industry. *Health Education Quarterly* 20 (1): 43-62.

Deyo RA. October 1991. Nonsurgical care of low back pain. *Neurosurgery Clinics of North America* 2 (4): 851-62.

Deyo RA, and AK Diehl. May 1988. Cancer as a cause of back pain: Frequency, clinical presentation, and diagnostic strategies. *Journal of General Internal Medicine* 3: 230-8.

Deyo RA, AK Diehl, and M Rosenthal. 23 October 1986. How many days of bed rest for acute low back pain? A randomized clinical trial. *New England Journal of Medicine* 315 (17): 1064-1070.

Deyo RA, J Rainville, and DL Kent. 12 August 1992. What can the history and physical examination tell us about low back pain? *Journal of the American Medical Association* 268 (6): 760-5.

Deyo RA, JD Loeser, and SJ Bigos. 15 April 1990. Herniated lumbar intervertebral disk. *Archives of Internal Medicine* 112 (8): 598-603.

Deyo RA, and JE Bass. 1989. Lifestyle and low-back pain: The influence of smoking and obesity. *Spine* 14 (5): 501-6.

Donchin M, O Woolf, L Kaplan, et al. 1990. Secondary prevention of low-back pain: A clinical trial. *Spine* 15 (12): 1317-20.

Evans C, JR Gilbert, W Taylor, et al. March 1987. A randomized controlled trial of flexion exercises, education, and bed rest for patients with acute low back pain. *Physiotherapy Canada* 39 (2): 96-101.

Gemignani G, I Olivieri, G Ruju, et al. June 1991. Transcutaneous electrical nerve stimulation in ankylosing spondylitis: A double-blind study. *Arthritis and Rheumatism* 34 (6): 788-9.

Gilbert JR, DW Taylor, A Heldebrand, et al. 21 September 1985. Clinical trial of common treatments for low back pain in family practice. *British Medical Journal* 291: 791-6.

Goodkin K, CM Gullion, and WS Agras. August 1990. A randomized, double-blind, placebo-controlled trial of trazodone hydrochloride in chronic low back pain syndrome. *Journal of Clinical Psychopharmacology* 10 (4): 269-78.

Graff-Radford SB, JL Reeves, RL Baker, et al. 1989. Effects of transcutaneous electrical nerve stimulation on myofascial pain and trigger point sensitivity. *Pain* 37: 1-5.

Gundewall B, M Liljeqvist, and T Hansson. 1993. Primary prevention of back symptoms and absence from work. *Spine* 18 (5): 587-94.

Hackett GI, D Seddon, and D Kaminski. February 1988. Electroacupuncture compared with paracetamol for acute low back pain. *The Practitioner* 232: 163-4.

Haimovic IC, and HR Beresford. December 1986. Dexamethasone is not superior to placebo for treating lumbosacral radicular pain. *Neurology* 36: 1593-4.

Jenkins DG, AF Ebbutt, and CD Evans. 1976. Tofranil in the treatment of low back pain. *Journal of International Medical Research* 4 (Suppl. 2): 28-40.

Kellett KM, DA Kellett, and LA Nordholm. April 1991. Effects of an exercise program on sick leave due to back pain. *Physical Therapy* 71 (4): 283-93.

Lahad A, AD Malter, AO Berg, et al. 26 October 1994. The effectiveness of four interventions for the prevention of low back pain. *Journal of the American Medical Association* 272 (16): 1286-91.

Larsson U, U Choler, A Lidstrom, et al. 1980. Auto-traction for treatment of lumbago-sciatica: A multicenter controlled investigation. *Acta Orthopaedica Scandinavica* 51: 791-8.

Lehmann TR, DW Russell, KF Spratt, et al. 1986. Efficacy of electroacupuncture and TENS in the rehabilitation of chronic low back pain patients. *Pain* 26: 277-90.

Lehmann TR, DW Russell, and KF Spratt. 1983. The impact of patients with nonorganic physical findings on a controlled trial of transcutaneous electrical nerve stimulation and electroacupuncture. *Spine* 8 (6): 625-34.

Linton SJ, LA Bradley, I Jensen, et al. 1989. The secondary prevention of low back pain: A controlled study with follow-up. *Pain* 36: 197-207.

Loeser JD, and E Volinn. October 1991. Epidemiology of low back pain. *Neurosurgery Clinics of North America* 2 (4): 713-8.

Malmivaara A, U Hakkinen, T Aro, et al. 9 February 1995. The treatment of acute low back pain--bed rest, exercises or ordinary activity? *New England Journal of Medicine* 332 (6): 351-5.

Mathews JA, and J Hickling. 1975. Lumbar traction: A double-blind controlled study for sciatica. *Rheumatology and Rehabilitation* 14: 222-5.

Mathews W, M Morkel, and J Mathews. 1988. Manipulation and traction for lumbago and sciatica: Physiotherapeutic techniques used in two controlled trials. *Physiotherapy Practice* 4: 201-6.

Mathews JA, SB Mills, VM Jenkins, et al. 1987. Back pain and sciatica: Controlled trials of manipulation, traction, sclerosant and epidural injections. *British Journal of Rheumatology* 26: 416-23.

McCauley M. May 1990. The effect of body mechanics instruction on work performance among young workers. *American Journal of Occupational Therapy* 44 (5): 402-7.

Meek JB, VW Guidice, JW McFadden, et al. October 1985. Colchicine confirmed as highly effective in disk disorders: Final results of a double-blind study. *Journal of Neurological and Orthopaedic Medicine and Surgery* 6 (3): 211-8.

Melzack R, P Vetere, and L Finch. April 1983. Transcutaneous electrical nerve stimulation for low back pain: A comparison of TENS and massage for pain and range of motion. *Physical Therapy* 63 (4): 489-93.

Million R, K Haavik Nilsen, MIV Jayson, et al. 1981. Evaluation of low back pain and assessment of lumbar corsets with and without back supports. *Annals of the Rheumatic Diseases* 40: 449-54.

Pal B, P Mangion, MA Hossain, et al. 1986. A controlled trial of continuous lumbar traction in the treatment of back pain and sciatica. *British Journal of Rheumatology* 25 (2): 181-3.

Postacchini F, M Facchini, and P Palieri. 1988. Efficacy of various forms of conservative treatment in low back pain: A comparative study. *Neuro-Orthopedics* 6: 28-35.

Reddell CR, JJ Congleton, RD Huchingson, et al. 1992. An evaluation of a weightlifting belt and back injury prevention training class for airline baggage handlers. *Applied Ergonomics* 23 (5): 319-29.

Schnebel BE, and JW Simmons. 1988. The use of oral colchicine for low-back pain: A double-blind study. *Spine* 13 (3): 354-7.

Simmons JW, WP Harris, CW Koulisis, et al. July 1990. Intravenous colchicine for low-back pain: A double-blind study. *Spine* 15 (7): 716-7.

Spengler DM, SJ Bigos, NA Martin, et al. 1986. Back injuries in industry: A retrospective study. I. Overview and cost analysis. *Spine* 11 (3): 241-5.

Sternbach RA. 1986. Pain and 'hassles' in the United States: Findings of the Nuprin Pain Report. *Pain* 27: 69-80.

Thorsteinsson G, HH Stonnington, GK Stillwell, et al. January 1977. Transcutaneous electrical stimulation: A double-blind trial of its efficacy for pain. *Archives of Physical Medicine and Rehabilitation* 58: 8-12.

Thorsteinsson G, HH Stonnington, GK Stillwell, et al. 1978. The placebo effect of transcutaneous electrical stimulation. *Pain* 5: 31-41.

Vallfors B. 1985. Acute, Subacute and Chronic Low Back Pain: Clinical Symptoms, Absenteeism and Working Environment. Goteborg, Sweden: Kompendietryckeriat-Kallered.

Volinn E, J Mayer, P Diehr, et al. 1992. Small area analysis of surgery for low-back pain. *Spine* 17 (5): 575-9.

Von Korff M, W Barlow, D Cherkin, et al. 1 August 1994. Effects of practice style in managing back pain. *Annals of Internal Medicine* 121 (3): 187-95.

Waddell G, CJ Main, EW Morris, et al. 22 May 1982. Normality and reliability in the clinical assessment of backache. *British Medical Journal* 284: 1519-23.

Walsh NE, and RK Schwartz. October 1990. The influence of prophylactic orthoses on abdominal strength and low back injury in the workplace. *American Journal of Physical Medicine and Rehabilitation* 69 (5): 245-50.

Weber H, AE Ljunggren, and L Walker. 1984. Traction therapy in patients with herniated lumbar intervertebral discs. *Journal of the Oslo City Hospitals* 34: 61-70.

RECOMMENDED QUALITY INDICATORS FOR LOW BACK PAIN (ACUTE)

These indicators apply to men and women age 18 and older. These indicators were not rated by this panel but were endorsed by a prior panel.

Diagnosis

Indicator	Quality of Evidence	Literature	Benefits	Comments
1. Patients presenting with acute low back pain should receive a focused medical history and physical examination. The history should include questions about "red flags" in at least one of the following areas:	III	Bigos et al., 1994; Deyo et al., 1992; Waddell et al., 1982	Prevent disability and potential premature mortality.	A thorough exam and history will increase the likelihood of identifying serious systemic disease that requires further testing and specialized treatment.
• Spine fracture: trauma, prolonged use of steroids;	III	Deyo et al., 1992; Waddell et al., 1982	Prevent debilitation. Reduce pain.	Plain film, CT, or MRI of the spine is recommended if spine fracture is suspected. Approximately 4% of patients in primary care will prove to have a spine fracture.
• Cancer: history of cancer, unexplained weight loss, immunosuppression;	III	Deyo et al., 1992; Waddell et al., 1982; Deyo and Diehl, 1988	Prevent debilitation. Reduce pain.	CT or MRI is recommended if cancer is suspected. Approximately 0.7% of patients presenting for acute low back pain have primary or metastatic bone cancer, which may be appropriately treated with radiation therapy.
• Infection: fever, IV drug use;	III	Deyo et al., 1992; Waddell et al., 1982	Prevent debilitation. Reduce pain.	Urinalysis recommended if infection is suspected. Approximately 0.01% of patients in primary care will prove to have an infection (e.g., urinary tract infection, skin infection), which may lead to epidermal abscess.
• "Red flags" for cauda equina syndrome (CES) or rapidly progressing neurologic deficit are: acute onset of urinary retention or overflow incontinence, loss of anal sphincter tone or fecal incontinence, saddle anesthesia, and global progressive motor weakness in the lower limbs.	III	Deyo et al., 1992; Waddell et al., 1982	Prevent permanent neurologic deficit. Reduce pain.	CT or MRI recommended if CES or neurologic deficit is suspected. Approximate prevalence of CES among patients with low back pain is 0.0004. A diagnosis of CES requires immediate surgery (or radiation therapy).

Indicator	Quality of Evidence	Literature	Benefits	Comments
2. For patients presenting with acute low back pain, the physical examination should include neurologic screening and straight leg raising.	III	Deyo et al., 1992; Waddell et al., 1982.	Prevent debilitation.	Neurologic screening includes ankle and knee reflexes, ankle and great toe dorsiflexion strength, and distribution of sensory complaints. These examination procedures are undertaken to identify lumbar disk herniations and facilitate appropriate course of treatment (e.g., NSAIDs, brief bed rest, surgery). Surgery is indicated in approximately 2-10% of patients. Multiple findings increase the likelihood that a herniated disk will be found at surgery.

Treatment

Indicator	Quality of Evidence	Literature	Benefits	Comments
3. Patients should NOT be taking any of the following medications for treatment of acute low back pain:				
a. Phenylbutazone;	III	Bigos et al., 1994.	Avoid aplastic anemia and agranulocytosis.	Increased risk for bone marrow suppression.
b. Dexamethasone;	I	Haimovic and Beresford, 1986.	Prevent side effects and complications.[1]	Effectiveness for pain relief has not been demonstrated.
c. Other oral steroids;	III	Bigos et al., 1994.	Prevent side effects and complications.[1]	Effectiveness for pain relief has not been demonstrated.
d. Colchicine;	I	Meek et al., 1985; Schnebel and Simmons, 1988; Simmons et al., 1990.	Prevent side effects such as gastro-intestinal irritation, chemical cellulitis from intravenous infiltration, skin problems, and bone marrow suppression.	Evidence on pain relief for persons with gout is conflicting.
e. Antidepressants.	I	Alcoff et al., 1982; Goodkin et al., 1990; Jenkins et al., 1976.	Prevent side effects such as urinary retention, ortho-static hypotension, constipation, and mania.	No studies have been done in patients with acute low back pain, and no significant differences have been found in studies of chronic low back pain.

Indicator	Quality of Evidence	Literature	Benefits	Comments
4. Patients should NOT be prescribed the following physical treatments for acute low back pain:				
a. Transcutaneous electrical nerve stimulation (TENS);	I	Melzack et al., 1983; Deyo et al., 1990; Gemignani et al., 1991; Graff-Radford et al., 1989; Hackett et al., 1988; Lehmann et al., 1983; Lehmann et al., 1986; Thorsteinsson et al., 1977; Thorsteinsson et al., 1978	Decrease time to recovery (benefits are inconclusive but the risks are low).	Evidence on effectiveness is inconclusive. Use of an ineffective treatment may delay recovery if more effective treatments are foregone.
b. Lumbar corsets and support belts;	I	Coxhead et al., 1981; Reddell et al., 1992; Walsh and Schwartz, 1990; Million et al., 1981	Decrease time to recovery.	No evidence of efficacy in patients with acute low back pain. Use of an ineffective treatment may delay recovery if more effective treatments are foregone.
c. Spinal traction.	I	Coxhead et al., 1981; Mathews et al., 1987; Mathews et al., 1988; Larsson et al., 1980; Mathews and Hickling, 1975; Pal et al., 1986; Weber et al., 1984	Prevent debilitation.	Prolonged traction may lead to debilitation.
5. Prolonged bed rest (> 4 days) should NOT be recommended for patients with acute low back pain.	I	Evans et al., 1987; Postacchini et al., 1988; Deyo et al., 1986; Gilbert et al., 1985	Prevent debilitation.	Evidence suggests that prolonged bed rest may lead to debilitation.

223

Definitions and Examples

[1] Side effects from long-term use include fluid and electrolyte disturbance, hyperglycemia, pituitary-adrenal function, demineralization of bone, and immunosuppression. High-dose complications include avascular necrosis of bone, myopathy, subcapsular cataract formation, and central nervous system disturbance.

Quality of Evidence Codes

I	RCT
II-1	Nonrandomized controlled trials
II-2	Cohort or case analysis
II-3	Multiple time series
III	Opinions or descriptive studies

16. ORTHOPEDIC CONDITIONS

Allison L. Diamant, MD, MSPH

The development of quality indicators for orthopedic conditions began with a MEDLINE search of the English language literature from 1985 to the present using subject headings for knee pain, shoulder pain, and various joint-specific disorders. Additional review articles and clinical trials were identified by reviewing the reference sections of articles previously identified.

Patients presenting with acute and subacute orthopedic complaints comprise a large proportion of all ambulatory care visits to primary care providers (Barker, 1991). The most common disorders not related to the back or neck involve the knee and the shoulder. This chapter provides an overview of important conditions for patients presenting with knee and shoulder complaints, including diagnosis, treatment, and follow-up. We have concentrated on the most common causes of acute or subacute knee and shoulder complaints. For that reason, screening, diagnosis, and treatment for osteoporosis, rheumatoid arthritis, or any of the crystalline-induced arthropathies will not be addressed in this chapter.

SHOULDER: OVERALL

IMPORTANCE

Shoulder discomfort is the third most common reason for visits to primary care physicians in ambulatory practice (Smith and Campbell, 1992) and is responsible for significant medical costs and time lost from work. The more common shoulder syndromes include subacromial bursitis/ supraspinatus tendinitis (i.e., impingement syndrome), bicipital tendinitis, supraspinatus tendon tear or rupture, adhesive capsulitis, and acromioclavicular joint osteoarthritis. Smith and Campbell (1992) estimated the prevalence of shoulder disorders based on a combination of three reports with a total of 160 patients who presented with shoulder complaints (see Table 16.1).

Table 16.1

Estimated Prevalence of Shoulder Disorders

Subacromial bursitis/supraspinatus tendinitis	60%
Bicipital tendinitis	4%
Supraspinatus tendon tear or rupture	10%
Adhesive shoulder capsulitis	12%
Acromioclavicular joint osteoarthritis	7%
Other/unclear	7%

Source: Smith and Campbell, 1992

SCREENING

There are no screening recommendations for shoulder disorders or shoulder pain.

DIAGNOSIS

Experts recommend the initial evaluation of a patient with a shoulder complaint should begin with a thorough history of the problem, including descriptions of each of the following: duration; onset (i.e., acute vs. chronic); activity or mechanism at the time of onset; activities that alleviate or exacerbate the condition; patient's age; past history of trauma or injury; past history of shoulder/arm surgery; therapeutic interventions attempted; and other medical conditions, especially diabetes mellitus, thyroid disease, coronary artery disease, alcohol abuse, and use of corticosteroids (Sigman, 1995; Smith, 1992) (Indicator 1).

Experts also recommend that the physical examination include the following diagnostic maneuvers: observation for anatomic abnormalities, range of motion testing (both passive and active), palpation, and neurologic and vascular evaluation (Sigman, 1995; Snyder, 1993) (Indicator 2). In addition, particular diagnostic maneuvers exist which help to focus the diagnostic possibilities. Many authors consider plain x-rays an essential part of the shoulder evaluation, but no RCTs exist to support this diagnostic strategy (Sigman, 1995; Snyder, 1993).

TREATMENT

Treatment modalities for shoulder disorders focus on relieving symptoms and returning the patient to an acceptable level of physical activity. The primary form of medical management for the conditions discussed in this chapter involves decreasing the inflammatory response through the use of various anti-inflammatory agents (White et al., 1986; Petri et al., 1987; Adebajo et al., 1990; Van der Heijden et al., 1996; Itzkowitch et al., 1996; Blair et al., 1996), in conjunction with physical therapy modalities. In some cases, surgical intervention may be necessary to repair damaged structures or to alleviate pain.

FOLLOW-UP

No studies were identified that support specific follow-up regimens for shoulder complaints. While follow-up is clearly important, we have recommended no quality indicators in this area for that reason.

IMPINGEMENT SYNDROME: SUBACROMIAL BURSITIS/SUPRASPINATUS TENDINITIS

IMPORTANCE

The impingement syndrome represents the most commonly diagnosed shoulder disorder (Smith and Campbell, 1992). It is characterized by recurrent or chronic shoulder pain brought on by repetitive trauma or vigorous overhead activities. Subacromial bursitis and supraspinatus tendinitis are grouped together in the diagnosis of impingement syndrome, because their physical findings may be difficult to differentiate.

DIAGNOSIS

Patients may present with complaints of acute (within hours or days) or more progressive (weeks to months) dull pain over the deltoid area, with radiation down the lateral aspect of the arm. In the orthopedic literature (Shapiro and Finerman, 1992; Smith and Campbell, 1992) a standard x-ray series of four views is commonly recommended to assess the presence of anatomic abnormalities as the etiology of the inflammation when evaluating a patient for impingement or rotator cuff

227

problems. However, no studies exist to support this diagnostic course of action.

TREATMENT

The principles of rehabilitation are to restore function and allow initial healing of inflamed tissue. The effectiveness of various antiinflammatory agents for treating impingement syndrome has been demonstrated in a number of RCTs (White et al., 1986; Petri et al., 1987; Adebajo et al., 1990; Itzkowitch et al., 1996). The goal of treatment is to reduce the inflammatory changes through the use of antiinflammatory agents, and the avoidance of repetitive and aggravating activities (Indicator 3). When the inflammatory changes are reduced or reversed, experts recommend range of motion exercises, either as formal physical therapy or through a home exercise program (Fu et al.,1991) (Indicator 4).

ROTATOR CUFF (SUPRASPINATUS TENDON) TEAR OR RUPTURE

IMPORTANCE

A rotator cuff tear or rupture results from two main etiologic mechanisms. In patients over age 50, decreased blood flow to the muscle may lead to degeneration and subsequent rupture. In younger patients, the most common causes of damage are repetitive use, overuse, and trauma.

DIAGNOSIS

It is difficult to differentiate a small supraspinatus tear from supraspinatus tendinitis or subacromial bursitis (i.e., impingement syndrome) on physical examination, but arm weakness is identifiable in the presence of a large rotator cuff tear or rupture. The drop arm sign is the accepted diagnostic maneuver when evaluating a patient for rotator cuff pathology. However, no study has prospectively assessed the usefulness or predictive value of the drop arm sign, motion weakness, or impaired abduction against resistance (Smith and Campbell, 1992). Magnetic resonance imaging (MRI) is performed if there is a question regarding the etiology of a shoulder disorder, but MRI is not required to make the diagnosis of a rotator cuff tear. Arthrography was previously the gold standard for rotator cuff imaging, but has been replaced by MRI where available (Snyder, 1993). In diagnosing rotator cuff tear, the sensitivity and specificity of MRI are 92 percent and 88-to-100 percent, respectively; for arthography, sensitivity is 92 percent and specificity is 98 percent. The sensitivity and specificity of ultrasound are only 63 percent and 50 percent, respectively (Snyder, 1993).

TREATMENT

Smith and Campbell (1992) suggest that the data support treatment with intraarticular steroids for small supraspinatus tendon tears, as none of the steroid injection trials revealed any deleterious effects. However, in a systematic review of randomized trials assessing the efficacy of intraarticular corticosteroid injections for shoulder disorders, Van der Heijden et al. (1996) concluded that evidence is scarce for supporting this treatment modality in small rotator cuff tears. Treatment of medium or large full-thickness tears requires early operative repair, as this has been shown to improve functional outcomes and decrease pain (Smith and Campbell, 1992; Adebajo et al., 1990; Levy, 1990) (Indicator 5). Recuperation may take six to nine months, during which recuperative passive shoulder exercises should be initiated early under orthopedic supervision and physical therapy guidance.

ADHESIVE CAPSULITIS

IMPORTANCE

Adhesive capsulitis is also known as frozen shoulder, periarthritis, and pericapsulitis. The incidence of this disorder in the general population is about two to five percent. It is more prevalent among diabetics (10-20%) than nondiabetics. Adhesive capsulitis affects women more than men, and commonly develops during middle age. An individual's nondominant shoulder is more likely to be involved, and approximately 12 percent of patients develop the condition bilaterally. Prophylactic measures for at-risk individuals include avoiding unnecessary immobilization of the shoulder joint, and range of motion exercises (Grubbs, 1993).

DIAGNOSIS

Symptoms of adhesive capsulitis frequently progress over several months. Early physical findings include lateral and anterior glenohumeral joint capsule tenderness, muscle spasms (usually in the scapular, pectoralis, and deltoid areas) as well as more diffuse pain (Smith and Campbell, 1992). Radiography rules out other shoulder conditions in adhesive capsulitis. Plain x-rays of the affected shoulder may be normal, or they may reveal calcium deposits, degenerative changes, diminished subacromial space, and osteoporotic or cystic changes.

TREATMENT

The goal of treatment is to alleviate pain and restore normal shoulder function. There are many treatments reported in the literature; however, the natural history of this condition is poorly understood, and no clinical studies have prospectively evaluated treatment outcomes. Nonsteroidal anti-inflammatory drugs (NSAIDs) and injectable corticosteroids are frequently used for the treatment of adhesive capsulitis (Smith and Campbell, 1992). Although intraarticular corticosteroid injection reportedly reverses the pain and fibrosis associated with adhesive capsulitis, it has not been shown to improve the rate at which function is restored to the shoulder (Grubbs, 1993). The use of exercises for treatment of this disorder has been associated with improved outcomes in observational trials (Grubbs, 1993) (Indicator 6).

BICIPITAL TENDINITIS

DIAGNOSIS

Anterior shoulder pain over the bicipital tendon, particularly with contraction of the biceps muscle, is the most prominent symptom of bicipital tendinitis. Inspection, rotation, and abduction of the shoulder are normal, but palpation of the bicipital tendon with elbow flexion causes exquisite tenderness.

TREATMENT

Optimal medical management for bicipital tendinitis has been difficult to determine because its natural course is unknown. In addition, it may be difficult to assess the response to treatment for bicipital tendinitis in the presence of co-existing subacromial bursitis and/or supraspinatus tendinitis. Patients are advised to avoid activities that provoke or aggravate shoulder pain. No studies have focused on the medical management of isolated bicipital tendinitis (Smith and Campbell, 1992). Non-surgical treatment includes the use of antiinflammatory medications including NSAIDs and local corticosteroid injections, to reduce the inflammatory response and improve normal shoulder function. Patients may be instructed to perform gentle range of motion exercises (e.g., "the pendulum") to avoid adhesive capsulitis and maintain range of motion (Indicator 8).

KNEE: OVERALL

IMPORTANCE

Knee disorders account for the most common orthopedic complaints among patients visiting primary care physicians. The major disorders that affect the knee are: meniscal injury; ligamentous injury (especially anterior cruciate and posterior cruciate ligaments); patellofemoral pain syndrome; osteoarthritis; inflammatory disorders/collagen vascular disease (i.e., gout, pseudogout, sarcoid, infection); and pain referred from the hip or back (Smith and Green, 1995). We cover four major acute knee syndromes: meniscal damage, cruciate and collateral ligament injuries, patellar instability, and septic arthritis.

SCREENING

There are no current recommendations on screening for knee pain or dysfunction.

DIAGNOSIS

Orthopedic expert opinion supports a detailed history and physical examination in making an accurate diagnosis for patients presenting with complaints of knee pain (Smith and Green, 1995; Litman, 1996; Neuschwander et al., 1996). The history should include the patient's age; duration of pain; onset of the disorder (i.e., recent vs. chronic); mechanism of injury; exacerbating and relieving factors; location of pain; functional disability; past history of injury or trauma; past history of surgery; evidence of swelling; time of onset; a sense of locking, popping, or catching; pain, weakness, or redness at the knee joint; medical conditions; and health behaviors such as smoking, alcohol use, recreational drug use, diet, and exercise (Smith and Green, 1995) (Indicator 7). The physical examination should include an assessment of all of the following: range of motion, palpation of the joint lines for evidence of tenderness, ligamentous stability, cartilaginous integrity, patellar irritability, and presence of effusions (Smith and Green, 1995; Davidson, 1993; Towheed and Hochberg, 1996). Maneuvers specific for particular knee disorders are also included in the physical exam. Lachman's test has a very high sensitivity and specificity for ACL tears. The pivot shift test also has a high sensitivity and specificity but may be difficult to perform due to patient discomfort. McMurray's test is the most sensitive and specific maneuver for meniscal tears. The posterior drawer test has the highest sensitivity for PCL tears (Indicator 8). Smith and Green (1995) advocate examining the uninjured knee first as a comparison prior to assessing the injured joint. The knee should be examined as soon after the injury as possible, before pain and swelling develop.

In the past, obtaining radiographic studies as part of the clinical work-up of a patient with a knee injury was generally accepted, although no data supported this process. Recently, physicians at the University of Ottawa developed and prospectively validated a set of guidelines for the use of radiography in the evaluation of acute knee injuries (Stiell et al., 1993, 1996), which are as follows:

The Ottawa Knee Rules - A knee x-ray is required only when acute knee injury is accompanied by one or more of the following findings related to age, tenderness, or function:

- Inability to bear weight for four steps both immediately after injury and in the emergency department (i.e., unable to transfer weight twice onto each lower limb);
- Age 55 years or older;
- Tenderness at the head of the fibula;
- Isolated tenderness of the patella (i.e., no bone tenderness of the knee other than the patella);
- Inability to flex to 90 degrees.

These guidelines have a sensitivity of 1.0 (95% CI 0.94-1.0), but a specificity of only 0.49 (95% CI 0.46-0.52) for clinically important knee fractures (Stiell et al., 1996). A clinically important fracture is defined as any bone fragment at least five millimeters in breadth or any avulsion fracture, regardless of size, that is associated with complete disruption of tendons or ligaments. These guidelines were written to discourage use of x-rays to evaulate knee pain and not necessarily to dictate when x-rays should be obtained. Thus, we have not written any indicator regarding use of x-rays.

TREATMENT

Initial treatment for acute soft tissue injuries should include rest, ice, compression, and elevation for the first 24 to 72 hours. Use of NSAIDs to reduce the inflammation is also indicated (Altchek, 1993; Smith et al., 1995). Treatment decisions are based on a number of variables including age, chronicity of symptoms, activity level, and the presence and characteristics of associated ligamentous and meniscal injuries.

FOLLOW-UP

No studies from the literature that support specific follow-up regimens for knee complaints were identified. While follow-up is clearly important, we have recommended no quality indicators in this area for that reason.

MENISCAL INJURIES

IMPORTANCE

Meniscal injuries are the most common reason for arthroscopy of the knee (Swenson and Harner, 1995). Injury to the menisci may be traumatic or degenerative. The medial meniscus is more commonly damaged than the lateral meniscus.

DIAGNOSIS

Maneuvers that can be performed to assist in diagnosing a meniscal injury include the bounce test, McMurray's test, and Apley's grind test; however none of these tests is 100 percent sensitive or specific (Indicator 8). MRIs have superseded arthroscopy as the most common diagnostic test (Smith and Green, 1995; Stone and Fu, 1997).

TREATMENT

There are no standard indications for surgical repair of isolated meniscal damage. Treatment in the acute phase relies on decreasing knee swelling through the use of ice and anti-inflammatory agents, although no specific studies address their utility. With the resolution of pain and swelling, patients are encouraged to participate in physical therapy that focuses on strengthening the flexors and extensors of the thigh.

LIGAMENTOUS INJURIES

IMPORTANCE

Injury to the anterior cruciate ligament (ACL) occurs most commonly. The posterior cruciate ligament (PCL) is injured less frequently than the ACL, and only accounts for 15 to 20 percent of all knee ligament injuries. Injuries to the PCL usually occur as a result of direct anterior trauma, often from athletic activities and motor vehicle accidents. The medial collateral ligament (MCL) and lateral collateral ligament (LCL) may also sustain injury, either isolated or in conjunction with other ligamentous or meniscal injuries.

DIAGNOSIS

Patients who damage their ACL may describe their knee as having "given out" or "buckled," and frequently report having noticed a popping sound at the time of injury. Swelling that occurs within a few hours is usually indicative of a hemarthrosis, and develops in 70 to 75 percent of cases. Three maneuvers exist that focus on evaluating the integrity of the ACL: the anterior drawer test, Lachman's test, and the pivot-shift test (Smith and Green, 1995; Katz and Fingeroth, 1986) (Indicator 8). In order to determine the sensitivity and specificity of these three tests in making the diagnosis of ACL damage, Katz and Fingeroth (1986) performed a retrospective study that compared findings from physical examination with those from arthroscopy performed within two weeks of the initial injury. All three tests had a specificity greater than 95 percent. The sensitivity of the pivot shift test was 89 percent, Lachman's test was 78 percent sensitive and the anterior drawer test was only 22 percent sensitive for ACL damage. Katz and Fingeroth concluded that when Lachman's test and the pivot-shift test are positive a correct diagnosis of an ACL tear can be made, and that when these tests are negative a medium or large ACL tear can be ruled out (Katz and Fingeroth, 1986). Because the pivot shift test is very painful to the patient, Lachman's test is the test of choice for evaluating ACL damage.

Injury to the PCL should be considered if a patient has suffered direct trauma to the anterior aspect of the knee. Diagnostic maneuvers that should be performed during the physical examination include the posterior drawer test and the posterior tibial sag test (Swenson and Harner, 1995) (Indicator 8). In a blinded RCT, the posterior drawer test was found to have a sensitivity of 90 percent and a specificity of 99 percent for isolated PCL injuries (Rubinstein et al., 1994). Identification of other ligamentous or meniscal injuries is important, because the treatment options differ if an isolated -- as opposed to combined -- PCL injury is present. Damage to the LCL usually occurs as a result of trauma to the medial aspect of the knee, or a twisting motion with a fixed foot. These injuries are less common but more severe than MCL damage, and are rarely isolated.

In order to evaluate and diagnose MCL injury or laxity, a valgus stress is applied to the knee. Injuries to the MCL are graded on the extent of laxity present.

TREATMENT

The goal of treatment for a patient with an ACL injury is to avoid re-injury that may lead to long-term complications. Deciding on the course of treatment depends on a number of factors, such as age, prior recreational and occupational activity levels, future expectations, ability and willingness to participate in a physical therapy program, degree of ligamentous laxity, and the presence of associated meniscal or ligamentous lesions (Swenson and Harner, 1995). In a prospective study, the factor that most strongly predicted whether a patient underwent reconstructive surgery was activity level prior to the injury (Johnson and Warner, 1993). Surgical repair for ACL injuries may be performed acutely (i.e., within 3 to 4 weeks) if necessary, but this may increase the risk for decreased loss of flexion, extension, or both, due to swelling, inflammation, and stiffness (Johnson and Warner, 1993; Swenson and Harner, 1995). No prospective studies have been performed comparing surgical and nonsurgical interventions, but patients should be referred for orthopedic evaluation at the time of diagnosis (Indicator 12). Nonsurgical interventions focus on quadriceps strengthening, proprioceptive exercises, and functional training. Surgical reconstruction of a torn PCL is usually reserved for situations in which there are combined ligament injuries, or when a patient is symptomatic from the damaged PCL (Swenson and Harner, 1995; Rubinstein et al., 1994).

Surgical intervention within three weeks of the initial injury is considered optimal treatment for injuries to the posterolateral corner of the knee, including the LCL (Swenson and Harner, 1995).

PATELLOFEMORAL PAIN SYNDROME

IMPORTANCE

Patellofemoral pain syndrome is a common diagnosis among people who participate in physical activities, and occurs most frequently among

236

adolescents and young adults. Women tend to have a higher incidence of patellofemoral syndrome than men. This disorder results from the repetitive microtrauma of overuse; either with normal anatomy and alignment, or with mild malalignment of the extensor mechanism.

DIAGNOSIS

The diagnosis of patellofemoral syndrome is usually based on the history and physical examination. Patients usually complain of a dull, aching pain that is peripatellar or retropatellar, occasionally becoming more severe during activities such as ascending or descending stairs, or with squatting or performing deep knee bends. Patients may also complain of pain after sitting with their legs bent for an extended period of time (known as the "theater sign"). Physical findings include tenderness with palpation of the patella; knee pain with compression of the patella, and pain provoked by quadriceps contraction (Davidson, 1993). Effusions are uncommon, and patients with patellofemoral pain syndrome frequently have normal knee x-rays (Davidson, 1993). There are no generally accepted guidelines or literature to support the use of knee radiography for the diagnosis of patellofemoral pain syndrome.

TREATMENT

Conservative treatment for patellofemoral pain syndrome is generally accepted, and includes NSAIDs, ice, and physical therapy (Davidson, 1993) (Indicator 13). These measures are successful for approximately 75 percent of patients, although some individuals may have recurrences of the disorder. Quadriceps strengthening exercises are recommended and may be provided in the context of formal physical therapy, or instruction of the patient by the provider in a home exercise regimen. Once patients have become asymptomatic, and have responded positively to leg-strengthening exercises, they may gradually increase their physical activity. Soft knee braces can be used to apply a medically directed force to counteract the abnormal tracking of the patella. Most experts agree that surgery should not be considered unless the patient has had no improvement after three to six months of conservative treatment. Surgery for those people with retropatellar pain not associated with significant subluxation or dislocation has not been reproducibly successful (Davidson, 1993).

SEPTIC JOINT

IMPORTANCE

The majority of nongonococcal joint infections are caused by gram-positive organisms, especially *Staphylococcus aureus*; although the proportion of cases attributable to gram-negative organisms has increased (Martens and Ho, 1995). Septic arthritis due to candida species in non-intravenous drug users is extremely rare (Martens and Ho, 1995). Adults over age 55 are most commonly affected by septic arthritis, as are individuals who have chronic joint diseases. Infectious arthritis has high morbidity and mortality rates in adults with chronic medical conditions such as rheumatoid arthritis and polyarticular infections (Martens and Ho, 1995). Most cases of enterococcal septic arthritis are reported in patients with prosthetic joint infections (Raymond et al., 1995).

DIAGNOSIS

Septic arthritis most commonly affects the large joints, but specific joint involvement does not impact on prognosis (Martens and Ho, 1995). Patients who present with a swollen knee should be asked about the following: onset and duration of the swelling, recent knee injury or trauma, presence of pain, history of crystal-induced arthropathy, fever, and other joint involvement (Indicator 9). The presence of a joint effusion is the most specific sign for joint inflammation, while the most sensitive sign is joint pain at the extreme range of motion (Towheed and Hochberg, 1996). If a patient presents with a non-traumatic effusion with onset within the prior three weeks, aspiration of the knee joint for synovial fluid should be performed to differentiate a septic arthritis from an exacerbation of a noninfectious etiology (Indicator 10). A sample of the joint fluid obtained should be evaluated for cell count and differential, examined on Gram stain, and sent for culture (Indicator 11). The results of the Gram stain will determine choice of antibiotics.

TREATMENT

The particular joint involvement affects the therapeutic management of the patient, specifically with regard to surgical versus non-surgical treatment. If the Gram stain is negative or inconclusive and the suspicion for septic arthritis is high, empiric antibiotic treatment should be instituted (Martens and Ho, 1995) (Indicator 14). According to Martens and Ho (1995), no consensus exists regarding the comparative effectiveness for easily accessible joints of arthrocentesis versus surgical drainage. No consensus exists regarding the treatment of septic arthritis due to candida species (Cuende et al., 1993).

REFERENCES

Adebajo AO, Nash P, and Hazleman BL. 1990. A prospective double blind dummy placebo cntrolled study comparing triamcinolone hexacetonide injection with oral diclofenac 50 mg TDS in patients with rotator cuff tendinitis. *The Journal of Rheumatology* 17 (9): 1207-1210.

Altchek D. July 1993. Diagnosing acute knee injuries. The office exam. *The Physician and Sports Medicine* 21 (7): 85-96.

Blair B, Rokito AS, Cuomo F, et al. November 1996. Efficacy of injections of corticosteroids for subacromial impingement syndrome. *The Journal of Bone and Joint Surgery* 78A (11): 1685-1689.

Cuende E, Barbadillo C, E-Mazzucchelli R, et al. February 1993. Candida arthritis in adult patients who are not intravenous drug addicts: report of three cases and review of the literature. *Seminars in Arthritis and Rheumatism* 22 (4): 224-41.

Davidson K. November 1993. Patellofemoral pain syndrome. *American Family Physician.* 48 (7): 1254-1262.

Fu FH, Harner CD, and Klein AH. August 1991. Shoulder impingement syndrome: A critical review. *Clinical Orthopaedics and Related Research.* 269: 162-73.

Grubbs N. September 1993. Frozen shoulder syndrome: a review of literature. *Journal of Orthopaedic and Sports Physical Therapy* 18 (3): 479-87.

Itzkowitch D, Ginsberg F, Leon M, et al. 1996. Peri-Articular injection of tenoxicam for painful shoulders: A double-blind, placebo controlled trial. *Clinical Rheumatology* 15 (6): 604-609.

Jensen JE, Conn RR, Hazelrigg G, et al. 1985. Systematic evaluation of acute knee injuries. *Clinics in Sports Medicine* 4 (2): 295-312.

Johnson DL, and Warner JJ. 1993. Diagnosis for anterior cruciate ligament surgery. *Clinics in Sports Medicine* 12: 671-84.

Katz JW, and Fingeroth RJ. 1986. The diagnostic accuracy of ruptures of the anterior cruciate ligament comparing the Lachman test, the anterior drawer sign, and the prvot shift test in acute and chronic knee injuries. *American Journal of Sports Medicine* 14: 88-91.

Litman K. March 1996. A rational approach to the diagnosis of arthritis. *American Family Physician* 53 (4): 1295-1309.

Martens PB, and Ho G Jr. September 1995. Septic arthritis in adults: clinical features, outcome, and intensive care requirements. *Journal of Intensive Care Medicine* 10 (5): 246-52.

Neuschwander D, Drez D Jr, and Heck S. January 1996. Pain dysfunction syndrome of the knee. *Orthopedics* 19 (1): 27-32.

Petri M, Dobrow R, Neiman R, et al. September 1987. Randomized, double-blind, placebo-controlled study of the treatment of the painful shoulder. *Arthritis and Rheumatism* 30 (9): 1040-1045.

Raymond NJ, Henry J, and Workowski KA. September 1995. Enterococcal arthritis: case report and review. *Clinical Infectious Diseases* 21 (3): 516-22.

Rubinstein RA, Shelbourne KD, McCarroll JR, et al. 1994. The accuracy of the clinical examination in the setting of posterior cruciate ligament injuries. *American Journal of Sports Medicine* 22: 550-7.

Shapiro MS, and Finerman GAM. 1992. Traumatic and overuse injuries of the shoulder. *Diagnostic Imaging of the Shoulder.* Seeger LL, Baltimore: Williams & Wilkins.

Sigman SA, and Richmond JC. 1995. Office diagnosis of shoulder disorders. *Physician and Sports Medicine* 23 (7): 25-31.

Sigman SA, and Richmond JC. 1995. Office diagnosis of shoulder disorders. *Physician and Sports Medicine* 23 (7): 25-31.

Smith BW, and Green GA. February 1995. Acute knee injuries: Part I. History and physical examination. *American Family Physician* 51 (3): 615-621.

Smith BW, and Green GA. March 1995. Acute knee injuries: Part II. Diagnosis and Management. *American Family Physician* 51 (4): 799-806.

Smith DL, and Campbell SM. 1992. Painful shoulder syndromes: Diagnosis and management. *Journal of General Internal Medicine* 7: 328-39.

Snyder SJ. 1993. Evaluation and treatment of the rotator cuff. *Orthopdic Clinics of North America* 24 (1): 173-92.

Stiell IG, et al. 26 October 1926. Derivation of a decision rule for the use of radiography in acute knee injuries. *Annals of Emergency Medicine* 4: 405-13.

Stiell IG, et al. 28 February 1996. Prospective validation of a decision rule for the use of radiography in acute knee injuries. *Journal of the American Medical Association* 275 (8): 611-705.

Stone JD, and Fu FH. 1997. Meniscal and Ligamentous Injuries of the Knee. , 2nd Edition ed. Principles of Orthopaedic Practice, Roger Dee, McGraw-Hill.

Swenson TM, and Harner CD. July 1995. Knee ligament and meniscal injuries. Current concepts. *Orthopedic Clinics of North America* 26 (3): 529-46.

Towheed TE, and Hochberg MC. 15 November 1996. Acute monoarthritis: A practical approach to assessment and treatment. *American Family Physician* 54 (7): 2239-2243.

Van der Heijden GJMG, Van der Windt DAWM, Kleijnen J, et al. May 1996. Steroid injections for shoulder disorders: a systematic review of randomized clinical trials. *British Journal of General Practice* 46 (406): 309-16.

White RH, Paull DM, and Fleming KW. 1986. Rotator cuff tendinitis: Comparison of subacromial injection of a long acting corticosteroid versus oral indomethacin therapy. *The Journal of Rheumatology* 13 (3): 608-613.

RECOMMENDED QUALITY INDICATORS FOR ORTHOPEDIC CONDITIONS

The following indicators apply to men and women age 18 and older.

Indicator	Quality of Evidence	Literature	Benefits	Comments
Shoulder: Diagnosis				
1. Patients presenting with new onset shoulder pain[1] should have a history obtained at the time of presentation that includes at least 4 of the following: • duration of pain; • location of pain; • activity at time the pain began; • activities that worsen the pain; • past history of injury; • past history of surgery; • therapeutic interventions attempted (e.g., NSAIDs, rest, physical therapy); • involvement of other joints.	III	Barker, 1991; Shapiro & Finerman, 1992	Prevent long-term disability through accurate diagnosis.	Evidence is based primarily on observational and anecdotal data. Accurate diagnosis of pain etiology is especially important if the patient sustained trauma to the shoulder prior to the onset of pain.
2. Patients who present with new onset shoulder pain[1] should have a physical examination performed at time of presentation that includes at least 3 of the following: • range of passive motion testing; • range of active motion testing; • the drop arm test; • testing for presence of impingement sign; • palpation to localize the site of pain; • cervical spine examination.	III	Barker, 1991; Shapiro & Finerman, 1992; Fu et al, 1991; Smith & Campbell, 1992	Prevent disability through accurate diagnosis.	Only observational evidence exists. No published prospective studies test the sensitivity and specificity of these maneuvers, but they are commonly used by orthopedic surgeons and primary care providers. Diagnostic accuracy of shoulder pain etiology is important in making the appropriate treatment decisions.

243

Indicator	Quality of Evidence	Literature	Benefits	Comments
Shoulder: Treatment				
3. Patients diagnosed with impingement syndrome[2] should be offered at least 1 of the following: • NSAIDs at time of presentation; • intra-articular steroid injection within 1 week of presentation.	III II-1 I	Fu et al, 1991; White et al, 1986; Petri et al, 1987; Adebajo et al, 1990; Itzkowitch et al, 1996; Blair et al, 1996	Decrease pain. Improve function.	RCTs have shown the benefits of using anti-inflammatory agents such as NSAIDs or intra-articular steroid injections
4. Patients diagnosed with impingement syndrome[2] should be offered 1 of the following within 2 weeks of diagnosis: • physical therapy referral; • instructions for a home exercise program.	III	Fu et al, 1991	Decrease pain. Improve function.	No RCTs exist that compare these modalities, but improved physical functioning has been noted in observational studies.
5. Patients diagnosed with a medium or large rotator cuff tear[3] who have not seen an orthopedist within 2 weeks before diagnosis, should be offered referral to an orthopedist at the time of diagnosis.	III I	Smith & Campbell, 1992; Adebajo et al, 1990; Levy,1990; Shapiro & Finerman, 1992	Improve function. Decrease risk of long-term disability.	No RCTs exist that compare surgical and non-surgical treatment for medium or large rotator cuff tears.
6. Patients diagnosed with adhesive capsulitis should receive education[4] regarding shoulder exercises at time of diagnosis.	III	Grubbs, 1993; Smith & Campbell, 1992	Decrease pain. Improve function. Decrease risk of long-term disability.	In patients at risk for adhesive capsulitis, predisposing factors should be reduced or removed. Observational studies show benefit from mobilization of the shoulder.
Knee: Diagnosis				
7. Patients presenting with new onset knee pain[5] should have a history taken at time of initial presentation that includes at least 3 of the following: • duration; • activity at time of onset; • exacerbating and relieving factors; • ability to ambulate; • history of prior trauma, surgery, or knee problems.	III	Smith & Green, 1995; Jensen et al, 1985	Prevent disability through accurate diagnosis.	When there is no clear-cut history of trauma and physical examination does not indicate injury to one or more anatomical structures, the following causes for spontaneous knee pain should be considered: nonarticular rheumatism, degenerative joint disease, crystal-induced arthritis, and rheumatoid arthritis.

244

Indicator	Quality of Evidence	Literature	Benefits	Comments
8. Patients presenting with new onset knee pain[5] after injury to their knee should undergo at least 2 of the following maneuvers during physical examination: • Lachman's test; • anterior drawer test; • posterior drawer test; • posterior sag test; • joint line palpation; • McMurray's test; • valgus stress; • varus stress.	III	Barker, 1991; Smith & Green, 1995; Katz & Fingeroth, 1986; Swenson & Harner, 1995	Prevent disability through accurate diagnosis.	Lachman's test has a very high sensitivity and specificity for ACL tears. The pivot shift test also has a high sensitivity and specificity but may be difficult to perform due to patient discomfort. McMurray's test is the most sensitive and specific maneuver for meniscal tears. The posterior drawer test has the highest sensitivity for PCL tears.
9. Patients presenting with new onset knee effusion[6] should have a history taken at time of initial presentation that includes: a. duration of swelling; b. history of trauma and injury; c. presence of pain; d. history of crystalline-induced arthropathies.	III	Martens & Ho, 1995; Towheed & Hochberg, 1996; Litman, 1996	Prevent disability through accurate diagnosis.	Accurate diagnosis of joint effusion etiology is important for instituting appropriate therapeutic interventions, especially in the case of a septic joint (where permanent joint damage may occur as a result of inappropriate treatment or delay). Various inflammatory processes have characteristic symptoms that aid in accurate diagnosis.
10. Patients presenting with new onset knee effusion[6] who do not have a history of recent trauma[7] should undergo arthrocentesis at time of presentation.	III	Towheed & Hochberg, 1996	Prevent disability through accurate diagnosis.	Repeat arthrocentesis may be indicated.
11. Patients who undergo an arthrocentesis for new onset knee effusion[6] should have the fluid analyzed for all of the following: a. cell count; b. culture; c. microscopic evaluation.	III	Towheed & Hochberg, 1996	Prevent disability through accurate diagnosis.	Cell count and culture are especially important when the suspicion for infection is very high. Microscopic examination is important in diagnosing a crystalline-induced arthropathy.
Knee: Treatment				
12. Patients diagnosed with an ACL rupture[8] who have not been seen an orthopedist within 2 weeks before diagnosis should be offered referral to an orthopedist at time of diagnosis.	III	Johnson & Warner, 1993; Swenson & Harner, 1995	Decrease pain. Improve function. Decrease risk for long-term disability.	Treatment will be based on severity of injury and individual patient characteristics (i.e., activity level prior to the injury, age, concomitant medical conditions).

Indicator	Quality of Evidence	Literature	Benefits	Comments
13. Patients newly diagnosed with patellofemoral syndrome should receive the following at time of diagnosis: a. prescription or recommendation for NSAIDs, unless contraindicated;[9] b. education[4] on quadriceps-strengthening exercises.	III	Davidson, 1993	Decrease pain. Improve function.	Surgery is rarely advised for this disorder, which has been shown to improve in most situations with focused strengthening exercises.
14. Patients diagnosed with a septic joint should be treated with intravenous antibiotics.	III	Towheed & Hochberg, 1996	Prevent disability through accurate diagnosis and treatment.	Antibiotics with broad spectrum coverage may be used initially; however, the culture results will determine the exact therapeutic regimen.

Definitions and Examples

[1] New onset shoulder pain: Shoulder pain existing for 3 weeks or less.

[2] Impingement syndrome: Supraspinatus tendinitis or bursitis.

[3] Medium or large rotator cuff tear: Diagnosis may be on physical exam or MRI, but must specify that rotator cuff has a medium or large tear.

[4] Education: May be done by the provider or by referral to physical therapy.

[5] New onset knee pain: Knee discomfort beginning within 3 weeks of presentation.

[6] New onset knee effusion: Effusion that has developed and been present for no more than 2 weeks.

[7] Recent trauma: Trauma within 6 weeks of presentation or 2 weeks before onset of effusion.

[8] ACL Rupture: Diagnosis may be by physical exam or MRI, but must specify that the ligament is ruptured.

[9] Contraindications to NSAID use: a history of gastrointestinal bleeding or current anticoagulant therapy.

Quality of Evidence Codes

I	Randomized controlled trials
II-1	Nonrandomized controlled trials
II-2	Cohort or case analysis
II-3	Multiple time series
III	Opinions or descriptive studies

246

17. OSTEOARTHRITIS TREATMENT

Alison Moore, MD

Several recent reviews provided the core references in developing quality indicators for the evaluation and management of osteoarthritis (OA) (Bálint and Szebenyi, 1996; Dearborn and Jergesen, 1996; Felson, 1996; Oddis, 1996; Puett and Griffin, 1994; Studenski et al., 1996). When these reviews referenced studies supporting individual indicators, we cited the original references.

IMPORTANCE

Osteoarthritis is the most common type of arthritis and the most common rheumatologic disease (Gabriel, 1996). Age is the strongest risk factor for OA. It is difficult to estimate the prevalence of OA because the diagnosis has been based on history, clinical examination, and radiography, alone or in combination. Based on data from the Tecumseh Community Health Study (Mikkelson, 1967), the prevalence of OA for persons aged 60 years or more when diagnosed by history is estimated at 17 percent for men and at 30 percent for women. When diagnosed by physical examination, the prevalence of OA is 20 percent for men and 41 percent for women.

Osteoarthritis causes pain or dysfunction in 20 percent of the elderly (Lawrence et al., 1989). More than 70 percent of hip and knee replacements are for OA. Symptoms most often occur in the weight-bearing joints of the lower extremities. Because there is currently no treatment to stop the degenerative process, therapeutic goals focus on reducing pain and improving function (Puett and Griffin, 1994).

SCREENING

There are no recommendations for screening for OA.

DIAGNOSIS

Clinical Features

Classically, patients with OA are older, deconditioned, and have joint motion restrictions and muscle weakness (Beals et al., 1985; Bunning and Materson, 1991; Minor et al., 1988). Other common complaints are: 1) pain that is worse with weight bearing or activity and relieved by rest; and 2) stiffness that is localized, generally of short duration, and relieved by exercise. The following joints are typically involved: the distal interphalangeal joints, proximal interphalangeal joints, first carpometacarpal joints, the hips, the knees, and the cervical and lumbar spine (Oddis, 1996). Typically, there is little or no joint effusion, but there may be bony swelling, localized tenderness, occasional secondary synovitis, and joint crepitus (Bálint and Szebenyi, 1996; Moskowitz, 1993). Other causes of pain that may be attributed to arthritis include intra-articular disease distinct from OA, periarticular sources of pain (e.g., tendonitis, bursitis, impingement, neoplasm), and referred pain from an adjacent or distant site (e.g., hip OA may refer pain to the knee; thigh or calf pain that is less severe when walking up stairs or inclines may indicate spinal stenosis) (Dearborn and Jergesen, 1996).

Initial evaluation should include a brief history to assess for typical symptoms of OA, presence or absence of limitations in daily activities, and to determine if there is a history or symptoms of a systemic or inflammatory disease (such as fever, malaise, weight loss, or stiffness lasting for more than 60 minutes). It is also important to ask about the effect of treatment modalities such as rest, ice, and nonsteroidal antiinflammatory drugs (NSAID) (Dearborn and Jergesen, 1996) (Indicator 1). A history of previous joint trauma or surgery and an assessment of the severity of pain and the degree of functional impairment should also be elicited (Dearborn and Jergesen, 1996) (Indicator 2).

The physical examination should focus on evidence of OA, including intra-articular pain, bony enlargement around the affected joints, limitation of motion, and presence or absence of effusion (Bálint and

Szebenyi, 1996; Block and Schnitzer, 1997; Dearborn and Jergesen, 1996; Griffin et al, 1995; Oddis, 1996; Perrot and Menkes, 1996; Puett and Griffin, 1994; Sack, 1995; Wollheim, 1996)(Indicator 3).

Laboratory Tests

Laboratory findings do not play an important role in the diagnosis of OA (Bálint and Szebenyi, 1996).

Radiography

Characteristic radiographic features of OA include degenerative changes such as marginal osteophyte formation along with sclerosis of the subchondral bone and the presence of subchondral cysts (Oddis, 1996). American College of Rheumatology classification criteria for knee, hip, and hand OA require radiographic evidence of disease for hip OA only (e.g., radiographic osteophytes or joint space narrowing) (Altman et al., 1986; Altman et al., 1990; Altman et al., 1991). An anteroposterior film of the affected hip is recommended for those persons who have a new presumptive diagnosis of OA of the hip (Altman et al., 1991) (Indicator 4). Although many older persons have radiologic features of OA, up to 40 percent of those with radiologically detectable OA have no symptoms (Claessens et al., 1990; Davis et al., 1992; Lawrence et al., 1966).

TREATMENT

Pharmacologic Therapies

NSAIDs are the mainstay of medical management for pain among persons with OA, but their use is associated with risks such as the development of peptic ulcer disease, renal insufficiency, hepatic toxicity, sodium retention, and loss of hypertension control on therapy (Bálint and Szebenyi, 1996; Block and Schnitzer, 1997; Dearborn and Jergesen, 1996; Gabriel et al., 1991; Griffin et al., 1991; Griffin et al., 1995; Oddis, 1996; Perrot and Menkes, 1996; Puett and Griffin, 1994; Sack, 1995; Wollheim, 1996; Studenski et al., 1996). Acetaminophen appears to have a much lower likelihood than aspirin or other NSAIDs of producing gastrointestinal side effects. In one randomized controlled trial in persons with symptomatic OA of the knee, acetaminophen was found to improve pain and function as much as ibuprofen (Bradley et al., 1991). Persons who have a new diagnosis of OA who wish to take medication for symptoms should be offered a trial of acetaminophen at approximately 4 g/day (Indicator 5). This regimen can be supplemented with other analgesics and anti-inflammatory agents for severe flares (Studenski et al., 1996). Misoprostol has been shown to reduce the prevalence of symptomatic gastrointestinal bleeding and perforation (Silverstein et al., 1995). This was shown in a multicenter private practice study in which misoprostol or placebo was added to patients' NSAID preparation. The misoprostol and placebo groups did not differ with regard to NSAID use over a six-month period, but 55 events of bleeding or perforation occurred in the placebo group as compared with 26 in the misoprostol-treated group. However, the cost-effectiveness of misoprostol in persons taking NSAIDs has not been evaluated.

Non-pharmacologic Therapies

Exercise for Knee, Hip and Hand OA

In 1994, Puett and Griffin reviewed all published trials that assigned patients with hip or knee OA to a treatment group of non-medicinal, noninvasive treatment or to a concurrent control group. The trials reviewed also included measures of pain or lower extremity function as outcomes. Exercise had the strongest evidence of benefit. In the three exercise trials with non-exercise controls (Chamberlain et al., 1982; Jan and Lai, 1993; Kovar et al., 1992), patients assigned to the exercise groups had greater pain reduction and more improved function than did the control groups. Exercise programs varied greatly from simple leg lifts done at home (Jan and Lai, 1993) to a sophisticated supervised program that included education, strengthening, and aerobics (Kovar et al., 1992). None of these exercise programs precipitated pain flares. Both studies that included aerobic exercise (Chamberlain et al., 1982; Kovar et al., 1992) showed that patients with moderate-to-severe knee OA can improve their aerobic capacity and exercise tolerance by participating in activities equivalent to 30 minutes of walking or swimming three times a week. The addition of aerobic exercise has been shown to improve the pain associated with OA to a greater degree than that achieved by stretching and strengthening alone; however, only one study specifically addressed this question.

The American College of Rheumatology recommends exercise as one of the mainstays of treatment for knee OA, based on several small, short-term studies that show that both aerobic and resistance exercise reduce pain and disability and improve physical fitness in people with knee OA (Chamberlain et al., 1982; Ettinger and Afable, 1994; Fisher et al., 1991; Fisher et al., 1993; Fisher and Pendergast, 1994; Jan and Lai, 1993; Kovar et al., 1992; Minor et al., 1989).

A randomized trial over an 18 month period was conducted to determine the effects of structured exercise programs on self-reported disability in older adults with knee OA (Ettinger et al., 1997). This trial had three arms: 1) an aerobic exercise program, 2) a resistance exercise program, and 3) a health education program. Compared with participants in the health education group, participants in both the aerobic exercise and resistance exercise groups had eight to ten percent lower mean scores on the physical disability scale, eight to twelve percent lower scores on the knee pain scale, and better ratings on a variety of physical performance tests.

A randomized trial of yoga and relaxation techniques was conducted for treatment of hand OA over a ten week period (Garfinkel et al., 1994). The yoga class included stretching and strengthening exercises emphasizing extension and alignment, group discussion, supportive encouragement, and a section for general questions and answers. The yoga participants improved significantly more than the control group in pain during activity, tenderness, and finger range of motion. Based on these studies, we recommend as a quality indicator that patients with hip or knee OA be advised to start a regular program of exercise (Indicator 6).

Other Non-Pharmacologic Therapies

Puett and Griffin also reviewed non-exercise therapies for hip and knee OA (Puett and Griffin, 1994). Diathermy (including ultrasound) before exercise is expensive and time consuming, and available evidence

251

suggests that this treatment provides no benefit in terms of pain reduction or functional improvement when added to an exercise program (Falconer et al., 1992; Jan and Lai, 1993; Svarcova et al., 1987). The data were insufficient to evaluate the efficacy of the other five non-medicinal, non-invasive therapies such as topical irritants (e.g., capsaicin), laser, acupuncture, transcutaneous electrical nerve stimulation, and pulsed electromagnetic fields. A single trial of topically applied capsaicin suggests that it may be useful to reduce pain associated with knee OA (Deal et al., 1991). Since Puett's review was published, a meta-analysis of placebo-controlled trials of capsaicin gels in OA showed superiority for the active drug, using intention-to-treat analysis (Zhang and Li Wan Po, 1994). In another study, laser treatment was found to be useful reducing the pain and disability associated the knee OA (Stelian et al., 1992).

Other physical modalities that may contribute to pain relief include the application of superficial heat (hot packs, heating pads, hot water bottles, or paraffin) and/or cold (cold packs or ice packs) (Block and Schnitzer, 1997; Studenski et al., 1996). Orthotic devices for shoes and short-term splinting of the hands can provide significant benefits in patients with OA (Block and Schnitzer, 1997; Sasaki and Yasuda, 1987; Studenski et al., 1996; Thompson et al., 1992). A number of assistive devices are available to help the individual with some of the more challenging activities of daily living, including opening jars and reaching for objects. The use of a cane or walker to give the individual more stability and to protect him or her from falling should be encouraged when appropriate (Block and Schnitzer, 1997; Fife, 1994; Perrot and Menkes, 1996; Studenski et al., 1996).

For women, weight accounts for OA more than any other known factor. For men, overweight is second to major knee injury as a preventable cause of knee OA (Anderson and Felson, 1988; Carman et al., 1994; Felson, 1996; Felson et al., 1988; Schouten et al., 1992; Tepper and Hochberg, 1993). In data from the first National Health and Nutrition Examination Survey, obese women -- those with a body mass index (BMI) greater than 30 -- had almost four times the OA risk of women whose BMI was less than 25. For men in the same overweight category, the risk was increased 4.8-fold (Anderson and Felson, 1988). The mechanism by which overweight causes OA is poorly understood; a contribution from both locally increased force across the joint and systemic factors is likely. Using data from the Framingham Study, Felson et al. (1992) evaluated the effect of weight loss or weight gain on the risk of later symptomatic knee OA. For women whose baseline BMI was 25 or greater, weight loss lowered the risk of knee OA by more than 50 percent for each two units of BMI lost (approximately 11 pounds). Weight gain was associated with a slightly increased rate of later knee OA by more than 25 percent for each two units of BMI gained. Based on these data, we recommend as a quality indicator that persons with knee OA whose BMI is greater than 25 be advised to lose weight (Indicator 6).

Invasive Therapies

Intra-articular steroid injections can provide relief in patients with painful flares. Patients who can be expected to have good responses to steroid injections are typically those who have OA flares involving only one or a few joints or pain that are unresponsive to optimal analgesic therapy (Block and Schnitzer, 1997). A given joint should not be injected more than three times a year (Block and Schnitzer, 1997; Fife, 1994).

Arthroscopic lavage with saline for osteoarthritic knees has been shown to alleviate pain and improve function in some patients with moderately severe OA, but the population most likely to benefit has yet to be clearly defined (Block and Schnitzer, 1997).

Surgical interventions, especially prosthetic joint replacement at the knee and hip, are most appropriate for the person whose symptoms are unrelieved (with consequent functional limitations) by rest or more conservative measures, and who has no other major functional limitations or surgical contraindications, such as severe cardiopulmonary or advanced neurologic disease. The person must also have sufficient cognition to cooperate with a postoperative rehabilitation program (Block and Schnitzer, 1997; Studenski et al., 1996). Given the complexity of structuring indicators to assess the appropriateness of joint replacement therapy, we are not currently proposing any indicators in this area.

FOLLOW-UP

Patients who are taking NSAIDs chronically should be evaluated regularly for therapeutic response and potential drug toxicity. Monitoring is especially important in patients at higher risk of renal abnormalities, including the elderly, those with hypertension, and those with an elevated baseline serum creatinine level or hepatic abnormalities (e.g., those receiving diclofenac). Evaluations should begin soon after initiation of NSAID therapy (Block and Schnitzer, 1997). All persons with OA should be seen for follow-up at least every six months (Indicator 7).

REFERENCES

Altman R, Alarcón G, Appelrouth D, et al. 1991. The American College of Rheumatology criteria for the classification and reporting of osteoarthritis of the hip. *Arthritis and Rheumatism* 34 (5): 505-514.

Altman R, Alarcón G, Appelrouth D, et al. 1990. The American College of Rheumatology criteria for the classification and reporting of osteoarthritis of the hand. *Arthritis and Rheumatism* 33 (11): 1601-1610.

Altman R, Asch E, Bloch D, et al. 1986. Development of criteria for the classification and reporting of osteoarthritis: Classification of osteoarthritis of the knee. *Arthritis and Rheumatism* 29 (8): 1039-1049.

Anderson J, and Felson DT. 1988. Factors associated with OA of the knee in the First National Health and Nutrition Examination Survey (NHANES I). *American Journal of Epidemiology* 128: 179-189.

Bálint G, and Szebenyi B. 1996. Diagnosis of osteoarthritis: Guidelines and current pitfalls. *Drugs* 52 (Suppl. 3): 1-13.

Beals CA, Lampman RM, Banwell BF, et al. 1985. Measurement of exercise tolerance in patients with rheumatoid arthritis and osteoarthritis. *Journal of Rheumatology* 12: 458-461.

Block JA, and Schnitzer TJ. 1997. Therapeutic approaches to osteoarthritis. *Hospital Practices* 32 (2): 159-64.

Bradley JD, Brandt KD, Katz BP, Kalasinski LA, and Ryan SI. 1991. Comparison of an antiinflammatory dose of ibuprofin, an analgesic dose of ibuprofen, and acetaminophen in the treatment of patients with osteoarthritis of the knee. *New England Journal of Medicine* 325: 87-91.

Bunning RD, and Materson RS. 1991. A rational program of exercise for patients with osteoarthritis. *Seminars in Arthritis and Rheumatism* 21: 33-43.

Carman WJ, Sowers MF, Hawthorne VM, and Weissfield LA. 1994. Obesity as a risk factor for osteoarthritis of the hand and wrist: A prospective study. *American Journal of Epidemiology* 139: 119-129.

Chamberlain MA, Care G, and Harfield B. 1982. Physiotherapy in osteoarthritis of the knees. *International Rehabilitative Medicine* 4: 101-106.

Claessens AAMC, Shouten JSAG, Ouweland FA, et al. 1990. Do clinical findings associate with radiographic osteoarthritis of the knee? *Annals of the Rheumatic Diseases* 49: 771-774.

Davis MA, Ettinger WH, Neuhaus JM, et al. 1992. Correlates of knee pain among US adults with and without radiographic knee osteoarthritis. *Journal of Rheumatology* 19: 1943-1949.

Deal CL, Schnitzer TJ, Lipstein E, et al. 1991. Treatment of arthritis with topical capsaicin: A double-blind trial. *Clinical Therapy* 13: 383-395.

Dearborn JT, and Jergesen HE. 1996. The evaluation and initial management of arthritis. *Orthopedics* 23 (2): 215-240.

Ettinger WH, and Afable RF. 1994. Physical disability from knee osteoarthritis: The role of exercise as an intervention. *Medicine and Science in Sports and Exercise* 26: 1435-1440.

Ettinger WH, Burns R, Messier SP, et al. 1997. A randomized trial comparing aerobic exercise and resistance exercise with a health education program in older adults with knee osteoarthritis: The Fitness Arthritis and Seniors Trial (FAST). *Journal of the American Medical Association* 277: 25-31.

Falconer J, Hayes KW, and Chang RW. 1992. Effect of ultrasound on mobility in osteoarthritis of the knee: A randomized clinical trial. *Arthritis Care Research* 5 (1): 29-35.

Felson DT. 1996. Weight and osteoarthritis. *American Journal of Clinical Nutrition* 63 (suppl): 430S-432S.

Felson DT, Anderson JJ, Naimark A, Walker AM, and Meenan RF. 1988. Obesity and knee osteoarthritis. *Archives of Internal Medicine* 109: 18-24.

Felson DT, Zhang Y, Anthony JM, Naimark A, and Anderson JJ. 1992. Weight loss reduces the risk for symptomatic knee osteoarthritis in women. *Archives of Internal Medicine* 116: 535-539.

Fife RS. 1994. Osteoarthritis. In *Principles of Geriatric Medicine and Gerontology*, Third ed. Eds Hazzard WR, Bierman EL, Blass JP, Ettinger WH, and Halter JB, 981-986. New York, NY: McGraw-Hill, Inc.

Fisher NM, Gresham GE, Abrams M, Hicks J, Horrigan D, and Pendergast DR. 1993. Quantitative effects of physical therapy on muscular and functional performance in subjects with osteoarthritis of the knees. *Archives of Physical Medicine and Rehabilitation* 74: 840-847.

Fisher NM, and Pendergast DR. 1994. Effects of a muscle exercise program on exercise capacity in subjects with osteoarthritis. *Archives of Physical Medicine and Rehabilitation* 75: 792-797.

Fisher NM, Pendergast DR, Gresham GE, and Calkins E. 1991. Muscle rehabilitation: Its effect on muscular and functional performance of patients with knee osteoarthritis. *Archives of Physical Medicine and Rehabilitation* 72: 367-374.

Gabriel SE. 1996. Update on the epidemiology of the rheumatic diseases. *Current Opinions in Rheumatology* 8: 96-100.

Gabriel SE, Jaakkimainen L, and Bombardier C. 1991. Risk for serious gastrointestinal complications related to use of nonsteroidal anti-inflammatory drugs: A meta-analysis. *Archives of Internal Medicine* 115: 787-796.

Garfinkel MS, Schumacher R, Husain A, Levy M, and Reshetar RA. 1994. Evaluation of a yoga based regimen for treatment of osteoarthritis of the hands. *Journal of Rheumatology* 21: 2341-2343.

Griffin MR, Brandt KD, Liang MH, Pincus T, and Ray WA. 1995. Practical management of osteoarthritis: Integration of pharmacologic and nonpharmacologic measures. *Archives of Family Medicine* 4: 1049-1055.

Griffin MR, Piper JM, Daugherty JR, Snowden M, and Ray WA. 1991. Nonsteroidal anti-inflammatory drug use and increased risk for peptic ulcer disease in elderly persons. *Archives of Internal Medicine* 114: 257-263.

Jan MH, and Lai JS. 1993. The effects of physiotherapy on osteoarthritic knees of females. *Journal of the Formosan Medical Association* 90: 1008-1013.

Kovar PA, Allegrante JP, MacKenzie R, Peterson MGE, Cutin R, and Charlson ME. 1992. Supervised fitness walking in patients with osteoarthritis of the knee: A randomized, controlled trial. *Archives of Internal Medicine* 116: 529-534.

Lawrence JS, Bremmer JM, and Bier F. 1966. Osteo-arthrosis. Prevalence in the population and relationship between symptoms and x-ray changes. *Annals of the Rheumatic Diseases* 25: 1-24.

Mikkelsen WM, Dodge HJ, Duff IF, et al. 1967. Estimates of the prevalence of rheumatic diseases in the population of Tecumseh, Michigan, 1959-1960. *Journal of Chronic Diseases* 20: 351-69.

Minor MA, Hewett JE, Webel RR, Anderson SK, and Kay DR. 1989. Efficacy of physical conditioning exercise in patients with rheumatoid arthritis and osteoarthritis. *Arthritis and Rheumatism* 32 (11): 1396-1405.

Minor MA, Hewett JE, Webel RR, Dreisinger TE, and Kay DR. 1988. Exercise tolerance and disease related measures in patients with rheumatoid arthritis and osteoarthritis. *Journal of Rheumatology* 15: 905-911.

Moskowitz RW. 1993. Clinical and laboratory findings in osteoarthritis. In *Arthritis and Allied Conditions*. Ed McCarty DJ, 1735-1760. Philadelphia, PA: Lea & Febiger.

Oddis CV. 1996. New perspectives on osteoarthritis. *American Journal of Medicine* 100 (Suppl. 2A): 2A-10S-2A-15S.

Perrot S, and Menkes C-J. 1996. Nonpharmacological approaches to pain in osteoarthritis: Available options. *Drugs* 52 (Suppl. 3): 21-26.

Puett DW, and Griffin MR. 1994. Published trials of nonmedicinal and noninvasive therapies of hip and knee osteoarthritis. *Archives of Internal Medicine* 121 (2): 133-140.

Sack KE. 1995. Osteoarthritis: A continuing challenge. *Western Journal of Medicine* 163: 579-586.

Sasaki T, and Yasuda K. 1987. Clinical evaluation of the treatment of osteoarthritic knees using a newly designed wedged insole. *Clinical Orthopaedics and Related Research* (221): 181-187.

Schouten JSAG, van den Ouweland F, and Valkenburg HA. 1992. A 12 year follow up study in the general population on prognostic factors of cartilage loss in osteoarthritis of the knee. *Annals of the Rheumatic Diseases* 51: 932-937.

Silverstein FE, Graham DY, Senior JR, et al. 1995. Misoprostol reduces serious gastrointestinal complications in patients with rheumatoid arthritis receiving nonsteroidal anti-inflammatory drugs: A randomized, double-blind, placebo-controlled trial. *Archives of Internal Medicine* 123: 241-249.

Stelian J, Gil I, Habot B, et al. 1992. Improvement of pain and disability in elderly patients with degenerative osteoarthritis of the knee treated with narrow-band light therapy. *Journal of the American Geriatric Society* 40: 23-26.

Studenski SA, Rigler SK, and Robbins JM. 1996. Musculoskeletal diseases and disorders. In *Geriatrics Review Syllabus: A Core Curriculum in Geriatric Medicine*, Third ed. Eds: Reuben DB, Yoshikawa TT, and Besdine RW, 234-251. New York, NY: American Geriatrics Society.

Svarcova J, Trnavsky K, and Zvarova J. 1987. The influence of ultrasound, galvanic currents and shortwave diathermy on pain intensity in patients with osteoarthritis. *Scandinavian Journal of Rheumatology (Suppl.)* 67: 83-85.

Tepper S, and Hochberg MC. 1993. Factors associated with hip osteoarthritis: Data from the First National Health and Nutrition Examination Survey (NHANES-I). *American Journal of Epidemiology* 137: 1081-1088.

Thompson JA, Jennings MB, and Hodge W. 1992. Orthotic therapy in the management of osteoarthritis. *Journal of the American Podiatric Medical Association* 82 (3): 136-139.

Wollheim FA. 1996. Current pharmacological treatment of osteoarthritis. *Drugs* 52 (Suppl. 3): 27-38.

Zhang WY, and Li Wan Po A. 1994. The effectiveness of topically applied capsaicin: A meta-analysis. *European Journal of Clinical Pharmacology* 46: 517-522.

RECOMMENDED QUALITY INDICATORS FOR OSTEOARTHRITIS

The following indicators apply to men and women age 18 and older.

Indicator	Quality of Evidence	Literature	Benefits	Comments
Diagnosis				
1. Providers caring for patients with symptoms of OA[1] should document all of the following at least once in 2 years:[2] a. the location of symptoms;[2] b. the presence or absence of limitations in daily activities; c. the presence or absence of a history or symptoms of systemic or inflammatory disease; d. the use and effectiveness of treatment modalities.[3]	III	Bálint and Szebenyi, 1996; Block and Schnitzer, 1997; Dearborn and Jergesen, 1996; Griffin, 1994; Griffin et al., 1995; Oddis, 1996; Perrot and Menkes, 1996; Puett and Griffin, 1994; Sack, 1995; Wollheim, 1996	Reduce disability and improve function.	Improves diagnosis and management of OA. Recommended by all articles reviewing this topic.
2. Providers caring for patients with incident symptoms of OA[1] should document at least one of the following: • the presence or absence of a history of any systemic or inflammatory disease that may mimic OA;[4] • the presence or absence of any current symptoms of systemic or inflammatory disease that may mimic OA;[5] • the presence or absence of a history of joint trauma or surgery.	III	Altman et al., 1986; Altman et al., 1990; Altman et al., 1991; Bálint and Szebenyi, 1996; Block and Schnitzer, 1997; Dearborn and Jergesen, 1996; Griffin, 1994; Griffin et al., 1995; Oddis, 1996; Perrot and Menkes, 1996; Puett and Griffin, 1994; Sack, 1995; Wollheim, 1996	Improve symptoms by making accurate diagnosis.	Improve diagnosis and management of OA. Recommended by all consensus developers and articles reviewing this topic.

	Indicator	Quality of Evidence	Literature	Benefits	Comments
3.	Providers caring for patients with symptoms of OA[1] should document the following for any one affected joint at least once in 2 years: a. the presence or absence of effusion; b. the presence or absence of bony enlargement; c. the presence or absence of tenderness; d. the presence or absence of limitations in range of motion.	III	Bálint and Szebenyi, 1996; Block and Schnitzer, 1997; Dearborn and Jergesen, 1996; Griffin, 1994; Griffin et al., 1995; Oddis, 1996; Perrot and Menkes, 1996; Puett and Griffin, 1994; Sack, 1995; Wollheim, 1996	Improve function.	Improve diagnosis and management of OA. Recommended by all consensus developers and articles reviewing this topic.
4.	Patients with incident symptoms of hip OA[1] should be offered an anteroposterior film of the affected hip.	III	Altman et al., 1991	Reduce disability.	Improve diagnosis of hip OA. Recommended by the American Rheumatism Association.
5.	Patients with a new diagnosis of OA who wish to take medication for joint symptoms should be offered a trial of acetaminophen.	I	Bradley et al., 1991	Decrease risk of complications associated with NSAIDs.	In a randomized controlled trial involving persons with symptomatic knee OA, acetaminophen (4 g/day) was found to improve pain and function as much as ibuprofen. Acetaminophen will not cause many of the complications that have been associated with the use of NSAIDs such gastrointestinal bleeding, renal insufficiency, sodium retention, and increased blood pressure.

Indicator	Quality of Evidence	Literature	Benefits	Comments
6. Providers caring for patients with symptoms of hip or knee OA[1] should recommend both of the following at least once in 2 years: a. exercise programs for persons with hip or knee OA; b. weight loss among persons with knee OA and a BMI >25.[6]	I, II, III	Anderson and Felson, 1988; Ettinger, 1997; Felson et al., 1992; Hochberg et al., 1995a; Hochberg et al., 1995b; Puett and Griffin, 1994	Improve symptoms and function.	Multiple trials, some employing randomization of subjects to treatment groups, have demonstrated benefits of exercise programs for hip and knee OA. For women with a BMI >= 25, weight loss has been shown to lower the risk of knee OA by more than 50% for each 2 units of BMI lost.
Follow-up				
7. Patients receiving care for symptoms of OA[1] should be seen in follow-up at least every 6 months.	III	Block and Schnitzer, 1997	Improve management of OA.	Recommended by all articles reviewing this topic.

Definitions and Examples

[1] Symptoms of osteoarthritis may occur in the hands, hips (manifested by symptoms in the groin, anterior thigh, buttocks, or knees), knees, neck, or lower back. Symptoms may consist of: a) pain that is worse with weight bearing or activity and relieved by rest; b) stiffness that is localized, generally of short duration, and relieved by exercise; and c) restrictions in motion that may interfere with daily activities.
[2] Joints commonly involved in osteoarthritis include the distal interphalangeal joints, proximal interphalangeal joints, and first carpometacarpal joints; hips; knees; and cervical and lumbar spine.
[3] Treatment modalities for OA include medications such as acetaminophen, NSAIDs, capsaicin, heat and/or ice, exercise, orthotics and splints, canes or walkers, weight loss, intra-articular steroid injections, and joint replacement surgery.
[4] Systemic or inflammatory disease that may mimic OA include psoriasis, gout, systemic lupus erythematosus, rheumatoid arthritis, sickle cell disease, and hemophilia.
[5] Symptoms of systemic or inflammatory diseases that may mimic OA include fever, malaise, weight loss, and prolonged stiffness (e.g., more than 60 minutes).
[6] Body mass index (BMI) = kg/meters^2

Quality of Evidence Codes

I	RCT
II-1	Nonrandomized controlled trials
II-2	Cohort or case analysis
II-3	Multiple time series
III	Opinions or descriptive studies

18. DYSPEPSIA AND PEPTIC ULCER DISEASE

Beatrice Golomb, MD, PhD

The development of quality indicators for dyspepsia and peptic ulcer disease (PUD) diagnosis and treatment was based on a MEDLINE search of the English language review literature published between 1992 and 1996. This was supplemented by identification of more specific review articles and clinical studies in areas of controversy, or in areas where benefit to selected diagnostic or therapeutic measures has been documented.

DYSPEPSIA

IMPORTANCE

Dyspepsia is a persistent symptom of epigastric discomfort or a feeling of gnawing hunger that is sometimes associated with meals, and with nausea, belching, or bloating (Barker et al., 1991). It may also be defined as pain or discomfort localized in the upper abdomen (Talley, 1993), or simply as symptoms that the physician believes are referable to the upper gastrointestinal (GI) tract (Pound and Heading, 1995). Figures on the prevalence of dyspepsia vary, with some citing a prevalence of seven percent in the U.S. (Barker et al., 1991), and others citing a six-month prevalence of over 35 percent (Pound and Heading, 1995). Differences in estimates probably depend on how dyspepsia is defined or elicited, and on the time window employed.

SCREENING

Only one in four of all patients with dyspepsia consult their general practitioner, and fewer than one in five of those age 20 to 40 do so (Pound and Heading, 1995). Because there are no data to indicate that all individuals with dyspepsia should consult their general practitioner. Our indicators do not address routine screening of individuals for dyspepsia.

DIAGNOSIS

Eliciting subjective details about the discomfort is not a highly reliable way to distinguish ulcer from nonulcer dyspepsia. Because ulcers are not the sole source of dyspepsia, the severity, timing, location of discomfort, and information on current bowel habits are often used to direct the diagnosis and guide use of further evaluative studies and treatment. Causes of nonulcer dyspepsia include: irritable bowel syndrome, which is classically associated with diffuse abdominal pain, altered bowel habits, and relief with defecation; cholelithiasis, which may be associated with discrete episodes of right upper quadrant pain; gastroesophageal reflux, which is associated with "heartburn" and a sensation of acid backwash; and chronic pancreatic disease, which is commonly associated with more severe pain and steatorrhea. Cases of nonulcer dyspepsia that defy these classifications are termed essential dyspepsia, in which approximately 50 percent will have *Helicobacter pylori* gastritis (Barker et al., 1991). Unfortunately, clinical diagnosis may not accurately predict endoscopic diagnosis in patients with dyspepsia (Muris et al., 1994). Although the majority of patients with chronic dyspepsia do not have concurrent ulceration, up to 40 percent of patients with chronic dyspepsia may have chronic peptic ulceration. However, symptoms alone are not sensitive and specific enough to make the diagnosis in most cases (Talley, 1993). One study suggests that 30 percent of patients with a major pathological lesion are misclassified, including 50 percent of ulcer patients. The chance-corrected validity of nonulcer dyspepsia was only slightly better than chance (Bytzer et al., 1996). Because of the questionable utility of symptom characteristics, no indicator requires that details of the character of the dyspeptic symptoms be elicited.

Use of current medications should be determined in patients with dyspepsia because this may influence the likelihood of diagnosing ulcer disease, ulcer complications, or drug-induced dyspepsia. Use of aspirin or nonsteroidal antiinflammatory drugs (NSAIDs) is particularly important, as these agents are widely used and may predispose patients to "NSAID gastritis" or ulcers (Griffin et al., 1988; Griffin et al., 1991; Clearfield, 1992; Walt, 1992; Rex, 1994; Lee, 1995). Each year, nearly 70 million prescriptions for NSAIDs are written (Lee, 1995) and more than 30 billion NSAID pills are consumed in the U.S. (Loeb et al., 1992). The global market for NSAIDs is estimated at $2 billion per year (Lee, 1995). An estimated 1.2 percent of the population take NSAIDs regularly, and many more take them intermittently (Loeb et al., 1992). One study found that upper GI symptoms occurred in 38 percent of patients within one month after assignment to a common NSAID (Bianchi Porro et al., 1991), and in 37 percent of chronic NSAID patients in the two months prior to questioning. The two to four percent overall risk of ulcers in patients taking NSAIDs is twice that of the general population (Ebell, 1992) and four to five times higher than that of age-matched controls in the elderly (Griffin et al., 1988; Griffin et al., 1991). The prevalence of gastric ulcers among NSAID users may be five to ten times higher than in the general population (Lee, 1995).

The risk of hospitalization or major adverse GI events is approximately three to ten times greater in patients who take NSAIDs than in those who do not (Clearfield, 1992; Ebell, 1992; Loeb et al., 1992). Patients who take NSAIDs are more likely to require emergency surgical intervention for hemorrhagic or perforated peptic ulcers, and one study found they had an increased mortality from PUD in comparison with a matched control group (Loeb et al., 1992). Although NSAIDs are not significantly associated with chronic duodenal ulcers, ulcer complications of duodenal or gastric origin are equally common (Loeb et al., 1992). Medical costs of GI complications from NSAIDs have been estimated at $3.9 billion per year (Loeb et al., 1992).

Drug-induced dyspepsia may also occur with corticosteroids (DePriest, 1995), theophylline, digoxin, oral antibiotics (especially ampicillin and erythromycin), or potassium or iron supplements (Pound and Heading, 1995). Use of Pepto Bismol or iron may lead to a history of black stools in a patient who is found to be hemoccult negative on physical examination. Because medications may influence the diagnosis and management of ulcer disease versus nonulcer dyspepsia (which may be more likely, for instance, if erythromycin was begun soon before symptom onset), the medical record should document medication use, or at least the presence or absence of NSAID use, in all patients newly presenting with dyspeptic symptoms (Indicator 1).

Ascertainment of smoking status is appropriate but not mandatory. Smoking has been shown to stimulate acid secretion, to impair mucosal defenses by reduction of blood flow and prostaglandin synthesis, and to provide an environment favorable to *H. pylori* (Bateson, 1993; Ziller and Netchvolodoff, 1993; Lanas et al., 1995). Cigarette smoking is believed by some to be an important risk factor for the development of PUD (Ebell, 1992; Bateson, 1993; Ziller and Netchvolodoff, 1993; Lanas et al., 1995). Smokers do indeed appear to be twice as likely as nonsmokers to develop PUD (Ebell, 1992), which may in turn induce symptoms of dyspepsia. Nonetheless, the evidence regarding a causal connection between smoking and PUD is not persuasive. Screening and treatment of smoking for all patients are discussed in Chapter 5 of the Cardiopulmonary Conditions book.

Ascertainment of alcohol use is appropriate but not mandatory. Alcohol use in itself has not been shown to be consistently associated with either dyspepsia (Talley et al., 1994) or peptic ulcers (Ebell, 1992; Chou, 1994), even though some recommend cessation or moderation of alcohol use in patients with ulcer disease (Loeb et al., 1992) and concurrent use of alcohol and NSAIDs may substantially increase the risk of upper GI bleeding (Ebell, 1992). Therefore, while it is probably appropriate to elicit an alcohol history, since this may influence the likelihood of diagnosing upper GI bleed (particularly with concurrent NSAIDs), no indicator has been formulated to require that alcohol use be elicited in the context of dyspepsia.

TREATMENT

Dyspepsia Not Associated With NSAID Use

H. pylori and Dyspepsia: *H. pylori* is common in the general population, and increases with age. More than 50 percent of asymptomatic persons over age 60 in North America show evidence of past or active *H. pylori* infection (Feldman and Peterson, 1993). A particularly high incidence of *H. pylori* is evident in patients with PUD, estimated at 90 to 95 percent of patients with duodenal ulcer and

70 percent of those with gastric ulcer (Cave, 1992). Furthermore, the eradication of *H. pylori* greatly lowers relapse rates of PUD (Feldman, 1993). In one study, relapse after six to twelve months of follow-up occurred in 85 percent of *H. pylori*-positive individuals, and in only ten percent of those with successful *H. pylori* eradication (Soll, 1996). Therefore, treatment of PUD has shifted emphasis from acid reduction to eradication of *H. pylori*, although traditional antiulcer treatment is still used to alleviate symptoms and promote ulcer healing. Finally, eradication of *H. pylori* can effectively reduce the re-bleeding rates for the two years following peptic ulcer hemorrhage, according to preliminary studies (Jiranek and Kozarek, 1996).

Management Options in Non-NSAID Dyspepsia

Guidelines from the Practice Parameters Committee of the American College of Gastroenterology recognize three approaches for management of new-onset dyspepsia not due to NSAIDs (Soll, 1996), most of which arise in association with *H. pylori* infection. Trial data are insufficient as yet to distinguish among these options. The first approach for management of new onset dyspepsia not due to NSAIDs is a single, short-term trial of empiric antiulcer therapy. If symptoms do not improve within two to four weeks, endoscopy should be pursued. If symptoms improve, the trial is discontinued after six weeks, and endoscopy is pursued if symptoms recur (Soll, 1996). The second option is a definitive diagnostic evaluation, including endoscopy with testing for *H. pylori* (Indicator 2). Endoscopy is performed immediately if there are "alarm" markers including anemia, GI bleeding, anorexia, early satiety, recurrent vomiting, dysphagia, jaundice, palpable mass, guaiac-positive stool, or weight loss (Talley, 1993; Soll, 1996). Because the diagnostic yield for organic pathology with endoscopy is 60 percent in patients over age 60, these patients should also receive early endoscopy, preferably within four to six weeks of presentation, if symptoms have occurred for the first time (Barker et al., 1991) (Indicator 3). Indeed, some recommend early endoscopy for those over age 45 (Talley, 1993). The third option for managing non-NSAID dyspepsia is noninvasive testing for *H. pylori* followed by antibiotics in *H. pylori*-positive patients. *H. pylori* treatment has potential side effects, and should only be undertaken if presence of *H. pylori* is confirmed. An exception may be made if *H. pylori* is highly probable, as in a person with dyspepsia with a history of duodenal ulcer and absence of NSAID use (Indicator 4). With empiric antibiotics in *H. pylori*-positive dyspeptic patients, the 15 to 30 percent who have an ulcer are likely to respond well, but nonulcer dyspeptic study subjects have been shown to have a variable response compared with subjects on placebo. The potential advantage of this approach lies in reserving definitive work-up and extended therapy for patients with recurrent symptoms after a course of antibiotics has been tried (Soll, 1996). However, the cost advantage of empiric therapy over prompt endoscopy is subject to debate. One decision analysis found the choice of optimal management strategy a "toss-up" (Silverstein et al., 1996), while another study reported frank cost savings and improved patient satisfaction with prompt endoscopy (Bytzer et al., 1994).

Management of Dyspepsia Associated With NSAID Use

In a patient with new dyspepsia who is taking NSAIDs, it is probably prudent to discontinue NSAIDs, if possible, and then reassess the patient (Soll, 1996). Although the incidence of dyspepsia is high, the incidence of dyspepsia leading to physician visits is substantially lower. If NSAIDs cannot be discontinued, dyspepsia or uncomplicated ulcers are often treated with H2 blockers twice a day. Although the use of H2 blockers may be appropriate, at present there is no convincing evidence that agents other than misoprostol protect against NSAID-induced ulcer disease; thus, no indicator will be formulated for use of prophylactic antiulcer medication in dyspeptic patients continuing to take NSAIDs.

FOLLOW-UP

The literature does not specify appropriate follow-up intervals for patients with dyspepsia. Management and follow-up for PUD are discussed below.

PEPTIC ULCER DISEASE

IMPORTANCE

Peptic ulcer disease is a major health problem in the United States. There are more than four million prevalent cases annually according to the National Institutes of Health (NIH, 1989), and 200,000 to 400,000 new cases each year (Barker et al., 1991; Ziller and Netchvolodoff, 1993). One in ten people in the U.S. will be affected by PUD at some time in their lives (Barker et al., 1991; NIH Consensus Panel, 1994). Although the disease has relatively low mortality, it results in substantial suffering (NIH Consensus Panel, 1994). There are approximately 150,000 nonfederal, short-stay hospitalizations each year in the U.S. for evaluation and treatment of bleeding ulcers (Laine and Peterson, 1994; Jiranek and Kozarek, 1996). The direct and indirect costs associated with PUD represent a large percentage of costs for the treatment of all diseases of the digestive system (Ziller and Netchvolodoff, 1993).

Peptic ulcer disease is the leading cause of acute hemorrhage of the upper GI tract, accounting for about 50 percent of all cases (Laine and Peterson, 1994). Hospitalization and surgery rates for uncomplicated ulcers have declined in the U.S. and Europe over the past 30 years; however, the number of admissions for bleeding ulcers is relatively unchanged (Laine and Peterson, 1994), with approximately 150,000 hospital admissions for bleeding ulcers in the U.S. each year (Jiranek and Kozarek, 1996). Despite advances in treatment, overall mortality has remained at approximately six to eight percent for the past 30 years, due in part to increasing patient age and prevalence of concurrent illness (Laine and Peterson, 1994).

Until recently, ulcers were thought to be related to stress and diet. It is now recognized that most ulcers are produced by NSAIDs or by *H. pylori*. Ninety percent of patients with bleeding ulcers are taking NSAIDs or have active *H. pylori* infection (Jiranek and Kozarek, 1996). Eradication of *H. pylori*, if it is present, and avoidance of NSAIDs have been proven to cure more than 95 percent of patients with PUD (Jiranek and Kozarek, 1996). A minority of patients with ulcers have etiologies distinct from NSAIDs and *H. pylori*, including gastrinoma and corticosteroid or "stress-related" ulcers.

SCREENING

Although *H. pylori* is strongly associated with PUD and highly prevalent in the population, screening asymptomatic individuals for ulcers and testing for *H. pylori* are not recommended.

PREVENTION

Treatment of *H. pylori*

Despite the strong association between *H. pylori* and PUD, treating asymptomatic patients who have *H. pylori* for primary prevention of ulcers is not recommended.

Discontinuation of NSAIDS

In patients with new dyspepsia taking NSAIDs, it is prudent to discontinue NSAIDs where possible (Soll, 1996). This may reduce the incidence of NSAID-associated ulcers in patients with NSAID-associated dyspepsia. However, dyspepsia is common in NSAID users in the absence of ulcers or ulcer complications, and ulcer complications of NSAIDs often occur in the absence of dyspeptic symptoms. Indeed, it is not known whether patients with NSAID-associated dyspepsia are at greater risk for serious NSAID-induced GI problems such as bleeding or perforation (Larkai et al., 1989). For this reason, we have not generated an indicator to discontinue NSAIDs if dyspepsia is present without documented ulcer disease, though this is probably appropriate.

Use of NSAIDs increases not only risk of ulcer but risk of hospitalization for ulcer and, in those patients with established ulcer disease, risk of major ulcer complications such as bleeding. Therefore, in patients treated with NSAIDs or aspirin who have endoscopically documented ulcers, the medical record should either state the reason for continuing NSAIDs or aspirin, or that the patient was advised to discontinue NSAIDs or aspirin (Indicator 5).

Prevention of NSAID-Induced Ulcers if NSAIDs are Continued

Misoprostol is the only drug approved by the FDA for prevention of NSAID-induced ulcers. Although proton pump inhibitors and H2 blockers have been used in practice and may be appropriate, no data are available to support this. Misoprostol co-therapy may be appropriate as secondary prevention in cases of continued NSAID use with prior clinical ulcer disease, or as primary prevention in cases with concurrent steroid or anticoagulant administration or with serious comorbid conditions that would increase risk for ulcer complications. Misoprostol is often difficult to tolerate because diarrhea and abdominal cramps limit patient compliance. In addition, cost effectiveness has not been established (Soll, 1996). No indicator is directed at use of misoprostol or other agents for prevention of NSAID-induced ulcers, though such an indicator may be appropriate in the future when more data are available.

Smoking Cessation

Smoking is associated with increased incidence and prevalence of PUD (Hixson et al., 1992; Ziller and Netchvolodoff, 1993; Rex, 1994; Soll, 1996); delayed ulcer healing (in the pre-*H. pylori* eradication era); and increased risk of refractory and recurrent ulceration (in the pre-*H. pylori* eradication era) (Ebell, 1992; Bateson, 1993; Ziller and Netchvolodoff, 1993; Lanas et al., 1995). All patients who smoke will benefit from quitting and should be strongly encouraged to do so; however, additional evidence of selective benefit to PUD with smoking cessation, under current conditions of PUD treatment (including *H. pylori* eradication treatment), is lacking. Therefore, although it is appropriate to counsel all patients with PUD who smoke cigarettes to quit (Loeb et al., 1992), no indicator was constructed for this.

Alcohol Cessation

The role of alcohol use in ulcer disease is ill-defined. Although some recommend discontinuation of moderate-to-heavy use of alcohol in patients with a history of ulcers, as a way to prevent ulcer recurrence (Loeb et al., 1992), a causal relationship between alcohol use and ulcers has not been convincingly demonstrated (Ziller and Netchvolodoff,

1993; Rex, 1994). While concurrent use of alcohol and NSAIDs may increase the risk of bleeding (Ebell, 1992), some studies show only modest or no increase in ulcer risk with alcohol use, and others actually suggest a possible protective effect. Therefore, while advice to curtail alcohol consumption is probably appropriate, no indicator will be directed at alcohol use in patients with PUD.

DIAGNOSIS

Endoscopy

Peptic ulcers are detected by the presence of a distinct crater that is visible on radiologic or endoscopic examination of the upper GI tract; they differ from erosions in that ulcers penetrate beyond the mucosa to the submucosa (Clearfield, 1992; Ziller and Netchvolodoff, 1993). Use of endoscopy to diagnose PUD is not recommended in the absence of symptoms, but may be appropriate in cases of dyspepsia or when evaluating GI bleeding. Indications for endoscopy to diagnose PUD are therefore listed in the management sections for dyspepsia and for GI bleeding.

Testing for *H. pylori* in PUD

Several tests are available for evaluating infection with *H. pylori*. Serological testing is sensitive and specific, and is the least expensive method (Walsh and Peterson, 1995). However, because serological testing does not distinguish between past and current *H. pylori* infection, it cannot be used to test for recurrence or for effect of treatment. Gastric mucosal biopsy -- by staining of biopsy materials, the Campylobacter-like organism test, or *H. pylori* culture -- and the ^{13}C-urea breath test may be used repeatedly to check for eradication of *H. pylori*. (*H. pylori* produces urease that hydrolyzes labeled urea, producing NH_3 and $^{13}CO_2$; $^{13}CO_2$ is identified in expired air by mass spectroscopy (Cave, 1992)). Culture is the least sensitive of the direct techniques (Walsh and Peterson, 1995). The urea breath test has the advantage of being noninvasive. These latter methods are sensitive to bacterial load and should be performed at least four weeks after use of bismuth or eradication therapy (Cave, 1992; Walsh and

Peterson, 1995), because recent *H. pylori* suppression without
eradication can lead to false negative results.

Testing for *H. pylori* may not be required in those ulcer patients
in whom the likelihood of *H. pylori* is very high.   In particular,
patients with previously diagnosed duodenal ulcers with no history of
NSAID use, no signs or symptoms of a hypersecretory state, and no
history of antimicrobial treatment that might have cured a past
infection, may not require testing for *H. pylori* (Walsh and Peterson,
1995) but may instead be candidates for empiric treatment.   In patients
with gastric ulcers, or those who are taking NSAIDs, however, the
prevalence of *H. pylori* is lower and testing to identify or exclude *H.
pylori* is indicated (Walsh and Peterson, 1995).

TREATMENT

Uncomplicated PUD

Management of uncomplicated PUD centers around removal of the
identified cause (usually *H. pylori* or NSAIDs) and antiulcer therapy.
Removal of contributing factors, such as cigarette smoking, has an
ancillary role.

Antiulcer Therapy

Regardless of specific treatment for *H. pylori* or cessation of
NSAID use, conventional ulcer therapy should be used for a minimum of
four weeks to facilitate symptom relief and healing in documented ulcers
(Indicator 6) (Soll, 1996).

There is no persuasive evidence to unequivocally favor one
antiulcer regimen over another.   Many randomized trials have shown
comparable efficacy in treatment of duodenal ulcer for antacids,
sucralfate, proton pump inhibitors (omeprazol or Prilosec), and H2
receptor antagonists such as cimetidine (Tagamet), ranitidine (Zantac),
famotidine (Pepsid), and nizatidine (Axid) (Soll, 1996).   Two meta-
analyses and one large multicenter trial have found statistically more
effective healing and a higher rate of symptom relief with omeprazole
than with H2 receptor antagonists used to treat duodenal ulcers (Parent,
1994); however, there is no consensus that a difference in clinical
efficacy is adequate to recommend omeprazole over other agents.   Full

doses of H2 receptor antagonists offer effective initial therapy for gastric ulcers. Proton pump inhibitors and probably sucralfate, while not approved for gastric ulcer treatment in the U.S., may be effective alternatives (Soll, 1996).

Four weeks is a reasonable minimum treatment duration. Twenty percent of duodenal ulcers fail to heal after four weeks of standard therapy. If treatment is continued for another four to eight weeks, ulcers will heal in 90 to 95 percent of patients. In patients who have failed *H. pylori* treatment, and perhaps in those who are *H. pylori* negative, treatment should probably be continued for six months, since most ulcer recurrences occur within this time (Soll, 1996).

NSAID-Associated Ulcers

In a patient with documented PUD who is taking NSAIDs, it is generally agreed that NSAIDs should be discontinued where possible, and the patient should be reassessed (Soll, 1996). This was reflected in Indicator 5 and no additional indicator is proposed.

H. pylori-Positive Ulcers

Recognition of the role of *H. pylori* in the pathogenesis of ulcer disease is recent, and new management strategies are in rapid flux. Broad spectrum antibiotic treatment is not without side effects (Hawkey, 1994). Therefore, in patients with peptic ulceration confirmed on endoscopy, *H. pylori* testing should be documented and recorded in the medical record before initiation of *H. pylori* treatment (Indicator 7). Because the presence of *H. pylori* predicts ulcer recurrence (Coghlan et al., 1987), and treatment of *H. pylori* hastens resolution of ulceration (Hosking et al., 1994) and reduces the ulcer relapse rate (Marshall et al., 1988) in randomized controlled trials, *H. pylori* eradication treatment should be initiated on endoscopic evidence of ulceration, and serological or pathologic evidence of *H. pylori* (Indicator 8). Many antibiotic regimens for treatment of *H. pylori* have been reported. These vary in cost, duration, side effects, and efficacy (Taylor et al., 1997). There is no evidence to support one regimen over all others (Taylor et al., 1997), and new regimens with adequate efficacy may soon be added to the list. At present, regimens should include at least two antibiotics with either colloidal bismuth (bismuth subsalicylate or

Pepto Bismol) or antisecretory agents (Soll, 1996). Common regimens include bismuth and metronidazole combined with either tetracycline or amoxicillin, with or without omeprazole; or omeprazole with any two out of the following three antibiotics: metronidazole, amoxicillin, or clarithromycin (Soll, 1996; Taylor et al., 1997).

Smoking Cessation

Data obtained in patients before the era of routine testing and treatment for *H. pylori* indicated that smoking impedes ulcer healing (Hixson et al., 1992; Ziller and Netchvolodoff, 1993; Rex, 1994; Soll, 1996). Healing rates in heavy smokers (those who smoke more than 1 1/2 packs per day) were about one-half the rates seen in nonsmokers after eight weeks of therapy with an H2 blocker (Rex, 1994). In addition, following standard antiulcer treatment (before *H. pylori* eradication therapy), nonsmokers not on maintenance therapy had an ulcer relapse rate of 40 to 50 percent at one year, whereas heavy smokers had a relapse rate of 100 percent at three months. However, there is no evidence that smoking cessation provides benefit (reduction of recurrence or complications) in patients for whom *H. pylori* eradication therapy is available. There is also no independent evidence of benefit for smoking cessation with NSAID-associated ulcers. Therefore, although it is appropriate to give strong recommendations to discontinue smoking to all patients, there is no evidence of selective benefit from smoking cessation in the context of current PUD management.

Gastric Ulceration

If gastric ulceration is noted on endoscopy, biopsy should be performed to exclude gastric cancer. Either multiple biopsies should be obtained at the time of initial endoscopy, or follow-up endoscopy for gastric ulceration is indicated to confirm healing. If the ulcer persists, multiple biopsies should again be obtained to exclude gastric cancer (Soll, 1996) (Indicators 9, 10).

Complicated PUD

Complicated PUD is defined to include PUD with associated bleeding, perforation, or obstruction. Gastrointestinal bleeding is the most common of these complications. Management in patients with complicated PUD should also include the following.

Diagnosis

Emergency endoscopy: Endoscopy should be performed on an emergent basis, that is, within 12 hours, if nasogastric or orogastric lavage indicates continuous bleeding. In five percent of cases, active bleeding continues and the mortality rate in these instances approaches 30 percent.

Urgent endoscopy: There is consensus that endoscopy should be performed in patients presenting with GI bleeding with evidence of marked or continuing hemodynamic instability, despite adequate resuscitation efforts. However, because it is difficult to ascertain continuing hemodynamic instability from medical records, we will not address this area specifically in an indicator. Endoscopy can be justified in most cases of upper GI bleed, on the grounds that: 1) superficial lesions may heal quickly, and be missed with later endoscopy; 2) multiple lesions are present in approximately 25 percent of cases, and early endoscopy can identify the lesion actually responsible for the bleeding; and, most important, 3) endoscopy can identify subjects likely to rebleed, allowing them to be treated more aggressively. Although bleeding from peptic ulcers ceases spontaneously and does not recur in 70 to 80 percent of cases, rebleeding does occur in approximately 25 percent of cases, with a mortality well above ten percent (Qureshi and Netchvolodoff, 1993).

Endoscopic Therapy

Several types of endoscopic treatment are available, including Nd:Yag laser, heater probe, bipolar (Bicap) electrode, or injection treatment with agents such as hypertonic saline, epinephrine, or pure ethanol (Sugawa and Joseph, 1992; Qureshi and Netchvolodoff, 1993). Injection treatment achieves permanent hemostasis in more than 80 percent of cases (Qureshi and Netchvolodoff, 1993); however, studies and meta-analyses comparing these techniques have not consistently shown any one to be superior (Sacks et al., 1990; Sugawa and Joseph, 1992).

Not all patients with internal bleeding require endoscopic treatment or, where endoscopic treatment is not available, surgery.

Whether or not patients require such treatment is based in part on the risk of recurrent upper GI bleeding, as assessed by endoscopic findings (Qureshi and Netchvolodoff 1993). The risk of recurrent bleeding is less than two percent for those with a clean ulcer base; less than 10 percent for those with a black or red spot; 35 percent for those with oozing from an adherent clot; 40 percent with a nonbleeding visible vessel or "sentinel clot" (a pigmented protuberance that represents a fibrin clot plugging a side hole in an artery that runs parallel to the base of the ulcer) (NIH Consensus Statement, 1989); 80 percent with a visible vessel and hypotension; and approximately 100 percent with active bleeding (Qureshi and Netchvolodoff, 1993). Endoscopic treatment was shown to reduce further bleeding, surgery, and mortality in patients with high-risk endoscopic features of active bleeding or nonbleeding visible vessels in two meta-analyses of 25 and 30 randomized controlled trials (Sacks et al., 1990; Cook et al., 1992). This has buttressed the belief, previously articulated in the 1989 NIH Consensus Statement on therapeutic endoscopy and bleeding ulcers, that endoscopic treatment is merited if there is active oozing or spurting of blood, or a visible vessel (Qureshi and Netchvolodoff, 1993) (Indicator 11). Surgery is an acceptable alternative where endoscopic therapy is not available. Data for ulcers with a clean base or for nonbleeding ulcers with an adherent clot do not show clear evidence of benefit with endoscopic treatment.

H. pylori Testing and Treatment

Bleeding ulcers differ from uncomplicated peptic ulcers in that up to 25 percent of patients with bleeding ulcers who are not taking NSAIDs may not be infected with *H. pylori*; therefore, the presence of infection should be documented before eradication is attempted (Laine and Peterson, 1994). Thus, in patients with ulcer complication not documented to be associated with NSAIDs, *H. pylori* testing should be performed. This may be done by obtaining specimens for histology at the time of endoscopy, or if this is not done, by serological testing (provided the patient has not received prior eradication therapy). *H. pylori* eradication in patients with complicated PUD has been shown to reduce the rate of rebleeding in randomized controlled trials (Graham et al., 1993; Rokkas et al., 1995). In those who test positive for *H.*

pylori, an eradication regimen for *H. pylori* should be initiated (Indicator 12).

FOLLOW-UP

Confirmation of *H. pylori* Eradication

Confirmation of successful *H. pylori* cure by endoscopic biopsy or urease breath test is important in patients with a history of ulcers complicated by bleeding, perforation, or obstruction, or ulcers that recur after *H. pylori* eradication therapy (Soll, 1996) (Indicator 13). Successful eradication of *H. pylori* has been clearly shown to reduce bleeding recurrences, while *H. pylori* persistence after therapy is associated with continued risk of rebleeding (Labenz and Borsch, 1994). Confirmation of eradication remains controversial in patients with uncomplicated ulcers who remain asymptomatic after antibiotic therapy (Soll, 1996).

Maintenance Therapy

Maintenance therapy with H2 receptor antagonists is indicated in high-risk patients with PUD who have *H. pylori*-negative ulcers or who fail *H. pylori* cure. Efficacy of maintenance therapy has not been explicitly tested in these groups, but is presumed to parallel that of patients evaluated before *H. pylori* testing was available, most of whom were likely to have been *H. pylori*-positive. Maintenance therapy has been shown to reduce duodenal ulcer recurrences at one year from 60 to 90 percent to 20 to 25 percent (Soll, 1996). The risk of subsequent recurrent ulceration after initial healing is not diminished after completing one year of maintenance therapy; however, continued maintenance therapy with H2 blockers remains effective in reducing ulcer recurrence for two to five years. Because no data are yet available in the populations for whom maintenance treatment would currently be considered, there is no consensus regarding duration of maintenance treatment. Because the relevant populations are a small subset of ulcer patients, no indicator has been generated regarding use of maintenance therapy.

Review of Follow-up Treatment

In subjects with an ulcer history requiring maintenance therapy, and in those with past ulcer complications, *H. pylori* identification should be pursued (Soll, 1996) (Indicator 14). As previously noted, *H. pylori* identification followed by *H. pylori* eradication reduces ulcer recurrence (Marshall et al., 1988), negates the need for maintenance treatment in most individuals, and reduces the rate of rebleeding in those with a history of bleeding ulcer (Graham et al., 1993; Labenz and Borsch, 1994; Jaspersen et al., 1995; Rokkas et al., 1995).

REFERENCES

Barker, L, J Burton, et al. 1991. Principles of Ambulatory Medicine. Baltimore: Williams and Wilkins.

Bateson M. 1993. Cigarette smoking and Helicobacter pylori infection. *Postgraduate Medical Journal* 69 (807): 41-44.

Bianchi PG, I Caruso, et al. 1991. A double-blind gastroscopic evaluation of the effects of etodolac and naptoxcen on the gastrointestinal mucosa of rheumatic patients. *Journal of Internal Medicine* 229: 5-8.

Bytzer P, J Hansen, et al. 1994. Empirical H2 blocker therapy or prompt endoscopy in the management of dyspepsia. *Gastrointestinal Endoscopy* 41 (5): 529-532.

Bytzer P, J Hansen, et al. 1996. Predicting endoscopic diagnosis in the dyspeptic patient: the value of clinical judgement. *European Journal of Gastroenterology and Hepatology* 8 (4): 359-63.

Cave D. 30 September 1992. Therapeutic approaches to recurrent peptic ulcer disease. *Hospital Practice* 33-49.

Chou S. 1994. An examination of the alcohol consumption and peptic ulcer association -- results of a national survey. *Alcoholism, Clinical and Experimental Research* 18 (1): 149-53.

Clearfield H. 1992. Management of NSAID-induced ulcer disease. *American Family Physician* 45: 255-258.

Coghlan J, D Gilligan, et al. 1987. Campylobacter pylori and recurrence of duodenal ulcers; a 12-month follow-up. *Lancet* 1109-1111.

Cook D, Guyatt G, et al. 1992. Endoscopic therapy for acute nonvariceal upper gastrointestinal hemoorhage; A meta-analysis. *Gastroenterology* 102: 139-148.

DePriest J. 1995. Stress ulcer prophylaxis: Do critically ill patients need it? *Postgraduate Medicine* 98 (4): 159-168.

Ebell M. 1992. Peptic ulcer disease. *American Family Physician* 46 (1): 217-227.

Feldman M and W Peterson. 1993. Helicobacter pylori and peptic ulcer disease. *Western Journal of Medicine* 159: 555-559.

Graham D, K Hepps, et al. 1993. Treatment of Helicobacter pylori reduces the rate of rebleeding in peptic ulcer disease. *Scandinavian Journal of Gastroenterology* 28: 939-942.

Griffin M, W Ray, et al. 1988. Nonsteroidal anti-inflammatory drug use and death from peptic ulcer in elderly persons. *Archives of Internal Medicine* 109: 359-363.

Griffin M, J Piper, et al. 1991. Nonsteroidal anti-inflammatory drug use and increased risk for peptic ulcer disease in elderly persons. *Archives of Internal Medicine* 114 (14): 257-263.

Hawkey C. 1994. Eradication of Helicobacter pylori should be pivotal in managing peptic ulceration. *British Medical Journal* 309: 1570-1571.

Hixson L, C Kelley, et al. 1992. Current trends in the pharmacotherapy for peptic ulcer disease. *Archives of Internal Medicine* 152: 726-732.

Hosking S, T Ling, et al. 1994. Duodenal ulcer healing by eradication of Helicobacter pylori without antacid treatment: randomised controlled trial. *Lancet* 343: 508-510.

Jaspersen D, T Koerner, et al. 1995. Helicobacter pylori eradication reduces the rate of rebleeding in ulcer hemorrhage. *Gastrointestinal endoscopy* 41 (1): 5-7.

Jiranek G, and R Kozarek. 1996. A cost-effective approach to the patient with peptic ulcer bleeding. *Surgical Clinics of North America* 76 (1): 83-103.

Labenz J and G Borsch. 1994. Role of Helicobacter pylori eradication in the prevention of peptic ulcer bleeding relapse. *Digestion* 55: 19-23.

Laine L and W Peterson. 1994. Bleeding peptic ulcer. *New England Journal of Medicine* 331 (11): 717-727.

Lanas A, Remacha B, et al. 1995. Risk factors associated with refractory peptic ulcers. *Gastroenterology* 109 (4): 1124-33.

Larkai E, J Smith, et al. 1989. Dyspepsia in NSAID users: the size of the problem. *Journal of Clinical Gastroenterology* 11 (2): 158-162.

Lee M. 1995. Prevention and treatment of nonsteroidal anti-inflammatory drug-induced gastropathy. *Southern Medical Journal* 88 (5): 507-513.

Loeb D, D Ahlquist, et al. 1992. Management of gastroduodenopathy associated with use of nonsteroidal anti-inflammatory drugs. *Mayo Clinic Proceedings* 67: 354-64.

Marshall B, C Goodwin, et al. 24 December 1988. Prospective double-blind trial of duodenal ulcer relapse after eradication of campylobacter pylori. *Lancet* 1437-1441.

Muris J, R Starmans, et al. 1994. Discriminant value of symptoms in patients with dyspepsia. *The Journal of Family Practice* 38 (2): 139-143.

NIH Consensus Development Panel on Helicobacter pylori in Peptic Ulcer Disease. 1994. Helicobacter pylori in peptic ulcer disease. *Journal of the American Medical Association* 272 (1): 65-69.

NIH Consensus Statement. 1989. Therapeutic endoscopy and bleeding ulcers. *Journal of the American Medical Association* 262: 1369-72.

Parent K. 1994. Acid reduction in peptic ulcer disease. *Postgraduate Medicine* 96 (4): 53-59.

Pound S and R Heading. 1995. Diagnosis and treatment of dyspepsia in the elderly. *Drugs & Aging* 7 (6): 347-354.

Qureshi W and Netchvolodoff C. 1993. Acute bleeding from peptic ulcers. *Postgraduate Medicine* 93 (4): 167-177.

Rex D. 1994. An etiologic approach to management of duodenal and gastric ulcers. *Journal of Family Practice* 38 (1): 60-67.

Rokkas T, A Karameris, et al. 1995. Eradication of Helicobacter pylori reduces the possibility of rebleeding in peptic ulcer disease. *Gastrointestinal Endoscopy* 41 (4): 1-4.

Sacks H, T Chalmers, et al. 1990. Endoscopic hemostasis: An effective therapy for bleeding peptic ulcers. *Journal of the American Medical Association* 264: 494-499.

Silverstein, M, T Petterson, et al. 1996. Initial endoscopy or empirical therapy with or without Helicobacter pylori for dyspepsia: a decision analysis. *Gastroenterology* 110: 72-83.

Soll A. 1996. Medical treatment of peptic ulcer disease: Practice guidelines. *Journal of the American Medical Association* 275 (8): 622-29.

Sugawa C and A Joseph. 1992. Endoscopic interventional management of bleeding duodenal and gastric ulcers. *Gastric Surgery* 72 (2): 317-333.

Talley N. 1993. Nonulcer dyspepsia: current approaches to diagnosis and management. *American Family Physician* 47 (6): 1407-1416.

Talley N, A Zinsmeister, et al. 1994. Smoking, alcohol, and analgesics in dyspepsia and among dyspepsia subgroups: lack of an association in a community. *Gut* 35 (5): 619-624.

Taylor J, M Zagari, et al. 1997. Pharmacoeconomic comparison of treatments for the eradication of Helicobacter pylori. *Archives of Internal Medicine* 157: 87-97.

Walsh J and W Peterson. 1995. The treatment of Helicobacter pylori infection in the management of peptic ulcer disease. *New England Journal of Medicine* 333 (15): 984-991.

Walt R. 1992. Misoprostol for the treatment of peptic ulcer and antinflammatory-drug-induced gastroduodenal ulceration. *New England Journal of Medicine* 327 (22): 1575-1580.

Ziller S and C Netchvolodoff. 1993. Uncomplicated peptic ulcer disease. *Postgraduate Medicine* 93 (4): 126-138.

RECOMMENDED QUALITY INDICATORS FOR DYSPEPSIA AND PEPTIC ULCER DISEASE

The following indicators apply to men and women age 18 and older with dyspepsia or PUD.

Indicator	Quality of Evidence	Literature	Benefits	Comments
Dyspepsia: Diagnosis				
1. Patients presenting with a new episode of dyspepsia[1] should have the presence or absence of NSAID[2] use noted in the medical record on the date of presentation.	II-2	Lee, 1995; Clearfield, 1992; Rex, 1994; Walt, 1992; Bianchi-Porro, 1991; Larkai, 1989; Ebell, 1992; Loeb, 1992; Griffin, 1991, 1988	Reduce dyspeptic symptoms. Reduce development of ulcers and ulcer complications.	Use of NSAIDs[2] increases symptoms of dyspepsia, risk of erosions and ulcers, and PUD complications.
Dyspepsia: Treatment of Non NSAID-Associated Dyspepsia				
2. Patients prescribed empiric antiulcer treatment[3] for dyspepsia who were not using NSAIDs[2] within the previous month should have at least one of the following within 8 weeks: • documentation in medical record that symptoms have improved; • endoscopy; • H. pylori test.[4]	III	Soll, 1996; NIH, 1994	Direct effective treatment. Reduce symptoms and complications of PUD.	To guide successful therapy (e.g., for *H. pylori*) and thereby prevent complications, identification of the cause is needed when empiric treatment fails.

284

Indicator	Quality of Evidence	Literature	Benefits	Comments
3. Patients with new dyspepsia[1] who have any of the following "alarm" indicators on the date of presentation should have endoscopy performed within 1 month, unless endoscopy has been performed in the previous 6 months: a. anemia;[5] b. early satiety; c. significant unintentional weight loss (exceeding 15 pounds in the past 3 months); d. guaiac-positive stool; e. dysphagia; f. over age 60.	II-2 III	Soll, 1996	Detect gastric cancer. Direct correct treatment. Reduce morbidity from ulcer complications.	Patients over age 60 and those with "alarm" symptoms have an increased incidence of positive findings on endoscopy. Older patients may be more likely to have gastric cancer, which can be treated if detected early.
4. Patients who are prescribed *H. pylori* eradication antibiotic treatment[6] within 3 months after presentation for a new episode of dyspepsia[1] should have one of the following noted in the medical record before start of antibiotic treatment: • prior positive test for H. pylori;[4] • both a history of documented duodenal ulcer and absence of NSAID[2] use.	III	Hawkey, 1994; Soll, 1996; Walsh, 1995	Prevent drug side effects.	Antibiotic treatment is not without risks, and treatment should not be given without prior testing except in cases where the probability of *H. pylori* as a causal agent is extremely high.

285

Indicator	Quality of Evidence	Literature	Benefits	Comments
Peptic Ulcer Disease: Secondary and Tertiary Prevention				
5. For patients with endoscopically documented PUD who have been noted to use NSAIDs[2] within 2 months before endoscopy, the medical record should indicate, within 2 months before or 1 month after endoscopy, one of the following: • a reason why NSAIDs[2] or aspirin will be continued; • advice to the patient to discontinue NSAIDs[2] or aspirin.	II-2	Clearfield, 1992; Lee, 1995	Reduce symptoms of dyspepsia. Reduce ulcer occurrence. Reduce hospitalization. Reduce mortality.	Use of NSAIDs[2] increases risk of ulcer, hospitalization for ulcer, PUD complications,[8] and delay of healing in existing ulcer.
Peptic Ulcer Disease: Treatment of Uncomplicated PUD				
6. Patients in whom peptic ulceration is confirmed on endoscopy should have antiulcer treatment[3] for a minimum of 4 weeks.	III	Soll, 1996	Assist ulcer healing. Reduce symptoms.	Antiulcer treatment[3] should be provided to assist ulcer healing even if specific therapy is given (e.g., H. pylori eradication treatment[6]).
7. Patients with endoscopically confirmed gastric or duodenal ulcer should have H. pylori testing[4] within 3 months before or 1 month after endoscopy, unless the medical record, in the same time period, documents a past positive H. pylori test[4] for which no H. pylori eradication treatment[6] was given.	III	Marshall, 1988; Graham, 1993	Prevent recurrence. Prevent side effects.	Testing allows identification or exclusion of H. pylori, which permits initiation of effective treatment to prevent recurrence, or avoidance of such treatment and its attendant side effects.
8. Eradication therapy for H. pylori should be offered within 1 month when all of the following conditions are met: • documentation of history of positive H. pylori test at any time in the past; • documentation of endoscopically confirmed ulceration of the duodenum at any time in the past.	I	Coghlan, 1987; Marshall, 1988	Prevent recurrence.	Recurrence of duodenal ulcer is predicted by presence of H. pylori. Recurrence of duodenal and gastric ulcer is markedly decreased after eradication of H. pylori infection.

286

Indicator	Quality of Evidence	Literature	Benefits	Comments
Peptic Ulcer Disease: Treatment				
9. Patients with a gastric ulcer confirmed by endoscopy should have one of the following: • a minimum of 3 biopsies during endoscopy; • follow-up endoscopy within 3 months.	III	Soll, 1996	Detect and treat gastric cancer.	Gastric ulceration and *H. pylori* are associated with increased incidence of gastric cancer. Failure to heal (identified on follow-up endoscopy) may indicate presence of gastric cancer, and biopsies should be obtained to exclude this possibility. It is preferable that follow-up endoscopy occur at least 4 weeks after discontinuing antibiotics, proton pump inhibitors, or bismuth if repeat *H. pylori* testing[4] will be performed.
10. Patients with endoscopically documented gastric ulcer who have follow-up endoscopy within 6 months should have one of the following at the follow-up endoscopy: • complete healing of the gastric ulcer noted; • a minimum of 3 biopsies of the ulcer.	III	Soll, 1996	Identify gastric cancer. Treat early gastric cancer.	Gastric ulceration that fails to heal may represent gastric carcinoma, which requires different treatment than does PUD alone. Gastric cancer may be cured if identified early.
Peptic Ulcer Disease: Treatment of Complicated Peptic Ulcer Disease				
11. Patients with endoscopically documented PUD should be offered endoscopic treatment[7] or surgery within the next 24 hours if either of the following are documented in the endoscopy note: a. continued oozing, bleeding, or spurting of blood; b. a visible vessel (or "pigmented protuberance").	I III	Sacks, 1990; Cook, 1992; NIH Consensus Statement, 1989	Reduce rebleeding. Reduce blood transfusions. Reduce need for emergency surgery. Improve survival.	A meta-analysis showed that endoscopic treatment reduced further bleeding, surgery, and mortality in patients with high-risk features of active bleeding or nonbleeding visible vessels.

287

	Indicator	Quality of Evidence	Literature	Benefits	Comments
12.	Patients with a documented PUD complication[8] who have had a positive H. pylori test[4] within 3 months after the complication should be started on an H. pylori eradication regimen[6] within 1 month of the positive test.	I	Marshall, 1988; Labenz, 1994; Graham, 1993; Rokkas, 1995; Jaspersen, 1995	Reduce symptoms. Reduce rebleeding.	Identification and treatment of H. pylori reduces recurrences of H. pylori-associated bleeding ulcers. Testing may be warranted even in the presence of NSAID use.

Peptic Ulcer Disease: Follow-up

	Indicator	Quality of Evidence	Literature	Benefits	Comments
13.	Patients with endoscopically confirmed PUD whose symptoms of dyspepsia or documented ulcers recur within 6 months after eradication therapy for H. pylori should receive confirmatory testing for successful H. pylori cure by endoscopic biopsy or urease breath test within 1 month of symptom recurrence.	II	Soll, 1996; Labenz, 1994	Reduce symptoms and complications from PUD.	Patients in whom symptoms recur may have continued H. pylori infection. Complications are reduced with successful H. pylori eradication.
14.	Patients with a history of PUD complications[8] in the past year should have results of H. pylori testing[4] documented in the medical record in the same time period.	I	Marshall, 1988; Labenz, 1994; Graham, 1993; Rokkas, 1995; Jaspersen, 1995	Prevent ulcer recurrence and rebleeding.	H. pylori treatment reduces rebleeding in PUD. Those with past complications should receive testing, and, where indicated, treatment for H. pylori.

Definitions and Examples

[1] New episode of dyspepsia: first visit for dyspepsia ever; or first visit for dyspepsia symptoms in the past year. Documentation of new onset or duration less than 3 months counts as a new episode.

[2] NSAIDs: Nonsteroidal antiinflammatory drugs. Selected short-acting NSAIDs include aspirin, diclofenac (Voltaren), ibuprofen (Advil, Motrin, Nuprin), indomethacin (Indocin), ketoprofen (Orudis), and tolmetin (Tolectin) (Clearfield, 1992). Selected long-acting NSAIDs include diflunisal (Dolobid), naproxen (Naprosyn), phenylbutazone (Butazolidin), piroxican (Feldene), and sulindac (Clinoril) (Clearfield, 1992).

[3] Antiulcer treatment may include sucralfate (Carafate); H2 receptor antagonists such as cimetidine (Tagamet), ranitidine (Zantac), famotidine (Pepsid), and nizatidine (Axid); proton pump inhibitors such as omeprazole (Prilosec); and antacids such as aluminum hydroxide, magnesium hydroxide, calcium carbonate, and sodium bicarbonate (Ebell, 1992).

[4] H. pylori test may include the following: serological test; 13-C or 14-C Urea breath test (may not be available commercially); endoscopy with gastic biopsy, followed by histological demonstration of organisms (Giemsa or Warthin-Starry stains or Hematoxylin and Eosin), direct detection of urease activity in the tissue specimen, or biopsy with culture of the H. pylori organism (NIH Consensus Conference, 1994).

[5] Anemia: Hematocrit less than 35 not due to other known cause.

[6] *H. pylori* eradication treatment: Antibiotic regimen including bismuth or omeprazole with at least two of the following: flagyl, ampicillin, tetracycline, or clarithromycin. Examples: BMT (1-2 wk); BMTO (1 wk); BMA (1-2 wk); MOA (1-2 wk); (B = Bismuth subsalicylate, 2 tab qid with meals and at bedtime; T = Tetracycline, 500 mg qid with meals and at bedtime; M = metronidazole, 250 or 500 mg qid with meals and at bedtime; C = clarithromycin, 500 mg bid or tid with meals; A = amoxicillin (not ampicillin), 500 mg or 1 gm qid with meals and at bedtime; O = 20 mg bid before meals).

[7] Endoscopic treatment may include laser treatment; injection treatment with saline, ethanol, epinephrine, or polidocanol; or thermal treatment such as heater probe or bicap (bipolar electrocoagulation)

[8] PUD complications are bleeding, perforation, or obstruction.

Quality of Evidence Codes

I	RCT
II-1	Nonrandomized controlled trials
II-2	Cohort or case analysis
II-3	Multiple time series
III	Opinions or descriptive studies

289

19. PREVENTIVE CARE[1]

Patricia Bellas, MD

For this chapter, we relied on the second edition of the *Guide to Clinical Preventive Services: A Report of the U.S. Preventive Services Task Force* (USPSTF, 1996) and the *CDC Prevention Guidelines: A Guide to Action* (CDC, 1997). A MEDLINE search was done on specific topics from 1993 to 1997. Additional references were obtained from the bibliographies of key articles.

IMPORTANCE

The importance of incorporating preventive care into health care practices has been supported by many medical authorities (USPSTF, 1996; USPHS, 1991). Primary prevention with immunizations has led to a reduction in many infectious diseases and their associated morbidity and mortality. Use of screening tests for early detection of diseases and or risk factors (such as cholesterol levels) have also been associated with substantial reductions in morbidity and mortality. The findings of the second USPSTF report (1996) highlight the promising role of assisting patients in changing personal health behaviors such as smoking, physical activity, poor nutrition, alcohol and other drug use, sexual practices and inadequate attention to safety precautions. These behaviors are risk factors for the leading causes of disease and disability in the United States (McGinnis and Foege, 1993). Although evidence to support the effectiveness of clinician counseling is limited, the USPSTF believes that "clinician counseling that leads to improved personal health practices may be more valuable to patients than conventional clinical activities such as diagnostic testing."

---

[1] This chapter is a revision of one written for an earlier project on quality of care for women and children (Q1). The expert panel for the current project was asked to review all of the indicators, but only rated new or revised indicators.

In deciding what constitutes necessary or inappropriate preventive care, experts have recommended evaluating three areas: 1) the burden of suffering associated with the condition, 2) the accuracy and acceptability of screening tests, and 3) the efficacy of treatment (or intervention) at the pre-clinical state versus treatment after the disease manifests itself (Hayward, 1991). In addition to these criteria, we have also evaluated the feasibility of operationalizing recommended indicators for this topic.[2] Topics to be included in this include immunizations, screening for tuberculosis (PPD screening), screening for hearing loss, screening for obesity, STD and HIV prevention counseling, seat belt use counseling, nutrition counseling, and counseling to promote physical activity. Other preventive services are covered elsewhere. Many of these preventive services can and should be included as part of visits that occur for other reasons than pure prevention. Each preventive service and indicator is examined in terms of its importance and efficacy/effectiveness.

IMMUNIZATIONS

The CDC and the American College of Physicians (ACP) Task Force on Adult Immunizations have published schedules and indications for adult vaccinations. Despite these recommendations, immunization compliance in adults is generally poor and many vaccine preventable deaths (see Table 19.1). We will review each vaccine below.

---

[2] Operationalization of a counseling indicator depends on documentation in a progress note unless a specific check list or computer field is used; we believe that in some cases appropriate counseling or risk assessment may be performed but not documented.

Table 19.1

Adult Vaccine Utilization and Preventable Deaths

Disease	Estimated Annual Deaths	Estimated Vaccine Efficacy*	Current Vaccine Utilization	Additional Preventable Deaths/Year
Tetanus-diphtheria	<25	99%	40%	<15
Influenza	20,000	70%	30%	9,800
Pneumococcal infection	40,000	60%	14%	20,640
Hepatitis B	5,000	90%	10%	4,050
Measles, mumps, rubella	<30	95%	variable	<30

*Efficacy in immunocompetent adults. Among elderly and immunocompromised patients, efficacy is estimated to be lower.
Source: Gardner and Schaffner, 1993.

Tetanus

Tetanus, an acute infectious disease of the nervous system, is caused by the bacillus *Clostridium tetani*. It is characterized by spasms of the voluntary muscles and painful convulsions and may eventually lead to death. Death occurs in 26 to 31 percent of all cases.

Serosurveys undertaken since 1977 indicate that many U.S. adults are not protected against tetanus, and most cases of tetanus occur in the elderly; primarily in those who never completed a primary immunization series (Gardner and Schaffner, 1993). Despite this, tetanus is relatively rare. The CDC and ACP recommendations are summarized below:

1. Ensure completion of a primary series: If the person was not immunized in childhood, two doses of Td (tetanus/diphtheria toxoid) IM are recommended four weeks apart, with a third dose six to 12 months after the second dose.

2. Follow primary series with a booster every ten years (CDC) and update at age 50 if the person completed the standard five dose series in childhood (ACP). According to the Preventive Service task force, intervals of 15 to 30 years between boosters are likely to be adequate if a primary series was completed.

3. Promote Td boosters for patients with tetanus-prone wounds. Persons with clean, minor wounds do not need another booster if

they have completed the primary series and their most recent booster was in the past ten years; those with other wounds do not need another booster if they have completed the primary series and their most recent booster was in the past five years (Gardner and Schaffner, 1993)(Indicator 3).

4. Tetanus vaccination should be combined with diphtheria (adult Td).

In order to facilitate these goals, we recommend as a quality indicator that notation of the date that a patient received a tetanus/diphtheria booster be included in the medical record (Indicators 1 and 2).

Local side effects of this vaccine are not uncommon, but severe reactions are relatively rare. Contraindications to receiving the vaccine include an immediate hypersensitivity reaction following a previous dose or history of a severe local (Arthus-type) reaction following a previous dose. Because Arthus-type hypersensitivity reactions occur most commonly after multiple boosters, Td boosters should not be given to anyone who, within the previous five years, has either completed a primary series or received a booster dose (Gardner and Schaffner, 1993) (Indicator 3b).

Diphtheria

Diphtheria is caused by the bacterium *Corynebacterium diphtheriae*. Both toxigenic and nontoxigenic strains of *C. diphtheriae* can cause disease, but only strains that produce toxin cause myocarditis and neuritis. From 1980 to 1989 only 24 cases of respiratory diphtheria were reported; two cases were fatal and 18 (75%) occurred in persons 20 years of age or older (CDC, 1991).

Limited serosurveys indicate that 22 to 62 percent of adults 18 to 39 years of age and 41 to 84 percent of those greater than 60 years of age may lack protective levels of circulating antitoxin against diphtheria. A complete vaccination series substantially reduces the risk of developing diphtheria and those vaccinated who develop the disease have milder illnesses (CDC, 1991). Complete vaccination is at least 85 percent effective in preventing diphtheria. Recommended frequency of vaccination is the same as for tetanus (Indicator 1).

Influenza

Influenza is responsible for significant morbidity and mortality during epidemics. In the past 25 years there have been ten different epidemics with 20,000 or more excess deaths. Approximately 80 to 95 percent of these excess deaths occur in persons aged 65 and older. In addition to the elderly, other individuals at high risk of lower respiratory-tract complications and death after influenza infection include persons with 1) chronic diseases of the cardiovascular, pulmonary, and/or renal systems, 2) metabolic diseases such as diabetes, 3) severe anemia and/or 4) compromised immune function including HIV infection. In nursing homes, residents suffer with very high attack rates and high fatality rates during influenza epidemics (CDC, 1997).

Influenza vaccine contains an inactivated (killed-virus) vaccine that is 70 to 80 percent effective in preventing influenza illness or reducing severity of infection in healthy children and adults younger than 65. In the elderly, the vaccine prevents only 30 to 40 percent of influenza episodes (Govaert, 1994), but it appears to lessen severity of disease resulting in a decrease in hospital admissions and death. There is one randomized placebo-controlled trial which evaluated the vaccine's efficacy in persons over age 60. In this study, the vaccine reduced illness, although the effect was less pronounced in those over age 70 (Nichol et al., 1994; USPSTF, 1996). While its side effects and adverse reactions are usually mild, persons with a history of anaphylactic hypersensitivity to eggs should not receive this vaccine.

Evidence of efficacy in other high risk populations, including those with HIV is limited, and rates of vaccination in high risk target groups have generally been poor. It is recommended that health care workers and those who live or work with high risk persons also be immunized. In addition, any adult who wishes to avoid influenza illness may be vaccinated.

We recommend as a quality indicator that all adults aged 65 and older be offered an annual influenza immunization (Indicator 4). In addition, adults under age 65 with the following high risk conditions should be offered annual immunization (Indicator 5):

- Residents of nursing homes and other chronic care facilities that house persons with chronic medical conditions;

- Adults with chronic disorders of the pulmonary or cardiovascular systems;

- Adults who have required regular medical follow-up or hospitalization during the preceding year because of chronic metabolic diseases, renal dysfunction, hemoglobinopathies or immunosuppression (CDC, 1997).

Pneumococcal Vaccine

Pneumococcal disease is a significant cause of morbidity and mortality in the U.S. Incidence rates are highest in the very young, those over age 65, African-Americans, Native Americans, nursing home residents, alcoholics, and those with underlying chronic medical or immunodeficient conditions. The highest case-fatality rates occur in elderly persons and those with co-morbid conditions (USPSTF, 1996). Emergence of antibiotic resistant strains of streptococcus pneumoniae are expected to increase the number of deaths due to invasive pneumococcal disease.

The current polysaccharide vaccine contains the 23 serotypes which are responsible for 88 percent of the isolates causing bacteremia in the U.S. It has an excellent safety record, although mild local reactions are not uncommon. The vaccine should be given once; although uncertainty regarding previous immunization status is not a reason to withhold vaccination from a high risk person.

Literature to support the efficacy of the pneumococcal vaccine has been conflicting. Meta-analysis of randomized controlled trials have failed to show a consistent beneficial effect in reducing either all cause mortality or mortality due to pneumonia, although there was a decrease in pneumococcal bacteremia (Fine, 1994). In other studies of varying quality, the vaccine has been found to be 47 to 70 percent effective in preventing pneumonia, although a large case control study by Shapiro et al (1991) found it much less effective in immunocompromised patients. Epidemiologic studies by the CDC also suggest an efficacy of 60 to 64 percent for vaccine type strains; again, this was lower in the elderly and for those with co-morbid conditions. However, many authorities, including the CDC, believe that the data continue to support the use of the pneumococcal vaccine for the following risk groups (CDC, 1997; USPSTF, 1996) (Indicator 6):

1. Immunocompetent adults who are at increased risk of pneumococcal disease or its complications because of chronic illnesses (cardiopulmonary disease, diabetes, anatomic asplenia, alcoholism[3], cirrhosis or CSF leaks) or who are age 65 or older, or institutionalized and over age 50.

2. Immunocompromised adults at increased risk of pneumococcal disease or its complications (Hodgkin's disease, lymphoma, multiple myeloma, chronic renal failure or nephrotic syndrome)

3. Adults with asymptomatic or symptomatic HIV infection.[4]

Hepatitis B

Each year approximately 300,000 persons, primarily young adults are infected with hepatitis B. About 5,000 persons die annually from hepatitis B related fulminant hepatitis, cirrhosis and liver cancer. There are estimated to be 1 to 1.25 million persons in the U.S. who are chronic HBV carriers. The sources of infection for most cases are intravenous drug use (28%), heterosexual contact with infected persons or multiple partners (22%), and homosexual activity (9%); however, 30 percent of infected persons deny any of these risks. Attempts to vaccinate high risk groups have failed and the United States now uses the strategy of universally immunizing of infants.

The current vaccines for hepatitis B licensed in the U.S. include a plasma derived vaccine and a recombinant vaccine. The recommended series

---

[3] Some studies have not found the vaccine effective in those with alcoholism or cirrhosis (Ortiz, 1994)

[4] There is limited information on efficacy of pneumococcal vaccine in HIV infected patients.

of three injections have been shown to be 80 to 95 percent effective in
preventing infection among susceptible persons. Hemodialysis and other
immunosuppressed patients need higher doses or increased number of doses to
obtain adequate antibody response. Those with HIV infection may also need
differing doses, but a specific recommended schedule has not yet been
defined (CDC, 1997). Testing for immunity is not routinely recommended,
but may be advisable for dialysis patients and staff, or those for whom a
suboptimal response may be anticipated or who may be at occupational risk.
Revaccination with one or more additional doses should be considered for
non-responders to the primary series, as up to 50 percent may subsequently
develop adequate antibody response. In the absence of serologic evidence
of immunity, the CDC and USPSTF recommend vaccinating the following high
risk groups (CDC, 1996; USPSTF, 1996) (Indicator 7):

- Those with occupational risk, such as health care or public safety
  workers;
- Clients of residential institutions for the developmentally
  disabled, and staff of residential and day-care programs for the
  developmentally disabled;
- Hemodialysis patients;
- Sexually active homosexual men;
- Intravenous drug users;
- Patients who receive clotting-factor concentrates;
- Household and sexual contacts of HBV carriers;
- Inmates of long term correctional facilities;
- Sexually active heterosexual persons with multiple sexual
  partners;
- Those with another sexually transmitted disease.

Measles, Mumps, and Rubella

Measles is a viral illness which can be quite severe, especially in
adults. Death occurs in one per 1,000 reported measles cases, with the
risk of death being higher in infants and adults than children and
adolescents. Since introduction of a vaccine for measles in the 1960s, the
number of cases has fallen dramatically. However, there have been

increases in recent years, primarily in unimmunized preschool children, but also in young adults. In 1990, adults aged 20 and older accounted for 22 percent of the 28,000 cases of measles, and 28 percent of deaths due to measles (Gardner and Schaffner, 1993). The number of cases of rubella and mumps has also increased in recent years, with a specific increase among young adults.

The current measles vaccine is a live attenuated strain which may be administered by itself or combined with mumps and rubella (MMR). Two doses at least one month apart are recommended. Contraindications include history of an anaphylactic reaction to eggs or neomycin. Persons who are severely immunocompromised (excluding HIV infection) should not receive this vaccine.

Based on serologic surveys, persons born before 1957 are generally considered immune. Persons born in or after 1957 may be considered immune if they have laboratory evidence of measles immunity, documentation of a physician-diagnosed case of measles, or evidence of two live measles vaccinations. All other persons born in or after 1957 should be offered measles vaccine, preferably MMR. Persons at high risk of exposure to measles such as college students, healthcare workers, and day-care providers should be targeted to receive two vaccines at least one month apart. We recommend as a quality indicator that providers ask high risk patients about their measles immunization status (CDC, 1997; USPSTF, 1996) (Indicator 8).

SCREENING

PPD Screening

It is estimated that 10 to 15 million persons in the U.S. are infected with *Mycobacterium tuberculosis*. There is considerable morbidity and mortality from tuberculosis, with 24,000 reported cases in 1994; the case fatality rate is highest in the elderly, who comprise 25 percent of active cases. Two thirds of all cases occur in ethnic minorities (African-Americans, Hispanics, Asians and Pacific Islanders). About 30 percent of new cases occur in foreign-born immigrants (USPSTF, 1996). Prevalence of active tuberculosis infections is higher in those with HIV, chronic renal disease, or diabetes.

The purpose of TB screening is to identify asymptomatic infected persons who can be treated with chemoprophylaxis (INH) to prevent active disease. Approximately five to ten percent of persons with latent TB infections progress to active disease. This percentage is much higher in HIV positive persons. In addition, screening may find persons with active clinical disease in need of treatment. Tuberculin skin testing is the only available method of screening for latent infection. The Mantoux test is the preferred technique; five tuberculin units of purified protein derivative (PPD) are intracutaneously administered into the forearm with a check for induration (delayed hypersensitivity reaction) in 48 to 72 hours (Indicator 11). Interpretation of a positive or reactive test varies by defined risk group and is based on a minimum number of millimeters of induration (Indicator 10) (see Table 19.2). These classifications are based on probabilistic epidemiologic assessments of positive predictive values of the test when applied to populations with differing prevalence, risk, and background infection with non-tuberculous organisms (Gonzalez-Rothi, 1997). A false positive test may result from faulty technique in test interpretation, or from cross-reactions with antigens such as atypical mycobacterium or Bacillus Calmette-Guerin (BCG). False negative tests are estimated to occur in five to ten percent of patients and may result from severe illness, anergy, improper handling of PPD solution, or waning delayed hypersensitivity response if many years have passed since initial infection. Some authorities have recommended skin testing for anergy in high risk groups, but this is considered optional in recent CDC guidelines (USPSTF, 1996).

Table 19.2

Classification of Induration Reactions to Tuberculin

Induration	Classification	Clinical Circumstances
None	Non-reactive (negative)	• No infection • Anergy • Does not exclude active TB
≥ 5 mm	Reactive (positive) if:	• Close contact of active case • Known or suspected HIV infection • Chest radiograph suggestive of previous TB • Intervenous drug users with unknown HIV status
≥ 10 mm	Reactive (positive) if:	• Medical conditions predisposing to active TB* • HIV-negative intervenous drug users • Children younger than 4 years • Foreign-born persons, high prevalence area • Residents of long-term care facilities such as nursing homes or prisons • Medically underserved, low-income groups • High risk racial and ethnic groups • High prevalence groups (homeless, migrants) • Health care workers who provide services to high risk groups
≥ 15 mm	Reactive (positive)	• Healthy, no known risk factors for TB

* This would include diabetes, renal failure, immunosuppressed, use of high dose steroids, silicosis, malnourished, certain malignancies.
Source: Adapted from Gonzalez-Rothi, 1997.
Abbreviations: TB: Tuberculosis
                      HIV: Human Immondeficiency Virus

All patients identified as having reactive or positive tuberculin tests should have a chest radiograph to rule out active disease (Indicator 12). Preventive therapy for those with latent infection has been shown to reduce the incidence of disease by 54 to 84 percent in controlled trials (CDC, 1990). The usual preventive therapy regimen is isoniazid (INH) administered daily for 12 months in HIV positive persons or those with abnormal chest radiographs, and at least six months for all others. A limitation in the use of INH is the potential of INH-induced hepatitis. This can occur in 0.3 to 2.3 percent of patients. It is estimated that fatal INH-induced hepatits occurs in 1 to 14 per 100,000 persons started on preventive therapy (USPSTF, 1996). The frequency of hepatitis increases with age and other factors such as alcohol use. Different treatment is recommended for those suspected to be infected with INH-resistant or multiple drug-resistant TB.

Table 19.3 lists the CDC criteria for recommending preventive therapy to persons with reactive tuberculin skin tests (CDC, 1990) (Indicator 13).

Table 19.3

CDC Criteria for Preventive Treatment for TB by Risk Factor

Patient Risk Factors	Criteria for Recommending Preventive Treatment	
	Age < 35	Age ≥ 35
• HIV infection/immunocompromised • Close contact of person with active disease • Fibrotic lesion on chest x-ray	PPD ≥ 5 mm	PPD ≥ 5 mm
• Medical condition predisposing to TB such as chronic renal failure, diabetes, leukemia, Hodgkin's Disease, immunosuppressive or high dose corticosteroid therapy. • Intravenous drug use • Recent converter	PPD ≥ 10 mm PPD ≥ 10 mm increase within a 2-year period	PPD ≥ 10 mm PPD ≥ 15mm increase within a 2-year period
• Foreign-born, high prevalence country • Medically underserved • Low-income populations and high risk minorities • Residents of long term care facilities • Children under age four • Homeless persons	PPD ≥ 10 mm	Do not treat
• Patients without risk factors	PPD ≥ 15mm	Do not treat

Source: Adapted from CDC, 1990
Abbreviations: PPD - Purefied Protein Derivative
             HIV - Human Immunodeficiency Virus
             CDC - Centers for Disease Control

PPD testing as a screening tool for latent infection should be directed at those high risk populations who would be considered for preventive therapy or who are at high risk of exposure (Indicator 9). This would include all HIV infected persons, and other patients at risk for developing TB disease because of comorbid medical conditions. Routine screening is not recommended for persons in low risk populations (CDC, 1997).

Special guidelines have been published by the CDC for persons in nursing homes. Because it is recommended that this group undergo screening/surveillance with PPD tests, new employees, volunteers, and residents of nursing homes should be tuberculin tested using a more sensitive but less specific two-step procedure, unless they have previously tested positive (Indicator 14). Tuberculin negative persons should periodically have repeat skin tests at a frequency dependent on the risk of tuberculosis specific to that facility (CDC, 1997).

Hearing Screening

In adults, the prevalence of hearing impairment increases with age. An objective hearing loss can be identified in over 33 percent of persons aged 65 and older and in up to half of patients aged 85 years and older. Hearing impairment has been correlated with social and emotional isolation, depression, and limited activity, particularly in the elderly (Bess, 1989).

Screening methods for detecting hearing loss include use of pure-tone audiometry, written patient questionnaires, clinical history taking, audiometry with a hand-held device, and simple clinical techniques designed to assess the presence of hearing impairment (such as the whispered voice test). Sensitivities range from 70 to 80 percent for self-assessment questionnaires (USPSTF, 1996).

There are no controlled studies evaluating the effectiveness of screening for hearing impairment in the adult population. However, hearing aid use in a group of hearing impaired elderly veterans led to improvement in social, cognitive, emotional, and communication function (Mulrow, 1990). The USPSTF (1996) recommends screening all older adults for hearing impairment by periodically questioning them about their hearing, counseling them about the availability of hearing aid devices, and making referrals for abnormalities when appropriate. The Canadian Task Force recommends screening the elderly for hearing impairment using a single question about hearing difficulty, a whispered-voice out of the field of vision, or audioscope. We recommend as a quality indicator that patients aged 65 and older with apparent functional hearing loss be referred for screening, including audiometric screening (Indicator 15).

Screening for Obesity

Obesity is an excess of body fat and has been defined by the National Center for Health Statistics as having a body mass index (BMI) greater than 27.3 for women and greater than or equal to 27.8 for men. Based on data from the NHANES III, approximately one-third of adults aged 20 and over are obese (USPSTF, 1996). Morbid obesity, defined as being 50 to 100 percent (or 100 pounds) above the recommended weight, has been correlated with increased mortality and morbidity. The prevalence of diabetes and hypertension is three times higher in overweight persons than in those of normal weight. There is a clear association between obesity and hypercholesterolemia and a possible independent relationship between obesity and coronary artery disease. In addition, obesity may influence the risk of cancer of the colon, rectum, gallbladder, biliary tract, breast, cervix, endometrium, and ovary. Finally, obesity affects quality of life by limiting mobility, physical endurance, and other functional areas.

While extremely overweight individuals can be easily identified in the clinical setting by their physical appearance, more precise methods are required to identify mildly or moderately obese persons. The most accurate methods of measuring body fat composition are underwater weighing, isotopic dilution measures, and other techniques not well suited to typical clinical practice. The most common clinical method for detecting obesity is the evaluation of body weight and height based on tables of average weights. However, this method only provides an approximate measure (USPSTF, 1996). Moreover, the criteria for desirable body weight are a matter of controversy among experts and vary considerably in different weight-height tables. An alternative is to calculate the BMI, a weight-height index (weight in kilograms divided by height in meters squared). This is a reliable measure and correlates fairly well with body fat content (USPSTF, 1996). Another method of measuring obesity is the measurement of body fat distribution by comparing the circumference or skinfold thickness of the trunk and limbs. Skinfold thickness has lower intra- and inter-observer reliability than weight and height measurements. The waist-hip ratio (the circumference of the waist divided by the circumference of the hips) has also been shown to predict complications from obesity, but has not been evaluated in all ethnic groups (USPSTF, 1996). Studies have shown that these measurements compare favorably with estimates obtained from hydrostatic weighing.

The purpose of screening for obesity is to convince the individual to lose weight thereby preventing the complications of obesity. Screening may also assist with counseling other patients regarding maintaining a healthy weight. Although there is little evidence from prospective studies that losing weight improves longevity, there is evidence that obesity increases mortality and that weight loss reduces important risk factors such as hypertension, elevated serum cholesterol, and impaired glucose tolerance (USPSTF, 1996).

Periodic height and weight measurements, although not proven to be effective in motivating patients to lose weight, are inexpensive, rapid and acceptable to most patients. There are inadequate data to determine the optimal frequency of obesity screening. The Institute of Medicine recommends height and weight measurements at least during each of five age intervals during adulthood: 18 to 24, 25 to 39, 40 to 59, 60 to 74, and over 75. The American Heart Association recommends body weight measurements every five years (USPSTF, 1996; Healthy People 2000, 1991). We recommend as a quality indicator that the medical record include measurements of height and weight at least once (Indicator 16).

COUNSELING

Seat Belt Use

Motor vehicle crash-related injuries were the eighth most common cause of death in the United States in 1993; and they are the leading cause of death before the age of 65 (USPSTF, 1996).

The effectiveness of safety belts has been demonstrated in a variety of study designs that include laboratory experiments (using human volunteers, cadavers, and anthropomorphic crash dummies), postcrash comparisons of injuries sustained by restrained and unrestrained occupants, and postcrash judgments by crash analysts regarding the probable effects of restraints had they been used (USPSTF, 1996). The proper use of lap and shoulder belts can decrease the risk of moderate to serious injury to front seat occupants by 45 to 55 percent and can reduce crash mortality by 40 to 50 percent (USPSTF, 1996).

The USPSTF, the AMA, the AAFP, and the ACP recommend that clinicians regularly urge their patients to use safety belts whenever driving or riding in an automobile. It is not known how effectively clinicians can alter behaviors regarding seat belt use. There have been a few controlled and uncontrolled trials in adults, but there were some methodological problems such as concerns with patient selection. There is stronger evidence that clinician counseling can be effective in promoting the use of infant and child safety seats. We recommend as a quality indicator that patients otherwise presenting for care receive counseling regarding the use of seat belts on at least one occasion (Indicator 17).

Sexually Transmitted Diseases and HIV Prevention

Almost 12 million cases of sexually transmitted diseases (STDs) occur annually. This includes about four million cases of *chlamydia trachomatis* infection; 800,000 cases of gonorrhea; over 110,000 cases of syphilis; several million cases of trichomonas vaginitis and nonspecific urethritis; one-half to one million cases of human papillomavirus (HPV) infection; 200,000 to 500,000 primary episodes of genital herpes; and 40,000 to 80,000 new infections with HIV (USPSTF, 1996). These diseases are associated with considerable morbidity. Chlamydia and gonorrhea produce mucopurulent cervicitis, pelvic inflammatory disease (PID), ectopic pregnancy and infertility in women and urethritis in men. Syphilis produces ulcers of the genitalia, pharynx, and rectum and can progress to secondary and tertiary syphilis if left untreated. Genital herpes causes painful vesicular and ulcerative lesions and recurrent infections due to latent infection. In addition, there are over one million chronic carriers of hepatitis B virus. Most people infected with HIV eventually develop AIDS. HIV infection is now the leading cause of death among men ages 25 to 44, and the fifth leading cause of years of potential life lost before age 65 (USPSTF, 1996). The total societal costs of STDs are estimated to be $3.5 billion annually (USPHS, 1991) and the medical costs of treating HIV and AIDS were projected to reach $15 billion in 1995 (USPSTF, 1996).

The most efficacious means of reducing the risk of acquiring STDs through sexual contact is either abstinence from sexual relations or maintenance of a mutually monogamous sexual relationship with an uninfected partner (USPSTF, 1996). However, accurately assessing a sexual partner's outside sexual activity and infection status may be difficult. Consistent and appropriate use of latex condoms reduces the risk of infection with HIV or other STDs. Spermacides and female barrier contraceptives appear to offer some protection against STDs although the effect on HIV infection is not consistent. Clinical experience with the female condom has been limited, and there are concerns that cost and inconsistent use limit its usefulness (USPSTF, 1996).

The primary purpose of HIV and STD counseling is to prevent further spread of infection. There is limited evidence that clinician counseling in the primary care setting is effective in reducing the incidence of STDs or in changing sexual behavior. However, counseling interventions delivered in a variety of settings can reduce specific STD risk behavior (e.g., HIV counseling in high-risk populations; condom promotion in at-risk heterosexual populations; interventions in non-clinical settings). A multi-center randomized controlled trial of three different counseling strategies to increase condom use and decrease new cases of STDs is currently being conducted among sexually transmitted disease clinic patients; this may help clarify which counseling methods may be the most efficacious (Kamb, 1996). Current CDC guidelines for HIV prevention messages and counseling stress that risk reduction messages be "client-centered", i.e., personalized and realistic, with a focused and tailored risk assessment which serves as the basis for assisting the client in formulating a plan to reduce risk (CDC, 1997). Physicians can play an important role in helping to promote behavior change by reinforcing and clarifying educational messages, identifying high risk behaviors, helping patients plan a feasible strategy to reduce risk, and providing literature and community resource references for additional information (USPSTF, 1996).

As part of an individual risk assessment, it is recommended that clinicians take a complete sexual and drug use history on all adult patients to identify risk factors for HIV (Indicators 18, 19, 20). In addition, clinicians should counsel at-risk patients on measures to prevent the spread of STDs and HIV (Indicator 21). Risk factors include: non-monogamous relationships; more than two sexual partners in the past six months; a history of STDs; a history of intravenous drug use; sexual relations with an infected partner; history of blood transfusion between 1978 and 1985; and hemophilia.

Early detection of asymptomatic HIV infection can reduce morbidity and mortality in infected persons, and there is some indirect evidence that screening reduces the incidence of new HIV infections (USPSTF, 1996). We recommend as a quality indicator that HIV testing be offered to all persons at increased risk for infection: those seeking treatment for sexually transmitted diseases; men who have had sex with men; past or present injection drug users; persons who exchange sex for money or drugs; women and men whose past or present sex partners were HIV-infected, bisexual, or injection drug users; and persons with a history of transfusion between 1978 and 1985 (USPSTF, 1996; CDC, 1997) (Indicator 22). Appropriate pre- and post-test counseling should be provided when testing is performed.

Promoting Physical Activity

Epidemiologic research has demonstrated an association with physical activity and decreased risk for several chronic diseases, including coronary artery disease, hypertension, non-insulin-dependent diabetes mellitus, osteoporosis, obesity, colon cancer, anxiety, and depression. Conversely, low levels of physical activity and fitness are associated with markedly increased all-cause mortality rates. As many as 250,000 deaths per year may be attributable to sedentary lifestyle (Pate, Pratt, and Blair 1995).

The CDC recommendation (Pate, Pratt, Blair 1995) is that "every US adult should accumulate 30 minutes or more of moderate-intensity physical activity on most, preferably all, days of the week". The health benefits gained depend on initial activity level; sedentary persons are expected to benefit most, however there is a dose-response effect with greater benefit at higher levels of energy expenditure. The report of the Surgeon General on physical activity (CDC, 1996) stresses the benefits of regular moderate-intensity activity rather than vigorous exercise and setting appropriate short term goals of small increases in activity level over time.

There is insufficient evidence that clinician counseling to promote increased physical activity will lead to long-term behavior change in asymptomatic primary care patients. However one of the *Healthy People 2000* (1991) risk reduction objectives is to increase to at least 50 percent the proportion of primary care providers who routinely assess and counsel their patients regarding the frequency, duration, type, and intensity of their physical activity practices. The USPSTF recommends that clinicians assess each patient's activity level (USPSTF, 1996) (Indicator 23).

REFERENCES

Bess F, et al. 1989. Hearing impairment as a determinant of function in the elderly. *Journal of the American Geriatrics Society* 37: 123-128.

CDC Prevention Guidelines. 1997. Friede A, O;Carroll P, Nicola R, Oberle M, Teutsch S, ed. Baltimore: Williams & Wilkins.

CDC Prevention Guidelines. 1997. Topic 5. Diphtheria, Tetanus, and Pertusis - original citation: *Morbidity and Mortality Weekly Report* 1991;40 (RR-10);1-28 in: Freide A, O'Carroll P, Nicola R, Oberle M, Teutsch S, ed. Baltimore: Williams & Wilkins.

CDC Prevention Guidelines. 1997. Topic 12. Hepatitis - original citation: Protection against viral hepatitis: Recommendations of the Immunization Practices Advisory Committee. *Morbidity And Mortality Weekly Report* 1990;39 (RR2):1-26 in: Freide A, O'Carroll P, Nicola R, Oberle M, Teutsch S, ed. Baltimore: Williams & Wilkins.

CDC Prevention Guidelines. 1997. Topic 14. Human immunodeficiency virus.aquired immunodeficiency syndrome . Original citations: Technical guidance on HIV counseling. *Morbidity And Mortality Weekly Report* 1993;42 (RR-02). Barrier protection against HIV infection and other sexually transmitted diseases. *Morbidity And Mortality Weekly Report* 1993;42 (30):589-591, 597. In: Freide A, O'Carroll P, Nicola R, Oberle M, Teutsch S, ed. Baltimore: Williams & Wilkins.

CDC Prevention Guidelines. 1997. Topic 15. Immunizations - General recommendations. original citation: Update on adult immunization: recommendations of the ACIP. *Morbidity And Mortality Weekly Report* 1991;40 (RR-12):1-52. In: Freide A, O'Carroll P, Nicola R, Oberle M, Teutsch S, ed. Baltimore: Williams & Wilkins.

CDC Prevention Guidelines. 1997. Topic 16. Influenza - original citation: Prevention and control of influenza - recommendations of the ACIP. *Morbidity And Mortality Weekly Report* 1995;44 (RR-3); 1-22. In: Freide A, O'Carroll P, Nicola R, Oberle M, Teutsch S, ed. Baltimore: Williams & Wilkins.

CDC Prevention Guidelines. 1997. Topic 23. Pneumococcosis. Original citation: Pneumococcal polysaccharide vaccine, recommendations of the ACIP. *Morbidity And Mortality Weekly Report* 1989;38 (5):64-68,73-76. In: Freide A, O'Carroll P, Nicola R, Oberle M, Teutsch S, ed. Baltimore: Williams & Wilkins.

CDC Prevention Guidelines. 1997. Topic 28. Sexually transmitted diseases in: Freide A, O'Carroll P, Nicola R, Oberle M, Teutsch S, ed. Baltimore: Williams & Wilkins.

CDC Prevention Guidelines. 1997. Topic 29. Tuberculosis - original citation: The use of preventive therapy for tuberculosis infection in the United States. Recommendations of the Advisory Committee for Elimination of Tuberculosis. *Morbidity And Mortality Weekly Report* 1990;39 (RR-8) 9-12. in: Freide A, O'Carroll P, Nicola R, Oberle M, Teutsch S, ed. Baltimore: Williams & Wilkins.

CDC Prevention Guidelines. 1997. Prevention and control of tuberculosis in U.S. communities with at-risk minority populations and prevention and control of tuberculosis among homeless persons. *Morbidity And Mortality Weekly Report* 1992;41 (RR-5):1. in: Freide A, O'Carroll P, Nicola R, Oberle M, Teutsch S, ed. Baltimore: Williams & Wilkins.

CDC Prevention Guidelines. 1997. Prevention and control of tuberculosis in facilities providing long-term care to the elderly. *Morbidity And Mortality Weekly Report* 1990;39 (RR-10):7-20. In: Freide A, O'Carroll P, Nicola R, Oberle M, Teutsch S, ed. Baltimore: Williams & Wilkins.

CDC Prevention Guidelines. 1997. Screening for tuberculosis and tuberculosis infection in high-risk population. *Morbidity And Mortality Weekly Report* 1995;44 (Rrr-11);18-34. In: Freide A, O'Carroll P, Nicola R, Oberle M, Teutsch S, ed. Baltimore: Williams & Wilkins.

CDC Prevention Guidelines. 1997. Topic 31. Varicella. In: Freide A, O'Carroll P, Nicola R, Oberle M, Teutsch S, ed. Baltimore: Williams & Wilkins.

CDC Prevention Guidelines. 1997. Topic 38. Exercise. (see ref Pate R, Pratt M, Blair S et al . Physical Activity and public health - a recommendation from the Centers for Disease Control and Prevention and the American College of Sports Medicine) *Geriatrrics and Soceity* 1989;37 (2):123-128. In: Freide A, O'Carroll P, Nicola R, Oberle M, Teutsch S, ed. Baltimore: Williams & Wilkins.

Centers for Disease Control and Prevention (CDC). July 1996. Physical Activity and Health: A report of the Surgeon General. US Department of Health and Huyman Services.

Fine M, et al. 1994. Efficacy of pneumococcal vaccination in adults. *Archives of Internal Medicine* 154: 2666-2677.

Gardner P, and Schaffner W. 1993. Immunization of adults. *New England Journal of Medicine* 328 (17): 1252-1257.

Gonzalez-Rothi R. May 1997. Resurgent TB: Stopping the spread. *Patient Care* 97-118.

Govaert T, et al. 1994. The efficacy of influenza vaccination in elderly individuals. *Journal of the American Medical Association* 272 (21): 1661-1665.

Kamb M, et al. 1996. Quality assurance of HIV prevention counseling in a multi-center randomized controlled trial. *Public Health Reports* 111 (s-1): 99-107.

McGinnis J, and Foege W. 1993. Actual Causes of Death in the United States. *Journal of the American Medical Association* 270 (18): 2207-2212.

Mulrow CD, Aguilar C, et al. 1990. Quality of life changes and hearing impairment, a randomized trial. *Archives of Internal Medicine* 113: 188-94.

Nicole K, et al. 1994. The efficacy and cost effectiveness of vaccination against influenza among elderly persons living in the community. *New England Journal of Medicine* 331 (12): 778-784.

Ortiz C, and LaForce F. 1994. Prevention of community-acquired pneumonia. *Medical Clinics of North America* 78 (5): 1173-1183.

Pate R, Pratt M, Blair S, et al. 1995. Physical Activity and public health - a recommendation from the Centers for Disease Control and Prevention and the American College of Sports Medicine. *Journal of the American Medical Association* 273: 402-407.

Shapiro E, et al. 1991. The protective efficacy of polyvalent pneumococcal polysaccharide vaccine. *New England Journal of Medicine* 325 (21): 1453-1460.

US Department of Health and Human Services. 1991. *Healthy People 2000: National Health Promotion and Disease Prevention Objectives*. Washington, DC: U.S. Government Printing Office.

US Preventative Services Task Force. 1996. *Guide to Clinical Preventative Services, 2nd ed*. Baltimore: Williams & Wilkins.

RECOMMENDED QUALITY INDICATORS FOR PREVENTIVE CARE

The following indicators apply to men and women age 18 and over. Only the indicators in bold type were rated by this panel; the remaining indicators were endorsed by a prior panel.

Indicator	Quality of Evidence	Literature	Benefits	Comments
Immunizations				
1. For patients under age 50, notation of the date that a patient received a tetanus/diphtheria booster within the last ten years should be included in the medical record.	I, II, III	USPSTF, 1996; CDC, 1997	Decrease morbidity and mortality from tetanus and diphtheria.	There is good evidence that the vaccine is effective. It is important to make sure all adults have received a primary series; there are differing recommendations for Td boosters. This indicator is operationalized to apply only to patients under age 50.
2. There should be documentation in the medical record that patients over the age of 50 were offered a tetanus/diphtheria booster after their 50th birthday.	I, II, III	USPSTF, 1996; CDC, 1997	Decrease morbidity and mortality from tetanus and diphtheria.	There is good evidence that t the vaccine is effective. It is important to make sure all adults have received a primary series; there are differing recommendations for Td boosters.
3. Patients receiving medical attention for any wound should receive Td injection under either of the following conditions: a. For clean minor wounds, if the last Td booster was greater than 10 years; b. For other/dirty wounds,[1] if the last Td booster was greater than 5 years.	III	USPSTF, 1996; CDC, 1997	Decrease morbidity and mortality from tetanus.	Persons with tetanus prone wounds need to be evaluated and immunized according to published guidelines.
4. All patients aged 65 and over should have been offered influenza vaccine in the past year.	I, II	USPSTF, 1996; CDC, 1997	Decrease morbidity and mortality from influenza and its complications.	In the elderly, the vaccine may be only 30-40% effective in preventing clinical disease. A randomized controlled trial showed a significant reduction in clinical illness and cohort and case control studies support a reduction in hospitalization rates and deaths.

314

Indicator	Quality of Evidence	Literature	Benefits	Comments
5. All patients under age 65 with any of the following conditions should have been offered influenza vaccination in the past year: a. Living in a nursing home; b. Chronic obstructive pulmonary disease [9]; c. Asthma; d. Chronic cardiovascular disorders; e. Renal failure; f. Immunosuppression; g. Diabetes mellitus; h. Hemoglobinopathies (e.g., sickle cell).	I-II	USPSTF, 1996; CDC, 1997	Decrease morbidity and mortality from influenza and its complications.	Persons with these conditions are at high risk of lower respiratory-tract complications and death after influenza infection. The influenza vaccine has been shown to have some efficacy in some of these populations, although the evidence is limited.
6. There should be documentation that all patients in the following groups and otherwise presenting for care were offered pneumococcal vaccine at least once: a. Patients aged 65 and older; b. Chronic cardiac or pulmonary disease; c. Diabetes mellitus; d. Anatomic asplenia; e. Persons over age 50 who are institutionalized.	II, III	USPSTF, 1996; CDC, 1997	Decrease morbidity and mortality from invasive pneumococcal disease.	Pneumococcal disease is a significant cause of morbidity and mortality in these populations. The current vaccine contains serotypes which are responsible for 88% of the isolates causing bacteremia. Evidence of efficacy of the vaccine in this population has been conflicting. Some authorities also recommend this vaccine for immunosuppressed patients, but there is limited evidence of efficacy in this group.

315

Indicator	Quality of Evidence	Literature	Benefits	Comments

7. There should be documentation that all patients identified as being in the following high risk groups were offered hepatitis B vaccination within one year after identification of the risk, unless the patient has serologic evidence of immunity:[2]
  a. Hemodialysis patients;
  b. Sexually active homosexual men;
  c. Household and sexual contacts of HBV carriers;
  d. Intravenous drug users;
  e. Persons with occupational risk;[3]
  f. Persons who have a history of sexual activity with multiple sexual partners in the past 6 months;
  g. Persons who have recently acquired another sexually transmitted disease.
	I, III	USPSTF, 1996; CDC, 1996	Decrease morbidity and mortality from hepatitis B infection.	There is good evidence that Hepatitis B vaccine is effective in these populations. Dosage and schedule may need to be modified for specific population groups as recommended (specific recommendations for hemodialysis patients are available). Although universal childhood immunization is now being implemented, there still is a large pool of susceptible adults in identified high risk groups.

8. All persons otherwise presenting for care in the following high risk groups should have documentation of measles immunization status:
  a. College students;
  b. Health-care workers;
  c. Day-care providers.
	I, III	USPSTF, 1996; CDC, 1997	Decrease morbidity and mortality from measles.	There is good evidence that the vaccine works. Persons in these groups are at greater risk of exposure to measles.

316

Screening

Indicator	Quality of Evidence	Literature	Benefits	Comments
9. There should be documentation of PPD reactivity status[4] for all patients otherwise presenting for care who are identified as being in the following risk groups in the year following identification of the risk:[5] a. Foreign born persons from countries of high TB prevalence (Asia, Africa, Latin America) who have been in the US less than 5 years;[5] b. Injection drug users; c. Persons with immunosuppression; d. Residents of long-term care facilities such as nursing homes; e. Homeless persons; f. Health care workers.	III	USPSTF, 1996; CDC, 1997	Decrease morbidity and mortality from tuberculosis; decrease spread of tuberculosis.	Early detection of tuberculosis infection is potentially beneficial because treatment with INH can prevent subsequent development of active TB disease. Chemoprophylaxis of latent infection is part of the national strategy to eliminate TB. PPD screening in HIV positive persons is covered in another chapter. The need to repeat PPD tests at regular intervals depends on the local or regional prevalence in these groups. Disease rates among the foreign born are highest in the first few years after arrival in the U.S. Diabetics and those with chronic renal failure have an increased risk of developing active tuberculosis if infected, however, given the wide geographic differences in tuberculosis infection prevalence, we do not recommend routine screening of these patients although it may be prudent to do so in some areas.
10. All Mantoux tests read as positive or reactive should document both of the following: a. The presence of induration; b. The diameter of the induration in millimeters.	III	American Thoracic Society, 1990; CDC, 1997	Prevent development of TB disease and its complications. Prevent toxicity of anti-TB medications.	Though a positive test requires induration, people often mistake erythema without induration for a positive. The diameter in millimeters is used to determine whether the test is positive according to risk stratification.
11. Mantoux tests should be read by a health professional or other trained personnel within 48-72 hours.	III	USPSTF, 1996	Prevent development of TB disease and its complications.	If the patient is seen at greater than 72 hours and significant induration is present, the test need not be repeated. In all other cases, if more than 72 hours have elapsed, the test should be repeated.

317

Indicator	Quality of Evidence	Literature	Benefits	Comments
12. Persons identified as having a newly positive or reactive PPD should have a chest radiograph performed within 1 month.[6]	III	USPSTF, 1996; CDC, 1997	Decrease morbidity and mortality from tuberculosis.	A chest radiograph is necessary to identify active TB disease, or evidence of old TB disease. Those with scarring are at higher risk of disease and should be offered preventive therapy.
13. Persons in the following risk groups who are identified as having TB infection (not disease) should be offered INH preventive therapy unless they have clear contraindications[7] : a. Patients with diabetes mellitus; b. Patients with chronic renal failure; c. Recent exposure to a case of active TB; d. Recent conversion of PPD (documented negative test in the previous 2 years); e. Immunocompromised or chronic high dose corticosteroids; f. Injection drug users g. Foreign born persons less than 35 years of age.	III	CDC, 1990	Decrease morbidity and mortality from TB.	Preventive therapy with INH decreases risk of developing active disease. Persons in these risk categories have a higher risk of developing TB disease than the general population.
14. If the initial PPD test on nursing home patients is negative, immediate retesting (two-step testing) should be performed.	III	CDC, 1990	Decrease morbidity and mortality from tuberculosis. Establish a reliable baseline. Prevent toxicity from anti-TB medication.	In the elderly, initial PPD testing may be negative due to waning immunity. In a population that is undergoing surveillance, subsequent testing may boost the immune response, causing the test to be positive. This should be distinguished from PPD test conversion which indicates recent exposure to the TB bacillus.

318

Indicator	Quality of Evidence	Literature	Benefits	Comments
15. Patients age 65 and older noted to have a hearing problem or complaint should be referred for a formal evaluation.[8]	II, III	USPSTF, 1996; Mulrow, 1990	Improve quality of life for those with hearing loss.	No studies show direct benefit from screening for hearing loss in the elderly although it has been recommended by some authorities (USPSTF); it is known that hearing loss is prevalent in the elderly and associated with adverse effects on quality of life. Use of hearing aids has been shown by a randomized clinical trial to lead to improved quality of life (Mulrow 1990). Screening may often be undocumented when no problem is found.
16. The medical record should include measurements of height and weight at least once.	III	USPSTF, 1996; Healthy People 2000, 1991	Prevention of complications of obesity.	This will serve to help identify individuals who are obese. However, it is debatable whether physician counseling for obesity is effective in adults.
Counseling				
17. Patients otherwise presenting for care should receive counseling regarding the use of seat belts on at least one occasion.	III	USPST, 1996	Prevention of motor vehicle injuries and fatalities.	Clinician suggestion may change this behavior.
18. Patients should be asked if they have ever been sexually active.	III	USPSTF, 1996	Prevent HIV. Prevent STDs.	Patients who have ever been sexually active may be at risk of HIV or STD infections.
19. Patients under the age of 50, who have ever been sexually active, should be asked the following questions: a. if they currently have a single sexual partner; b. if they have had more than 2 sexual partners in the past 6 months; c. if they have a history of any STDs.	III	USPSTF, 1996	Prevent HIV. Prevent STDs.	Non-monogamous relationships, more than 2 sexual partners in the past 6 months and past history of STDs are risk factors for HIV and other STDs. Men and women under 25 account for two-thirds of all cases of chlamydia and gonorrhea, and men and women under 35 account for two-thirds of newly reported HIV infection.
20. Patients should be asked about current or past use of intravenous drugs at least once.	III	USPSTF, 1996	Prevent HIV. Prevent STDs.	Intravenous drug use is a risk factor for HIV infection.

319

	Indicator	Quality of Evidence	Literature	Benefits	Comments
21.	Patients who are sexually active and not in a monogamous relationship, have had more than 2 sexual partners in the past six months, have a history of STDs or have used intravenous drugs should be counseled regarding the prevention and transmission of HIV and other STDs.	III	USPSTF, 1996	Prevent HIV. Prevent STDs.	Persons with risk factors for HIV or other STDs should receive appropriate counseling.
22.	Testing for HIV should have been offered in the past year to all persons in the following groups at increased risk for HIV infection: a. Those seeking treatment for sexually transmitted diseases (chlamydia, GC, syphilis, trichomonas, genital herpes, condyloma, or chancroid); b. Men who have sex with men; c. Past or present injection drug users; d. Persons who exchange sex for money or drugs; e. Women and men whose past or present sex partners were HIV-infected, bisexual, or injection drug users; f. Persons with a history of transfusion between 1978 and 1985.	III	USPSTF, 1996; CDC, 1997	Decrease morbidity from HIV infection. Prevent spread of HIV infection.	Early identification of HIV infection and treatment with anti-viral therapy and prophylaxis of some opportunistic infections may help reduce morbidity and mortality from HIV infection. There is some evidence that persons identified as HIV infected and counseled regarding high risk sexual practices may change their behavior (USPSTF, 1996)

Indicator	Quality of Evidence	Literature	Benefits	Comments
23. There should be documentation that patients' level of physical activity was assessed on at least one occasion.	III	USPSTF, 1996; Healthy People 2000, 1991	Reduce mortality from all causes associated with sedentary lifestyle.	There is good evidence that physical activity is associated with reduced mortality and there is a protective effect of physical activity on the risk of several chronic diseases, such as diabetes, coronary heart disease, hypertension, colon cancer, obesity, anxiety and depression. There is insufficient evidence that clinician counseling is effective in motivating asymptomatic patients to change their level of physical activity. However, it seems prudent that counseling to promote physical activity be included in continuity care for all patients. Documentation of counseling practices are often missing, whereas, documentation of risk assessment is more likely to be present.

Definitions and Examples

[1] Failure to document Td status will be considered failure to comply with this indicator.

[2] HBAg+, HBSAb+, HBCoreAb+, or HBeAb+.

[3] Health care providers; staff of residential institutions or day care centers for the developmentally disabled.

[4] If there is no previous documentation, a PPD test should be performed using intermediate strength PPD. If a patient has a clear history of a previous positive PPD, it need not be repeated unless the patient is being considered for INH prophylaxis.

[5] This criterion will be applied only if there is documentation of number of years in the US.

[6] This assumes the test was a screening test of an asymptomatic person. Definition of a reactive test should follow recommended guidelines based on risk category.

[7] Contraindications may include previous INH toxicity, current alcohol use, liver disease with abnormal liver function tests.

[8] Formal audiogram including speech discrimination and hearing aid evaluation.

[9] Excluding asthma.

Quality of Evidence Codes

I	RCT
II-1	Nonrandomized controlled trials
II-2	Cohort or case analysis
II-3	Multiple time series
III	Options or descriptive studies

20. VAGINITIS AND SEXUALLY TRANSMITTED DISEASES[5]

Allison L. Diamant, MD, MSPH, and Eve Kerr, MD, MPH

The approach to developing quality indicators for vulvovaginitis and sexually transmitted diseases (STDs) began with reviewing a general text on ambulatory medicine (Barker et al., 1991) and a text of diagnostic strategies for common medical problems (Panzer et al., 1991). Specific treatment recommendations were derived from the Centers for Disease Control (CDC) 1993 Treatment Guidelines for Sexually Transmitted Diseases (CDC, 1993). The guidelines were based on systematic literature reviews by CDC staff and consensus opinions by experts. The literature reviews are summarized, in part, in the April 1995 Supplement to *Clinical Infectious Diseases*, which was reviewed to add greater detail to treatment controversies. Pertinent articles published since 1993 were also reviewed for additional recommendations regarding screening and treatment of vaginitis and STDs in non-pregnant, non-HIV infected women and non-HIV infected men.

VULVOVAGINITIS

IMPORTANCE

The most common causes of vulvovaginal infections are *Gardnerella vaginalis*, *Candida albicans*, and *Trichomonas vaginalis*. An estimated 75 percent of women will experience at least one episode of vulvovaginal candidiasis in their lifetimes, and 40 to 45 percent will experience two or more episodes (CDC, 1993). There are an estimated 10 million visits to

---

[5] This chapter is a revision of one written for an earlier project on quality of care for women and children (Q1). The expert panel for the current project was asked to review all of the indicators, but only rated new or revised indicators.

physicians' offices each year for vaginitis (Reef et al., 1995). Vulvovaginal candidiasis and bacterial vaginosis (*G. vaginalis*) are not considered STDs in the heterosexual population, and women who are not sexually active are rarely affected by bacterial vaginosis (CDC, 1993). However, recent nonrandomized studies suggest that vulvovaginal candidiasis and bacterial vaginosis (*G. vaginalis*) may be transmitted between women who participate in same sex relations (Berger et al., 1995). *T. vaginalis* is transmitted through sexual activity. Gonococcal and chlamydial infections, although not causative of vulvovaginitis, may sometimes cause women to present with an abnormal discharge. In fact, as many as 25 percent of women with abnormal discharge have cervical infections (Panzer et al., 1991).

Candida vaginitis does not have important medical sequelae but does cause discomfort that may impair the patient's quality of life. Bacterial vaginosis may be associated with pelvic inflammatory disease (PID) (Joesoef and Schmid, 1995). A recent randomized controlled trial (RCT) found that women with bacterial vaginosis who were treated with metronidazole before abortion had a three-fold decrease in PID after abortion, compared with untreated women (Joesoef and Schmid, 1995).

SCREENING

There is no indication for screening the general population for vaginitis.

DIAGNOSIS

The approach to diagnosis is well summarized by Panzer et al. (1991). The history and physical examination have poor predictive value. For example, approximately 35 percent of symptomatic patients had no evidence of infection, 32 percent of asymptomatic patients had infection, and approximately 15 percent of infected patients had normal pelvic examinations. However, risk factors for STDs -- such as the number and gender of sexual partners in the past month, history of STDs, presence of genitourinary symptoms, and sexual contact with an infected partner -- increase the prior probability of a sexually transmitted cause for vaginal discharge (Indicator 1).

Table 20.1 displays the variability in the operating characteristics of diagnostic tests for vaginitis. For *T. vaginalis*, the wet mount is highly specific (70 to 98 percent) but not particularly sensitive (50 to 75 percent). For *Candida albicans*, the potassium hydroxide preparation is highly specific (90 to 99 percent), but has varied sensitivity (30 to 84 percent) compared with culture. For bacterial vaginosis (*G. vaginalis*), Amsel et al. (1983) developed diagnostic criteria that are widely accepted (Panzer et al., 1991; Joesoef and Schmid, 1995). The diagnosis in a symptomatic patient is based on the presence of at least three of the following four criteria; 1) pH greater than 4.5; 2) positive whiff test; 3) clue cells on wet mount; and 4) thin homogeneous discharge.

Diagnostic strategy in the evaluation of acute vulvovaginitis is often governed by the need to initiate antimicrobial therapy. The first decision lies in determining whether the infection is cervical or vaginal (Indicator 2). An assessment of risk factors for STDs and a careful pelvic examination will help determine this. If the discharge is thought to be vaginal in origin, then a saline wet mount, potassium hydroxide wet mount, and the application of Amsel's criteria should be used to determine the etiology of the vaginitis (Indicator 3).

A small proportion of women have recurrent vulvovaginal candidiasis (i.e., three or more annual episodes of symptomatic vulvovaginal candidiasis). These women should be evaluated for predisposing conditions such as diabetes, immunosuppression, concomitant corticosteroid use, and HIV infection. However, the majority of women with recurrent vulvovaginal candidiasis have no identifiable risk factors (Reef et al., 1995).

Table 20.1

Operating Characteristics of Common Diagnostic Tests for Vaginal and Cervical Infection

Infection Type/ Test	Sensitivity (%)	Specificity (%)
Vaginal Infection		
Trichomonas vaginalis	–	–
Saline wet mount	50-75	70-98
Direct fluorescent antibody	80-86	98
Vaginal candidiasis (*C. albicans*)	–	–
Potassium hydroxide preparation	30-84	90-99
Bacterial vaginosis (*G. vaginalis*)	–	–
Vaginal pH	81-97	–
Clue cells	85-90	80
"Whiff" test	38-84	–
Thin homogeneous discharge	80	–
Gram stain of vaginal wash	97	79
Abnormal amines by chromatography	98	–
Cervical Infection	–	–
Chlamydia trachomatis	–	–
Direct fluorescent antibody	70-87	97-99
Enzyme immunoassay	80-85	80-85
Culture (single cervical swab)	70-80	98
Neisseria gonorrhoeae	–	–
Cervix Gram stain	50-79	98
Culture (single cervical swab)	85-90	98
Herpes Simplex Virus	–	–
Tzanck smear: vesicular; pustular; crusted	67; 54; 17	85

Source: Panzer et al., 1991

TREATMENT

Bacterial Vaginosis (*G. vaginalis*)

These recommendations are based, in part, on randomized controlled studies and meta-analyses reviewed by the CDC (Joesoef and Schmid, 1995). According to the CDC review, a seven-day treatment regimen of metronidazole is preferred over a single dose regimen of the same, but all appropriate treatments for non-pregnant women are listed below. The CDC report notes that further evaluation of the topical formulations is required (CDC, 1993) (Indicator 4):

- Metronidazole 500 mg orally twice a day for seven days (95 percent overall cure rate);
- Metronidazole 2 g orally in a single dose (84 percent overall cure rate);
- Clindamycin 300 mg orally twice a day for seven days;
- Clindamycin cream at night for seven days; or
- Metronidazole cream twice a day for five days.

T. vaginalis

For people infected with *T. vaginalis*, it is necessary to treat both patients and their sex partner(s) with:

- Metronidazole 2 g orally in a single dose; or
- Metronidazole 500 mg twice daily for seven days.

Both regimens have been found to be equally effective in RCTs, with a cure rate of approximately 95 percent (CDC, 1993) (Indicator 5).

Candida albicans

A number of topical formulations in the azole class (e.g., butoconazole, clotrimazole, miconazole, tioconazole, terconazole) provide effective treatment for vulvovaginal candidiasis, with symptom relief and negative cultures after completion of therapy in approximately 90 percent of patients (CDC, 1993). These treatment recommendations are based on clinical trials reviewed by the CDC (Reef et al., 1995) (Indicator 6). In addition, several trials have demonstrated that oral azole drugs (e.g., fluconazole, ketoconazole, and itraconazole) may be as effective as topical

327

agents. The FDA has approved single-dose fluconazole for the treatment of vulvovaginal candidiasis (Wall Street Journal, July 7, 1994). Practicing physicians report this regimen to be an effective treatment (Inman et al., 1994). Use of fluconazole is contraindicated for treatment of vulvovaginal candidiasis in pregnancy. Optimal treatment for recurrent vulvovaginal candidiasis is not well established, but a role for oral agents is being investigated (Reef et al., 1995).

FOLLOW-UP

Follow up care, including cultures, is unnecessary for women whose symptoms resolve after treatment (CDC, 1993).

DISEASES CHARACTERIZED BY CERVICITIS/URETHRITIS

IMPORTANCE

Mucopurulent cervicitis is most often caused by *Neisseria gonorrhea* and *C. trachomatis* -- two sexually transmitted infections. *C. trachomatis* is the most common cause of cervical infection, with a prevalence ranging from approximately five to 15 percent in asymptomatic women and 20 to 30 percent in women treated at STD clinics. The incidence of chlamydial infection in 1988 was 215 per 100,000 women (DHHS, 1990). The most common cause of nongonoccocal urethritis in men is *C. trachomatis* (23-55%), although a large number of cases are caused by *Ureaplasma urealyticum* (20-40%). The prevalence of chlamydia among men tends to decline with age. Approximately 13 percent of women with a chlamydial infection have a concurrent gonococcal infection, and an estimated 30 percent of women with a gonococcal infection have a chlamydial infection (Panzer et al., 1991). Transmission of gonorrhea from infected men to uninfected women occurs in 90 percent of exposures. In 1989, the incidence of gonococcal infection among women aged 15 to 44 was 501 per 100,000 (DHHS, 1990), with approximately one million new infections occurring each year (CDC, 1993).

Initially, both gonococcal and chlamydial infections may be asymptomatic in men and women, or may present with a variety of symptoms.

Women may complain of vaginal symptoms (e.g., mucopurulent vaginal discharge, vaginal itching, dyspareunia, dysuria, and vague lower abdominal pain), anorectal symptoms, and pharyngeal symptoms. Both organisms have the potential to cause PID in women, with possible sequelae such as ectopic pregnancy and infertility. Men may notice penile discharge, dysuria, testicular or epididymal pain, or may be asymptomatic. Women and men who engage in fellatio may contract a gonococcal pharyngitis characterized by a white pharyngeal exudate, and pharyngeal discomfort. Anorectal gonococcal disease may occur in men or women who participate in receptive anal intercourse and may present as rectal pain and/or discharge, constipation, and tenesmus.

SCREENING

Screening for both *N. gonorrhea* and *C. trachomatis* should be performed at the annual pelvic examination for all women with multiple male sexual partners (Indicator 7), the presence of other STDs (Barker, 1991), and a history of unprotected sexual intercourse -- and perhaps for all sexually active women 24 years of age or younger (CDC, 1993). There is no currently recommended screening for older women or men of any age.

DIAGNOSIS

The presence of symptoms such as mucopurulent vaginal discharge, vaginal itching, dyspareunia, dysuria, and vague lower abdominal pain in a heterosexual sexually active woman should lead one to suspect cervicitis. The physical examination may reveal a red, edematous, and friable cervix with mucopurulent cervical discharge. For men with a history of penile discharge and/or dysuria, a diagnosis of urethritis due to *C. trachomatis* or *N. gonorrhea* should be considered, although asymptomatic infections are common (CDC, 1993). If a sexually active male patient presents with penile discharge he should be tested for both chlamydia and gonorrhea at the time of presentation (Indicator 9).

C. trachomatis

Diagnosis in patients with symptoms of cervicitis or urethritis is confirmed by direct fluorescent antibody testing, which has a 70 to 87 percent sensitivity and a 97 to 99 percent specificity; or by enzyme immunoassay, which has a 80 to 86 percent sensitivity and a 98 percent specificity (Panzer et al., 1991).

N. gonorrhea

Suspected gonococcal infections may be initially confirmed by Gram stain, which has a 50 to 79 percent sensitivity and a 98 percent specificity (Panzer et al., 1991).

TREATMENT

In patients with symptoms or physical exam that are inconclusive, one must consider the pre-test probabilities of infection when assessing the need for treatment. In populations with a high prevalence of STDs, in those patients with known or suspected exposures, or in patients who might be unlikely to return for treatment, medical therapy should be provided without waiting for the confirmatory results of cultures. In other cases, according to the CDC, one may wait for the test results to determine the need for treatment (CDC, 1993). Treatment for mucopurulent cervicitis or urethritis should include the following:

- Treatment for gonococcal and chlamydial infections in patient populations with a high prevalence of STDs, such as patients seen at many STD clinics;
- Treatment for chlamydia only, if the prevalence of N. gonorrhea is low but the likelihood of chlamydia is significant;
- Await test results if the prevalence of both infections is low, and if compliance to return for further treatment if necessary is low (CDC, 1993). Patients should be advised to refer their sexual contacts for evaluation and appropriate treatment.

C. trachomatis

Based on the CDC review of RCTs (Weber and Johnson, 1995), either of the following treatment regimens is recommended:

- Doxycycline 100 mg orally twice a day for seven days; or
- Azithromycin 1 g orally in a single dose.

Other effective treatments include: ofloxacin, erythromycin, or sulfisoxazole. The patient's sexual partner(s) should also be referred for treatment.

N. gonorrhea

The treatment for gonorrhea also follows CDC recommendations based on reviews of RCTs (Moran and Levine, 1995). All patients treated for gonorrhea should also be treated for chlamydia (Indicator 8). Any of the following regimens are considered appropriate treatment for gonorrhea:

- Ceftriaxone 125 mg IM in a single dose;
- Cefixime 400 mg orally in a single dose;
- Ciprofloxacin 500 mg orally in a single dose; or
- Ofloxacin 400 mg orally in a single dose.

A clinical trial showed a cure rate of greater than 95 percent for anal and genital infections with one of the above treatment regimens, whereas treatment with either ceftriaxone or ciprofloxacin in the above-listed doses cured 90 percent of pharyngeal infections. Other effective antibiotics are available and may be used, such as spectinomycin, other cephalosporins, and other fluoroquinolones.

FOLLOW-UP

Follow-up cultures for chlamydia are not necessary for patients who completed treatment with doxycycline or azithromycin, unless symptoms persist or re-infection is suspected (CDC, 1993). If an alternative antibiotic regimen was selected (e.g., erythromycin, sulfisoxazole, or amoxicillin), re-testing should be performed three weeks after completion of the therapeutic course. Patients treated for gonorrhea who are symptom-free after completion of an appropriate antibiotic regimen do not need follow-up cultures (CDC, 1993).

Patients treated for gonorrhea should undergo screening for syphilis at the time of diagnosis.

PELVIC INFLAMMATORY DISEASE

IMPORTANCE

PID represents a spectrum of upper genital tract inflammatory disorders, including endometritis, salpingitis, tubo-ovarian abscess, and pelvic peritonitis. In the U.S., more than one million cases of PID are diagnosed and treated annually (DHHS, 1990). PID and its associated complications of ectopic pregnancy and infertility are estimated to cost more than $2.7 billion per year, with the total as high as $4.2 billion when all direct and indirect costs are included (Walker et al., 1993). The most common etiologic agents are *C. trachomatis* and *N. gonorrhea*.

DIAGNOSIS

The diagnosis of PID is usually made on the basis of clinical findings, including both speculum and bi-manual examinations (Indicator 10). In some cases, women may have an atypical presentation with abnormal bleeding, dyspareunia, or vaginal discharge. In the absence of an established cause other than PID (such as ectopic pregnancy or acute appendicitis) the CDC (1993) suggests that empiric treatment for PID should be initiated when all of the following clinical criteria for pelvic inflammation are present (Indicator 11):

- Lower abdominal tenderness;
- Adnexal tenderness; and
- Cervical motion tenderness.

The specificity of the diagnosis is increased if the following signs are also present (CDC, 1993):

- Oral temperature greater than 38.3C;
- Abnormal cervical or vaginal discharge;
- Elevated erythrocyte sedimentation rate;
- Elevated C-reactive protein; and
- Laboratory documentation of cervical infection with *N. gonorrhea* or *C. trachomatis*.

Algorithms based only on clinical criteria fail to identify some women with PID, and may misclassify others. Assessment by endometrial biopsy and laparoscopy, either separately or in combination, is more specific but less sensitive (Walker et al., 1993)

TREATMENT

Primarily on the basis of expert opinion, the CDC (1993) recommends hospitalization for parenteral antibiotic therapy under any of the following circumstances (Indicator 12):

- The diagnosis is uncertain and potential surgical emergencies such as acute appendicitis and ectopic pregnancy cannot be excluded;
- A pelvic abscess is suspected;
- The patient is pregnant;
- The patient is an adolescent;
- The patient is seropositive for HIV;
- There is severe illness or intractable nausea and vomiting that preclude outpatient management; or
- Clinical follow-up within 72 hours of initiating antibiotic therapy cannot be arranged.

Based on RCTs and extensive study of inpatient antimicrobial treatment for PID, the CDC recommends therapy with two antibiotics in either of the following regimens (Indicator 13):

Regimen 1:

- Cefoxitin 2 g IV every 6 hours or Cefotetan 2 g IV every 12 hours (for at least 48 hours); and
- Doxycycline 100 mg IV or orally every 12 hours (for 14 days).

Regimen 2:

- Clindamycin 900 mg IV every 8 hours; and
- Gentamicin.
- This regimen should be continued for at least 48 hours, followed by oral doxycycline or clindamycin.

No specific comparisons of inpatient and outpatient treatment have been performed, and there is limited information from clinical trials regarding outpatient management for PID (Walker et al., 1993). Patients who do not respond to outpatient therapy within 72 hours should be hospitalized, because it is expected that they would be afebrile and improved in terms of subjective complaints by that time (Peterson et al., 1990). For patients who do not respond to outpatient treatment, either of the following regimens is appropriate:

Regimen 1:

- Cefoxitin 2 g IM plus probenecid, 1 g orally in a single dose concurrently, or ceftriaxone 250 mg IM or any other parenteral third-generation cephalosporin; and
- Doxycycline 100 mg orally twice a day for 14 days.

Regimen 2:

- Ofloxacin 400 mg orally twice a day for 14 days; and
- Either clindamycin 450 mg orally 4 times a day OR metronidazole 500 mg twice a day for 14 days.

FOLLOW-UP

Patients who receive outpatient therapy should be followed up within 72 hours to assess clinical improvement (Indicator 14), and should also undergo microbiologic re-examination seven to ten days after completing antibiotic therapy.

Patients who require hospitalization for antimicrobial therapy should also have repeat cultures performed, seven to ten days after completion of the course of treatment to determine cure. Some patients may warrant further microbiologic re-examination after four to six weeks (CDC, 1991a). The male sexual partners of all patients should be empirically treated for *C. trachomatis* and *N. gonorrhea* (CDC, 1993).

DISEASES CHARACTERIZED BY GENITAL ULCERS

IMPORTANCE

The majority of persons with genital ulcers in the U.S. have genital herpes simplex virus (HSV), syphilis, or chancroid, with genital herpes being the most common. Three to ten percent of patients with genital ulcers may have more than one infection present. All of these infections are associated with an increased risk for HIV infection (CDC, 1993).

GENITAL HERPES SIMPLEX VIRUS

Screening

The literature does not suggest a useful role for screening for genital HSV infection.

Diagnosis

Based on serologic studies, the prevalence of genital HSV infection in the U.S. is 30 million people (CDC, 1993). The diagnosis is most often made on the basis of the history and physical examination, and is confirmed by HSV culture or antigen test. The sensitivity of the culture decreases with the duration – that is, with the age of the lesion(s). The sensitivities for vesicular, pustular, and crusted lesions are 70 percent, 67 percent, and 17 percent, respectively (Panzer et al., 1991). Specimens from primary and cutaneous lesions are most likely to grow HSV in culture.

Treatment

RCTs have demonstrated the effectiveness of acyclovir in decreasing the symptoms and signs of HSV during the initial and subsequent episodes, as well as when used for suppressive daily therapy (CDC, 1993; Stone and Whittington, 1990). The CDC does not generally recommend treatment with acyclovir for recurrent episodes of HSV infection because early therapy can rarely be initiated. The CDC does recommend that after one year of continuous suppressive therapy, acyclovir should be discontinued to allow re-assessment of the patient's recurrence of disease. If the recurrence rate for HSV is low, suppressive therapy may be discontinued either permanently or temporarily.

Other Management Issues

Patient education is very important in preventing the transmission of HSV. Patients should be advised to abstain from sexual activity while lesions are present, and to use condoms during all sexual exposures

(Indicator 15). All patients with genital ulcers should undergo serologic testing for syphilis, and HIV testing should be offered for those patients with known or suspected HSV (Indicator 16).

CHANCROID

Screening

Screening for chancroid is not indicated.

Diagnosis

The causative agent of chancroid is the bacterium *Haemophilus ducreyi*. As many as ten percent of patients with chancroid may be co-infected with *Treponema pallidum* or HSV (CDC, 1993). Because of the lack of a readily available method of testing for *H. ducreyi*, the diagnosis is made primarily on clinical grounds. The CDC supports the probable diagnosis of chancroid based on the following: 1) The presence of one or more painful genital ulcers; 2) The absence of evidence of *T. pallidum* infection on dark field exam or via a serologic test for syphilis performed at least seven days after the onset of the ulcers; and 3) The clinical presentation of the ulcer(s) is not typical of HSV and/or the HSV test results are negative.

Treatment

The CDC recommendations for treatment include single-dose azithromycin or IM ceftriaxone, or a seven-day course of erythromycin (Indicator 17). Patients with chancroid should be tested for HIV and syphilis, and if the initial test results are negative, they should be advised to undergo re-testing in three months (CDC, 1993). All persons with whom the patient had sexual contact within ten days before the onset of symptoms should be examined and treated.

Follow-Up

Patients should be re-examined within 10 days after initiation of antimicrobial treatment to assess clinical response (Indicator 18).

PRIMARY AND SECONDARY SYPHILIS

Syphilis is a systemic disease caused by *T. pallidum*. The incidence of primary and secondary syphilis in the U.S. has been rising steadily, with 118 cases per 100,000 population reported in 1989 (USDHHS, 1990). There appears to be an association between genital ulcer disease and the spread of HIV via sexual contact.

Screening

Screening of the general population is not indicated, except in the pregnant population. Those populations at risk for infection with *T. pallidum* (i.e., those with other STDs) should be screened using a nontreponemal test (CDC, 1993).

Diagnosis

Primary syphilis should be diagnosed based on the presence of a usually nonpainful genital ulcer (or recurrent history of a genital ulcer), and a positive laboratory test for syphilis. Twenty percent of patients will have a negative nontreponemal test (VDRL or RPR) at the time of presentation, but direct examination of the chancre via dark-field microscopy or direct fluorescence antibody will be positive (Panzer et al., 1991).

Secondary syphilis is a systemic illness characterized by a prominent rash which develops six weeks to several months after the initial exposure. According to the CDC recommendations, persons sexually exposed to individuals with any stage of syphilis should be evaluated clinically and serologically.

Treatment

Treatment of primary and secondary syphilis should be initiated with Benzathine penicillin G (2.4 million units IM in a single dose), in the absence of a penicillin allergy (Indicator 19). The decision to treat should not rely on waiting for the test results, but on the history, physical examination, and index of suspicion (Indicator 20).

Follow-up

Treatment failures occur in approximately five percent of patients treated with penicillin-based regimens, and more frequently in other regimens (Rotls, 1995). The CDC recommendations for follow-up include re-examination clinically and serologically at three and six months for assessment of successful response to therapy (CDC, 1993) (Indicator 21).

DISEASES CHARACTERIZED BY GENITAL WARTS (HUMAN PAPILLOMA VIRUS)

IMPORTANCE

The prevalence of infection with human papilloma virus (HPV) is increasing, with over one million new cases each year (Mayeaux, 1995). Although over 60 different types of HPV have been identified, only a relative few have a moderate risk (types 33, 35, 39,40, 43, 45 and 51) or high risk (types 16 and 18) of oncogenic potential (Mayeaux, 1995; CDC, 1993). There is usually a very long latency period between infection with the virus and any manifestation of cervical cancer. Individuals of all ages may contract HPV through sexual contact, although sexually active young adults have the highest prevalence and incidence of infection. HPV infection occurs at mucosal surfaces where micro-abrasions have caused epithelial disruption. Individuals, not knowing that they are infected with HPV, may transmit the virus to their sexual partners. Various viral strains of HPV have been strongly associated with the development of cervical cancer in women. The risk for contracting HPV increases with a woman's number of lifetime male sexual partners.

SCREENING

There is no indication for general population screening for HPV in either men or women, and no widely accepted screening tests exist.

DIAGNOSIS

HPV may be diagnosed in the presence of genital warts, condyloma accuminata, which have a hypertrophic appearance. Application of five-

338

percent acetic acid to small flat lesions suspicious for condyloma accuminata produces characteristic acetowhite changes. The differential diagnosis of HPV includes other sexually transmitted diseases condyloma latum (syphilis), HSV, and molluscum contagiosum, as well as common benign skin lesions, and dermatologic neoplasms. (Mayeaux, 1995). Lesions may be found in many genito-anal locations on both men and women. Single or multiple lesions may exist, as well as sub-clinical infection that is not apparent without the application of acetic acid. HPV lesions are rarely found on other non-genital mucosal surfaces such as the oral mucosa, larynx, and trachea (Mayeaux, 1995). Mucosal changes indicative of HPV infection may be noted on Pap smears (Indicator 22), although viral typing using recombinant DNA techniques is not routinely performed.

TREATMENT

It is not possible to eradicate HPV with the currently available treatment regimens. Therefore, the goal of treatment is to reduce the symptoms and signs of infection. Treatment of external genital warts is not likely to influence the development of cervical cancer (CDC, 1993). The results of many RCTs and other treatment studies have shown a wide range of 22 to 94 percent in the effectiveness of available therapies for clearing exophytic genital warts, and a very high recurrence rate of 25 percent at three months (CDC, 1993). The recurrence of genital warts is believed to be most commonly due to activation of sub-clinical infection rather than re infection. Genital warts due to HPV may resolve, remain unchanged, or grow if they are left untreated. Providers should inform patients of the necessity of practicing safe sexual habits such as the use of condoms, abstinence, or monogomy in order to reduce the spread of HPV.

A number of treatments for genital warts due to HPV exist, and RCTs have been conducted to assess the various treatment modalities (CDC, 1993). Some of the treatments are site-specific and include cryotherapy with liquid nitrogen or cryoprobe, Podofilox, Podophyllin, Trichloroacetic acid, and electrodesiccation or electrocautery.

FOLLOW-UP

Regularly scheduled follow-up is not necessary after the warts have responded to therapy. Annual cytologic screening is recommended for women with a history of genital warts. Recommendations for cervical cancer screening are covered in Volume II of this series, which covers ocologic conditions and HIV (see Chapter 3: Cervical Cancer Screening).

REFERENCES

Amsel R, Totten PA, Spiegel CA, et al. January 1983. Nonspecific vaginitis: Diagnostic criteria and microbial and epidemiologic associations. *American Journal of Medicine* 74: 14-22.

Barker LR, Burton JR, and Zieve PD. 1991. *Principles of Ambulatory Medicine, 3rd Edition*. Baltimore, MD: Williams and Wilkins.

Barker, L Randol, Burton, John R, Zieve, and Philip D, Editors. 1991. *Principles of Ambulatory Medicine*, Third ed. Baltimore, MD: Williams and Wilkins.

Berger J, Kolton S, Zenilman J, et al. 1995. Bacterial Vaginosis in Lesbians: A Sexually Transmitted Disease. *Clinical Infectious Diseases* 21: 1402-5.

Centers for Disease Control. September 1993. 1993 Sexually Transmitted Diseases Treatment Guidelines. *Morbidity and Mortality Weekly Report* 42 (RR-14): 1-102.

Centers for Disease Control. April 1991. Pelvic inflammatory disease: Guidelines for prevention and management. *Morbidity and Mortality Weekly Report* 40 (RR-5): 1-25.

Centers for Disease Control. May 1991. Sexually Transmitted Diseases: Clinical Practice Guidelines. *U.S. Department of Health and Human Services*

Centers for Disease Control and Prevention. 1997. *Sexually Transmitted Diseases: Guidelines for Health Education and Risk Reduction Activities*. Baltimore, MD: Williams and Wilkins, pp. 636-753.

Department of Health and Human Services. 1991. *Healthy People 2000: National Health Promotion and Disease Prevention Objectives*. Washington, DC: U.S. Government Printing Office; (PHS) 91-50212.

Hatch KD. April 1995. Clinical appearance and treatment strategies for human papillomavirus: A gynecologic perspective. *American Journal of Obstetrics and Gynecology* 172 (4 (Part 2)): 1340-1344.

Hoffman IF and Schmitz JL. September 1995. Genital ulcer disease - Management in the HIV era. *Postgraduate Medicine* 98 (3): 67-82.

Inman W, Pearce G, and Wilton L. 1994. Safety of fluconazole in the treatment of vaginal candidiasis: A prescription-event monitoring study, with special reference to the outcome of pregnancy. *European Journal of Clinical Pharmacology* 46: 115-118.

Joesoef MR and Schmid GP. 1995. Bacterial Vaginosis: Review of treatment options and potential clinical indications for therapy. *Clinical Infectious Diseases* 20(suppl. 1): S72-79.

Mayeaux EJ Jr, Harper MB, et al. September 1995. Noncervical Human Papillomavirus Genital Infections. *American Family Physician* 52 (4): 1137-1146.

Moran JS and Levine WC. 1995. Drugs of choice for the treatment of uncomplicated gonococcal infections. *Clinical Infectious Diseases* 20 (suppl. 1): S47-65.

Panzer RJ, Black ER, Griner PF, Editors. 1991. *Diagnostic Strategies for Common Medical Problems*. Philadelphia, PA: American College of Physicians.

Peterson HV, Walker CK, Kahn JF, et al. November 1991. Pelvic Inflammatory Disease: Key treatment issues and options. *Journal of the American Medical Association* 266 (18): 2605-2611.

Preventive Services Task Force. 1989. *Guide to Clinical Preventive Services: An Assessment of the Effectiveness of 169 Interventions*. Baltimore, MD: Williams and Wilkins.

Reef SE, Levine WC, McNeil MM, et al. 1995. Treatment options for vulvovaginal candidiasis, 1993. *Clinical Infectious Diseases* 20(suppl 1): S23-38.

Rolfs RT. 1995. Treatment of syphilis, 1993. *Clinical Infectious Diseases* 20 (1): S23-38.

Skolnik NS. March 1995. Screening for chlamydia trachomatis Infection. *American Family Physician* 51 (4): 821-826.

Stone KM and Whittington WL. July 1990. Treatment of genital herpes. *Reviews of Infectious Diseases* 12 (suppl. 6): S610-619.

Walker CK, Kahn JF, Washington EA, et al. October 1993. Pelvic inflammatory disease: Meta-analysis of antimicrobial regimen efficacy. *The Journal of Infectious Diseases* 168: 969-978.

Weber JT and Johnson RE. 1995. New treatments for chlamydia trachomatis genital infection. *Clinical Infectious Diseases* 20 (suppl. 1): S66-71.

Zenilman JM. February 1993. Gonorrhea: Clinical and Public Health Issues. *Hospital Practice* 29-50.

RECOMMENDED QUALITY INDICATORS FOR VAGINITIS AND SEXUALLY TRANSMITTED DISEASES

The following indicators apply to men and women age 18 and older. Only the indicators in bold type were rated by this panel; the remaining indicators were endorsed by a prior panel.

Indicator	Quality of Evidence	Literature	Benefits	Comments
Vaginitis - Diagnosis				
1. A sexual history should be obtained at the time of presentation from all women with a chief complaint of vaginal discharge. The history should include: a. Number of male partners in the previous 6 months; b. Absence or presence of symptoms in partners; c. Prior history of sexually transmitted diseases.	III	Panzer et al, 1991; CDC, 1993	Decrease discharge, itching, and dysuria. Decrease PID and abdominal pain. Decrease infertility. Decrease mortality from ectopic pregnancy.	In patients with one or more risk factors, there is an increased prior probability of an STD (i.e., chlamydia or gonorrhea) as a cause of discharge, and a culture for the causative organisms may be appropriate. This is important because cervicitis has more significant long-term consequences than vaginitis, such as PID, infertility, and ectopic pregnancy.
2. In women presenting with a chief complaint of vaginal discharge, the practitioner should perform a speculum exam at the time of the initial presentation to determine if the source of the discharge is vaginal or cervical.	III	Panzer et al, 1991	Decrease discharge, itching, and dysuria.	Since implications of and treatment for cervicitis and vaginitis differ substantially, physical exam must be performed.
3. If three of the following four criteria are met, a diagnosis of bacterial vaginosis, or gardnerella vaginitis should be made: • pH greater than 4.5; • positive whiff test; • clue cells on wet mount; and • thin homogeneous discharge.	III	Panzer et al, 1991	Decrease discharge, itching, and dysuria.	pH determination is also sensitive, but its specificity is unknown. Therefore, at a minimum, the two wet mounts should be performed.
Vaginitis - Treatment				
4. Treatment for bacterial vaginosis should be with metronidazole (orally or vaginally) or clindamycin (orally or vaginally) at the time of diagnosis.	I	CDC, 1993	Decrease discharge, itching, and dysuria.	These are the only proven effective regimens; RCTs reviewed by the CDC show that the evidence for efficacy of oral treatment is better than that for topical treatment.

343

Indicator	Quality of Evidence	Literature	Benefits	Comments
5. Treatment for T. vaginalis should be with oral metronidazole, if the patient does not have an allergy to metronidazole or is not in first trimester of pregnancy at the time of diagnosis.	I	CDC, 1993	Decrease discharge, itching, and dysuria.	Based on RCTs reviewed by the CDC this is the only known effective treatment.
6. Treatment for non-recurrent (< 3 episodes in the previous year) yeast vaginitis should be with topical 'azole' preparations (e.g. clotrimazole, butoconazole, etc.) or fluconazole at the time of diagnosis.	I	CDC, 1993	Decrease discharge, itching, and dysuria.	Based on RCTs reviewed by the CDC. These regimens are approved by the FDA.
Cervicitis - Diagnosis				
7. Routine testing for gonorrhea (culture) and chlamydia trachomatis (antigen detection), should be performed with the routine pelvic exam for women with multiple male sexual partners (more than 1 during the previous 6 months).	III	CDC, 1993; ACOG, 1993 (The Obstetrician Gynecologist Primary Preventive Healthcare)	Alleviate pain. Alleviate fever. Decrease infertility. Decrease mortality from ectopic pregnancy.	This recommendation is based on epidemiologic studies of transmission and prevalence, as summarized by the CDC. Women with multiple sexual partners are at higher risk for STDs, and these may be asymptomatic.
Cervicitis - Treatment				
8. Women treated for gonorrhea should also be treated for chlamydia at the time of presentation.	II-2; III	CDC, 1993	Prevent PID. Decrease infertility. Decrease mortality from ectopic pregnancy.	Women with gonorrhea are likely to be coinfected with chlamydia. Since the sensitivity of chlamydia assays are variable, concurrent treatment is recommended.
Urethritis - Diagnosis				
9. If a sexually active male patient presents with penile discharge he should be tested for both chlamydia and gonorrhea at the time of presentation.	III	CDC, 1993	Decrease infertility. Provide accurate diagnosis and treatment.	This is based on epidemiologic studies of transmission and prevalence, as summarized by the CDC.

Indicator	Quality of Evidence	Literature	Benefits	Comments
Pelvic Inflammatory Disease (PID) - Diagnosis				
10. Patients with the diagnosis of PID should receive all of the following at the time of diagnosis: a. Speculum exam; b. Bi-manual exam.	III	CDC, 1993	Alleviate pain. Alleviate fever. Decrease infertility. Decrease mortality from ectopic pregnancy.	The diagnosis of PID is based primarily on physical exam. In addition, one should obtain cervical specimens for culture. Therefore, a physical exam is mandatory before treatment can be initiated.
11. If a patient is given the diagnosis of PID, at least 2 of the following signs should be present on physical exam: • lower abdominal tenderness; • adnexal tenderness; and • cervical motion tenderness.	III	CDC, 1993	Alleviate pain. Alleviate fever. Decrease infertility. Decrease mortality from ectopic pregnancy.	It is important to correctly identify PID since symptoms may mimic appendicitis and ovarian torsion. The CDC states that all 3 signs should be present. We have stated that at least 2 must be present and documented.
Pelvic Inflammatory Disease - Treatment				
12. Women with PID and any of the following conditions should receive parenteral antibiotics at the time of diagnosis: a. Pelvic abscess is present or suspected; b. Pregnancy; c. HIV infection; d. Uncontrolled nausea and vomiting; e. Lack of clinical improvement within 72 hours of beginning therapy.	III	CDC, 1993	Alleviate pain. Alleviate fever. Prevent sepsis. Decrease infertility. Decrease mortality from ectopic pregnancy.	Although other reasons for hospitalization may exist (i.e., cannot rule out appendicitis), these conditions have been recommended by the CDC and should be discernible by chart review. The purpose of hospitalization is to ensure effective treatment in persons at risk of complications (e.g., HIV infection) or poor follow-up (e.g., adolescents).
13. Duration of total antibiotic therapy for PID should be no less than 10 days (inpatient, if applicable, plus outpatient).	III	CDC, 1993; Peterson et al, 1991	Alleviate pain. Alleviate fever. Prevent sepsis. Decrease infertility. Decrease mortality from ectopic pregnancy.	The standard of care is 10-14 days, although RCTs have not specifically addressed duration of treatment. Shorter treatment periods may result in lower cure rates.

345

Indicator	Quality of Evidence	Literature	Benefits	Comments
Pelvic Inflammatory Disease - Follow-Up				
14. Patients receiving outpatient therapy for PID should receive follow-up contact within 72 hours of diagnosis.	III	CDC, 1993; Peterson et al, 1991	Alleviate pain. Alleviate fever. Prevent sepsis. Decrease infertility. Decrease mortality from ectopic pregnancy.	Early effective treatment is important in preventing complications.
Genital Ulcers - Diagnosis				
15. All patients with genital herpes should be counseled on reducing the risk of transmission to a sexual partner.	III	CDC, 1993	Prevent spread of genital herpes.	Genital herpes is can be transmitted even in the absence of current outbreak. Unlike most other STDs, there is not an effective cure for herpes. Therefore, prevention of transmission is of primary importance.
16. If a patient presents with the new onset of genital ulcers then all of the following should be offered at the time of presentation: a. Cultures for HSV b. Blood test for HIV c. Blood test for syphilis.	III	CDC, 1993	Prevention of complications of untreated syphilis and HIV. Limit transmission of genital herpes.	There has been an increase in the prevalence of genital herpes in association with HIV. Effective treatment for syphilis is available with a single IM injection of penicillin. There is no effective cure for herpes; therefore preventing transmission of the virus is of prime importance.
Genital Ulcers - Chancroid - Treatment				
17. Patients with chancroid should be treated with azithromycin, ceftriaxone, or erythromycin (in the absence of allergy to these medications).	I	CDC, 1993	Decrease pain. Heal ulcer. Limit transmission of chancroid.	These have been shown to be effective in RCTs reviewed by the CDC.
Genital Ulcers - Chancroid - Follow-up				
18. Patients receiving treatment for chancroid should be re-examined within 10 days of treatment initiation to assess clinical improvement.	III	CDC, 1993	Prevent complications of untreated syphilis. Prevent transmission of chancroid, syphilis, and herpes.	Most patients will have improved by 7 days.

346

Indicator	Quality of Evidence	Literature	Benefits	Comments
Genital Ulcers - Syphilis - Treatment				
19. Patients with primary and secondary syphilis who do not have a penicillin allergy should be treated with IM-administered benzathine penicillin G.	I	CDC, 1993	Prevent late complications of syphilis.	Penicillin is the best studied of all regimens and is known to be effective through single IM administration. This recommendation is based on RCTs reviewed by the CDC.
20. If a patient has a primary ulcer consistent with syphilis, treatment for syphilis should be initiated before laboratory test results are available.	III	CDC, 1993	Prevent late complications of syphilis.	Not all patients will return for follow-up. Because effective treatment exists and consequences of untreated syphilis are serious, treatment should be initiated at the time of first presentation.
Genital Ulcers - Syphilis - Follow-up				
21. Patients with primary or secondary syphilis should be re-examined clinically and serologically within 6 months after treatment.	III	CDC, 1993	Prevent complications of untreated syphilis.	If a treatment failure has occurred, the patient requires re-treatment.
Genital Warts - Diagnosis				
22. Women with an initial diagnosis of HPV should have a speculum examination and a pap smear (if not performed during the preceding year).	III	CDC, 1993; CDC, 1997	Identify cervical dysplasia and exophytic warts.	Based on RCTs, effective treatment for cervical dysplasia exists. Effective treatments are available to remove exophytic warts which can cause discomfort to patients.
STDs (General) - Diagnosis				
STDs include herpes, syphilis, genital warts, gonorrhea, chlamydia, trichomoniasis, HPV, and chancroid				
23. If a patient presents with an initial infection of any STD, HIV testing should be discussed and offered at the time of presentation.	III	CDC, 1993	Prevent progression and reduce transmission of HIV.	Persons with one STD are at high risk for another. Treatment to slow the disease course of HIV and prophylaxis against opportunistic infections are available.
24. If a patient presents with any STD, a non-treponemal test (VDRL or RPR) for syphilis should be performed at the time of presentation	III	CDC, 1993	Prevent late complications of syphilis.	Persons with one STD are at high risk for another. Since there is effective treatment to prevent late complications of syphilis, testing is recommended.

347

Indicator	Quality of Evidence	Literature	Benefits	Comments
STDs (General) - Treatment				
25. Sexual partners of patients with new diagnoses of gonorrhea, chlamydia, chancroid, and primary or secondary syphilis should be referred for treatment as soon as possible.	III	CDC, 1993	Prevent complications from PID and syphilis.	Persons with one STD are at high risk for another. Since there is effective treatment to prevent late complications of syphilis, testing is recommended. Women with untreated gonococcal and chlamydial infections are at increased risk for PID and ectopic pregnancy.

Quality of Evidence Codes

I	RCT
II-1	Nonrandomized controlled trials
II-2	Cohort or case analysis
II-3	Multiple time series
III	Opinions or descriptive studies

21. URINARY TRACT INFECTION[6]

Eve A. Kerr, M.D., M.P.H.

The general approach to urinary tract infections (UTIs) was obtained from two ambulatory medical text chapters (Barker et al., 1991; Goroll et al, 1996), a textbook of diagnostic strategies (Panzer et al., 1991), and review articles which dealt with diagnosis and management of urinary tract infections. The review articles were chosen from a MEDLINE search which identified all English language review articles on urinary tract infection between the years of 1990 and 1997. Further, since the main controversy in UTIs concerns laboratory testing and therapy, we selected and reviewed references from the review articles which related to laboratory testing and antibiotic therapy. Finally, we performed another MEDLINE search (1990-1997) to identify any randomized controlled trials (RCTs) regarding treatment of UTIs. This chapter focuses on diagnosis and treatement of acute upper and lower tract infections. It does not specifically cover diagnosis or treatment of prostatitis nor of bacteriuria caused by indwelling catheters.

IMPORTANCE

UTIs are among the most common bacterial infections seen by physicians and are the most common bacterial infection in women (Winickoff et al., 1981). They affect ten to 20 percent of women in the United States annually and account for over five million office visits per year. The prevalence of UTI increases with increasing age, and the prevalence of bacteriuria in elderly men approaches that in women (i.e., 20-30%) (Lipsky

---

[6] This chapter is a revision of one written for an earlier project on quality of care for women and children (Q1). The expert panel for the current project was asked to review all of the indicators, but only rated new or revised indicators.

et al., 1987). Outpatient expenditures for patients with UTIs in the United States approach $1 billion (Powers, 1991).

SCREENING

There is no role for screening for UTIs or bacteriuria in otherwise healthy men and non-pregnant women (Pels et al., 1989; US Preventive Task Force, 1996). Treatment of asymptomatic bacteriuria has not been shown consistently to affect outcomes (Childs and Egan, 1996; Baldassarre and Kaye, 1991). Consequently, we will not address screening for UTI, nor treatment for asymptomatic bacteriuria, in this chapter.

DIAGNOSIS

The diagnosis of UTI is typically derived from the patient's history. An uncomplicated UTI is suggested by symptoms of bladder irritation and occasionally hematuria. An upper tract infection is suggested by the concomitant presence of fever, chills, and/or back pain (Indicator 1). In addition, vaginal infections (due to candida and trichomonas) and urethritis (due to *Chlamydia trachomatis, Neisseria gonorrhoeae,* or herpes simplex virus) could present with UTI-type symptoms. Therefore, a history of vaginal (Indicator 2) or penile discharge and sexual activity should be sought. However, data on the positive predictive value of dysuria for urinary tract infection in men are limited. Work-up of penile discharge is covered in the chapter on sexually transmitted diseases. Since those with diabetes and immunosuppression are treated differently, the history should specifically include these questions (Barker et al., 1991).

In men, acute and chronic prostatitis may also present with symptoms of dysuria (Lipsky, 1989). Men with acute prostatitis are often systemically ill and have pelvic pain and/or a tender prostate. Chronic prostatitis and prostatic hypertrophy may be underlying causes for recurrent UTI in men.

The urinalysis is the most important initial study in the evaluation of a patient suspected of having a UTI by history (Indicator 3). A negative urinalysis makes the diagnosis of UTI extremely unlikely (Barker et al., 1991). In women, a specimen should be collected by the "clean-catch" method to minimize likelihood of contamination (Barker et al.,

1991), or by catheterization when the "clean-catch" method is impossible. A "clean-catch" is thought to be unnecessary in men (Lipsky, 1989). A finding by microscopic examination using a high-power lens of bacteria of more than seven white cells/mm^3 in unspun urine or more than two white cells per high-power field in spun urine is consistent with an UTI in women. The leukocyte esterase test has a sensitivity for defining UTI (if the test is positive) of between 62 and 68 percent, with a positive predictive value of only 46 to 55 percent and a negative predictive value of 88 to 92 percent (Pfaller and Koontz, 1985). A nitrite test has a sensitivity of 35 to 85 percent and specificity of 92 to 100 percent for the presence of bacteria (Pappas, 1991). The leukocyte-esterase nitrite combination has a sensitivity of 79.2 percent, a specificity of 81 percent and a negative predictive value of 94.5 percent for specimens with greater than 10^5 CFU/ml (Pfaller and Koontz, 1985). A combination of findings (i.e., bacteriuria, pyuria and a positive nitrite test) is more highly predictive for UTI (Bailey, 1995). The three or four-glass test for localizing source of infection in men has generally fallen out of favor due to high costs and low specificity (Goroll, 1995 Lipsky , 1989)

Most experts agree that a routine urine culture is not warranted in women who present with non-recurrent acute dysuria without symptoms of upper tract infection and with a positive urinalysis (Hooten and Stamm, 1991; Forland, 1993). Some experts do recommend routine culture in men presenting with dysuria, and in the elderly (Lipsky, 1989; Baldassare and Kaye, 1991; Childs and Egan, 1996). However, we were unable to find any studies that demonstrate the usefulness of cultures versus empiric treatment in these populations, and have not created an indicator requiring cultures for all men and elderly patients. However, all authors agree that certain criteria for appropriate use of a culture exist for both genders and all age groups (Indicator 4). A summary of these criteria are shown in Table 21.1.

Table 21.1

Criteria for Appropriate Use of Culture

A culture should be obtained in patients who have:

- "Several" (three or more) infections in the past year
- Diabetes or immunocompromised state
- Fever, chills and/or flank pain
- Acute pyelonephritis
- Structural or functional anomalies of the urinary tract
- Symptoms for more than 7 days before presentation
- Pregnancy
- A relapse of symptoms after initial treatment
- Hospital acquired infection
- Indwelling foley catheter
- Recent instrumentation of the urinary tract

Sources: Powers, 1991; Barker et al., 1991; Panzer et al., 1991; Hooton and Stamm, 1991.

TREATMENT

Treatment currently rests with the appropriate use of antibiotics (Indicator 5). A single-dose or a three-day course of an oral antimicrobial has been shown to eradicate approximately 90 to 95 percent of cases of uncomplicated UTI in young women. However, therapy for three days or longer was more effective than single-dose therapy in most trials and in a meta-analysis (Stamm and Hooton, 1993; Elder, 1992; Johnson and Stamm, 1989; Norrby, 1990). Baldassare and Kaye (1991) recommend a similar approach to treatment for elderly women, although some recommend seven days of treatment in elderly patients with uncomplicated UTI (Stamm and Hooten, 1993). There are no good studies on the appropriate duration of treatment for men with acute lower tract infection, although some authors recommend seven days instead of the shorter three day regimens (Hooten and Stamm, 1991). Our indicator specifies that treatment of uncomplicated lower tract infection in women under age 65 should not exceed seven days (Indicator 7).

However, patients of both genders, regardless of age, who have "complicated lower tract infections"[7] should receive antibiotic treatment for at least seven days (Indicator 10). Patients with mild to moderate acute uncomplicated pyelonephritis should be treated for 10 to 14 days as outpatients (Stamm et al., 1987) (Indicator 8). Severe pyelonephritis, with nausea and vomiting, or possible urosepsis, may require parentral antibiotics, as does pyelonephritis in pregnancy (Indicator 9).

In general, trimethoprim/sulfamethoxazole double strength (160 mg/800 mg) is the most effective first-line agent for acute uncomplicated lower UTI in women under age 65, with resistance in five to 15 percent of cases (Indicator 6). It should be used unless there is documented resistance, allergy, or pregnancy. Amoxicillin and nitrofurantoin have higher rates of failure (Stamm and Hooton, 1993; Johnson and Stamm, 1989; Elder, 1992; Norrby, 1990). The use of quinolones, while effective (Stein et al., 1987; Hooton et al., 1991), should be reserved for patients with known resistance or allergy to other first-line agents to avoid unnecessary expense and the promotion of resistant strains (Sable and Scheld, 1993).

Empiric selection of antibiotics in men and the elderly is more complicated, because the causative agents of urinary tract infections are more diverse. More frequent use of catheterization, incontinence, and debilitation in the elderly, and concomittant prostatitis in men, makes the selection of antibiotics more dependent on the clinical situation. Therefore, our indicators will only suggest the use of trimethoprim/sulfamethoxazole double strength as the first line agent in non-elderly women.

FOLLOW-UP

Experts disagree on necessity for follow-up in lower tract infection. Some feel a follow-up culture is unnecessary if symptoms of uncomplicated UTI have resolved within three days of starting treatment (Stamm and

---

[7] Complicated lower tract infections: Diabetes or immunocompromised state; functional or structural anomaly of the urinary tract; symptoms for longer than seven days; recent urinary tract infection; acute pyelonephritis or more than 3 urinary tract infections in past year; pregnancy (Stamm and Hooton, 1993; Johnson and Stamm, 1989).

Hooton, 1993; Patton et al., 1991; Winickoff et al., 1981; Schultz et al., 1984). Barker et al. (1991) stipulate that the urinalysis should be re-evaluated within seven days if a single-dose regimen was utilized or within four weeks if a seven to ten day course was used, even if symptoms have cleared. Most experts agree, however, that follow-up culture is indicated within two weeks of complicated cystitis or pyelonephritis (Stamm and Hooton, 1993)(Indicators 11 and 12).

The issue of when to do further work-up in men with recurrent UTIs remains unresolved. Prostatic involvement accounts of the majority of instances of infection relapse (Goroll, 1995), and usually responds to a prolonged course of antibiotics. Previous recommendations for men with even one UTI have centered around urologic evaluation. However, there is considerable uncertainty about the clinical and prognostic significance of abnormalities detected by roentgenographic and urodynamic tests in men with one or more UTIs, and it is not clear which test is the most appropriate, even for men with recurrent infections or pyelonephritis (Lipsky, 1989; Goroll, 1995). Therefore, we have not included any specific indicators on testing or referral in men with UTIs.

REFERENCES

Bailey BL. January 1995. Urinalysis predictive of urine culture results. *Journal of Family Practice* 40 (1): 45-50.

Baldassarre JS and Kaye D. 1991. Special problems of urinary tract infection in the elderly. *Medical Clinics of North America* 75 (2): 375-390.

Barker LR, Burton JR, and Zieve PD, Editors. 1991. *Principles of Ambulatory Medicine*, Third ed.Baltimore, MD: Williams and Wilkins.

Carlson KJ, and Mulley AG. 1985. Management of acute dysuria. *Archives of Internal Medicine* 102 (2): 244-9.

Childs SJ and Egan RJ. 1996. Bacteriuria and urinary infections in the elderly. *Urologic Clinics of North America* 23 (1): 43-54.

Childs SJ. 1991. Current concepts in the treatment of urinary tract infections and prostatitis. *American Journal of Medicine* 91 (suppl 6A): 6A-120S-123S.

Elder NC. 1 November 1992. Acute urinary tract infection in women: What kind of antibiotic therapy is optimal. *Postgraduate Medicine* 92 (6): 159-72.

Fihn SD, Johnson C, Roberts PL, et al. March 1988. Trimethoprim-sulfamethoxazole for acute dysuria in women: A single-dose or 10-day course. *Archives of Internal Medicine* 108 (3): 350-7.

Forland M. 1993. Urinary tract infection. How has its management changed? *Postgraduate Medicine* 93 (5): 71-86.

Goroll AH, Lawrence A, and Melley AG. 1995. *Primary care medicine: Office evaulation and management of the adult patient. 3rd Edition.* Philadelphia: JB Lippincott Company.

Hooton TM and Stamm WE. 1991. Management of acute uncomplicated urinary tract infection in adults. *Medical Clinics of North America* 75 (2): 339-357.

Hooton TM, Johnson C, Winter C, et al. 1991. Single-dose and three-day regimens of ofloxacin versus trimethoprim-sulfamethoxazole for acute cystitis in women. *Antimicrobial Agents and Chemotherapy* 35 (7): 1479-83.

Jaff M and Paganini EP. 1989. Meeting the challenge of geriatric UTIs. *Geriatrics* 44 (12): 60-69.

Johnson JR, and Stamm W. 1 December 1989. Urinary tract infections in women: Diagnosis and treatment. *Archives of Internal Medicine* 111 (11): 906-17.

Lipsky BA. 1989. Urinary tract infections in men. *Archives of Internal Medicine* 110: 138-150.

Lipsky BA, Ireton RC, Fihn SD, et al. 1987. Diagnosis of bacteriuria in men: specimen collection and culture interpretation. *Journal of Infectious Diseases* 155 (5): 847-854.

Nicolle LE, Henderson E, Bjornson J, et al. 1987. The association of bacteriuria with resident characterisitcs and survival in elderly institutionalized men. *Annals of Internal Medicine* 106 (682-686):

Norrby SR. May 1990. Short-term treatment of uncomplicated lower urinary tract infections in women. *Reviews of Infectious Diseases* 12 (3): 458-67.

Panzer RJ, Black ER, and Griner PF, Editors. 1991. *Diagnostic Strategies for Common Medical Problems.* Philadelphia, PA: American College of Physicians.

Pappas PG. March 1991. Laboratory in the diagnosis and management of urinary tract infections. *Medical Clinics of North America* 75 (2): 313-25.

Patton JP, Nash DB, and Abrutyn E. March 1991. Urinary tract infection: Economic considerations. *Medical Clinics of North America* 75 (2): 495-513.

Pels RJ, Bor DH, Woolhandler S, et al. 1 September 1989. Dipstick urinalysis screening of asymptomatic adults for urinary tract disorders. *Journal of the American Medical Association* 262 (9): 1221-4.

Pfaller MA, and Koontz FP. May 1985. Laboratory evaluation of leukocyte esterase and nitrite tests for the detection of bacteriuria. *Journal of Clinical Microbiology* 21 (5): 840-2.

Powers RD. May 1991. New directions in the diagnosis and therapy of urinary tract infections. *American Journal of Obstetrics and Gynecology* 164 (Volume 5, Part 2): 1387-9.

Ronald AR and Pattullo AL. 1991. The natural history of urinary infection in adults. *Medical Clinics of North America* 75 (2): 299-312.

Sable CA, and Scheld WM. June 1993. Fluoroquinolones: How to use (but not overuse) these antibiotics. *Geriatrics* 48 (6): 41-51.

Schultz HJ, McCaffrey LA, et al. June 1984. Acute cystitis: A prospective study of laboratory tests and duration of therapy. *Mayo Clinic Proceedings* 59: 391-7.

Stamm, WE, McKevitt M, and Counts GW. May 1987. Acute renal infection in women: Treatment with trimethoprim-sulfamethoxazole or ampicillin for two or six weeks. *Archives of Internal Medicine* 106 (3): 341-5.

Stamm WE, and Hooton TM. 28 October 1993. Management of urinary tract infections in adults. *New England Journal of Medicine* 329 (18): 1328-34.

Stein GE, Mummaw N, et al. October 1987. A multicenter comparative trial of three-day norfloxacin vs ten-day sulfamethoxazole and trimethoprim for the treatment of uncomplicated urinary tract infections. *Archives of Internal Medicine* 147: 1760-2.

Winickoff RN, Wilner SI, et al. February 1981. Urine culture after treatment of uncomplicated cystitis in women. *Southern Medical Journal* 74 (2): 165-9.

Zhanel GG, et al. 1990. Asymptomatic bacteriuria. Which patients should be treated? *Archives of Internal Medicine* 150: 1389-1396.

RECOMMENDED QUALITY INDICATORS FOR URINARY TRACT INFECTIONS

The following indicators apply to men and women age 18 and older without diabetes or immunocompromise. Only the indicators in bold type were rated by this panel; the remaining indicators were endorsed by a prior panel.

Indicator	Quality of Evidence	Literature	Benefits	Comments
Diagnosis				
1. In patients presenting with dysuria, presence or absence of fever and flank pain should be elicited.	III	Barker et al., 1991; Powers, 1991	Alleviate pain and fever. Prevent sepsis. Prevent abscess formation.	Fever and flank pain increase probability of upper tract infection (pyelonephritis).
2. In women presenting with dysuria, a history of vaginal discharge should be elicited.	III	Panzer et al., 1991; Barker et al., 1991	Alleviate dysuria. Prevent allergic reactions from antibiotics. Prevent antibiotic associated diarrhea and yeast vaginitis.	Dysuria may be caused by vaginitis (and rarely cervicitis) as well as UTI. By evaluating cause for dysuria, treatment for vaginitis may be initiated and avoidance of antibiotics for non-UTI causes can be accomplished.
3. Patients who present with dysuria and are started on antimicrobial treatment for urinary tract infection should have had a urinalysis or dipstick evaluation on the day of presentation.	III	Johnson and Stamm, 1989; Panzer et al., 1991	Prevent allergic reactions from antibiotics. Prevent antibiotic-associated diarrhea and yeast vaginitis.	Urinalysis, if negative for white blood cells, rules out UTI and antibiotics do not need to be used.
4. A urine culture should be obtained for patients who have dysuria and any one of the following: a. "several" (three or more) infections in the past year; b. diabetes or immunocompromised state; c. fever, chills and/or flank pain; d. suspected diagnosis of pyelonephritis; e. structural or functional anomalies of the urinary tract; f. a relapse of symptoms, if no culture previously obtained; g. a recent invasive procedure.	III	Powers, 1991; Barker et al., 1991; Panzer et al., 1991	Alleviate dysuria. Prevent pyelonephritis. Prevent UTI recurrence.	Appropriate and prompt treatment in these instances can prevent complications and recurrences. However, there is little empiric evidence to support the timing for obtaining a urine culture.

358

Treatment

Indicator	Quality of Evidence	Literature	Benefits	Comments
5. If a diagnosis of UTI (upper or lower tract) has been made, the patient should be treated with antimicrobial therapy.	III; II-2	Stamm and Hooton, 1993; Johnson and Stamm, 1989; Powers, 1991	Prevent complications of untreated infection.	Both upper and lower tract infections respond to a number of antimicrobial agents. Trimethoprim-sulfa is usually chosen as a first line agent. While no RCTs have shown benefits of treatment, it is recognized that treatment of both lower and upper tract infections is beneficial (see above).
6. Trimethoprim-sulfamethoxazole should be used as a first-line agent in women under age 65 with uncomplicated lower tract infection[1] unless there is documented history of allergy or pregnancy	II-2; III	Johnson and Stamm, 1989; Carlson, 1985; Sable, 1993	Decrease dysuria. Prevent drug resistance.	This recommendation is based on studies of susceptibility of urinary tract infections to various antibiotics and costs, primarily reviewed in the Johnson and Stamm article. TMP-SMZ is the most effective antibiotic (least resistance, lower rates of recurrence). Flouroquinolones, while equally effective, have a broader spectrum and casual use promotes resistance in the individual and population.
7. Treatment with antimicrobials for uncomplicated lower tract infections[1] in women under age 65 should not exceed 7 days.	I; III	Stamm and Hooton, 1993; Johnson and Stamm, 1989; Elder, 1992; Fihn et al., 1988	Decrease dysuria. Prevent antibiotic allergic reactions. Prevent antibiotic associated diarrhea. Prevent antibiotic associated superinfections.	Several studies, summarized in the review articles cited, have shown that one day therapy is effective but that it may increase relapse. A well-conducted RCT by Fihn et al using TMP-Sulfa showed that although a 10 day tx yielded superior cure rate at 2 weeks, by 6 weeks the advantage had diminished. The adverse effects were higher in the 10 day group. Therefore, several experts advocate the 3 day regimen in absence of RCT data on the 3 day regimen. There is no evidence that the benefit of prolonged therapy outweighs the risk of antibiotic allergies, superinfection, diarrhea and constitutional symptoms.

Indicator	Quality of Evidence	Literature	Benefits	Comments
8. At least 10 days of antimicrobial therapy should be prescribed for a suspected upper tract infection (pyelonephritis).	III	Johnson and Stamm, 1989; Stamm and Hooton, 1993; Stamm et al., 1991	Decrease pain. Decrease fever. Prevent recurrence of UTI. Prevent complications (such as sepsis and abscess).	In general, it is agreed that longer treatment is necessary for upper tract than lower tract infections. There is some controversy about the need for 10 vs. 14 days of treatment and studies have reached varying conclusions. Johnson and Stamm indicate that there is not enough evidence to warrant treatment for less than 14 days, based on recurrence of infection. As this is an area of controversy, we propose at least 10 days of treatment.
9. A patient with known or suspected upper tract infection who has uncontrolled vomiting in the office or ER should receive parenteral antibiotics.	III	Stamm and Hooton, 1993	Decrease pain. Decrease fever. Prevent sepsis.	If vomiting cannot be controlled in the office or ER, it is unlikely that the patient will be able to take oral medications at home. Some hospitals have provisions to administer IV antibiotics in the home.
10. Regimens of at least 7 days should be used for patients with complicated lower tract infections: that is, those with: a. diabetes, b. functional or structural anomaly of the urinary tract, c. symptoms for longer than 7 days, d. urinary tract infection in the past month, e. pregnancy.	III	Stamm and Hooton, 1993	Prevent recurrence of UTI. Prevent sepsis. Prevent abscess formation. Prevent spontaneous abortion.	While there are no RCTs that demonstrate the optimal duration of treatment in these situations, a longer duration of treatment than for an uncomplicated lower tract infection is recommended because eradication is more difficult (i.e., in structural anomalies) and/or potential complications secondary to incomplete eradication are more serious (i.e, diabetes, pregnancy).
Follow-up				
11. For upper tract infection a repeat culture should be obtained within 2 weeks of finishing treatment.	III	Barker et al., 1991; Stamm and Hooton, 1993	Prevent recurrence of UTI.	Since eradication of organism is sometimes difficult in pyelonephritis and complicated lower tract infections, and incomplete eradication may lead to complications, a repeat culture is indicated.
12. For complicated lower tract infection,[2] a repeat culture should be obtained within 2 weeks of finishing treatment.	III	Barker et al., 1991; Stamm and Hooton, 1993	Prevent recurrence of UTI.	Since eradication of organism is sometimes difficult in pyelonephritis and complicated lower tract infections, and incomplete eradication may lead to complications, a repeat culture is indicated.

360

Definitions and Examples

[1] An uncomplicated infection includes episodes of acute cystitis in women who are otherwise healthy and who have none of the risk factors that are known to increase the risk of treatment failure listed in definition 2.

[2] Complicated UTI includes cystitis in women and men who have the following risk factors for treatment failure:

- a. three or more infections in the past year;
- b. diabetes or immunocompromised state;
- c. fever, chills and/or flank pain;
- d. acute pyelonephritis;
- e. structural or functional anomalies of the urinary tract;
- f. symptoms for more than seven days before presentation;
- g. pregnancy;
- h. a relapse of symptoms after initial treatment;
- i. hospital acquired infection;
- j. indwelling foley catheter;
- k. recent instrumentation of the urinary tract.

Quality of Evidence Codes

I	RCT
II-1	Nonrandomized controlled trials
II-2	Cohort or case analysis
II-3	Multiple time series
III	Opinions or descriptive studies

22. VERTIGO AND DIZZINESS

Douglas S. Bell, MD

Review articles and cohort studies were found through MEDLINE searches covering 1985 to the present. Text words and keywords used included dizziness, vertigo, Meniere's disease, and labyrinthitis. Guidelines for the use of MRI were found by MEDLINE searching for keywords magnetic resonance, sensitivity, and specificity, and articles on the use of Holter monitoring were found by searching on ambulatory ECG monitoring, and cost-benefit analysis. Initial quality indicators were based on approaches outlined in the general medicine literature (McGee, 1995; Ruckenstein, 1995; Froehling et al., 1994a), and a textbook chapter on dizziness (Reilly, 1991). Indicators were then reviewed with Robert W. Baloh, a leading expert on vestibular disorders. Many additional references were identified for diagnosis and therapy of vestibular disorders, leading to the sub-classification of vertigo recommended in this review.

Unlike most conditions for which quality indicators may be developed, vertigo and dizziness are symptom complexes rather than specific diagnoses. Because a large number of disorders may cause a presentation with dizziness and because the diagnosis is often uncertain, quality indicators must be organized around this presenting complaint rather than the final diagnosis. Table 22.1 lists the most important disorders that may present with dizziness and that were considered for this review. This review will address steps that should be taken by generalist physicians to diagnose the cause of dizziness. It will also address therapy that should be carried out by a generalist, and the situations that should trigger specialty referral for further diagnosis or therapy. Diagnosis will be considered in less detail for conditions that usually present with frank syncope or with symptoms beyond isolated dizziness, such as seizure disorders, arrhythmias, and sepsis.

IMPORTANCE

Dizziness is a common presenting complaint, accounting for one percent of all office visits in 1989 (McGee, 1995). It is among the ten most frequent presenting complaints for women age 65 to 74 and men age 75 and older. Although most patients presenting with dizziness in primary care improve on their own, a significant minority of patients (44%) in one study had the same or worse symptoms at one-year follow-up (Kroenke et al., 1994). Ten percent of patients in that study had central vertigo that "may have" been due to cerebrovascular disease, though none had died at one year. Among patients presenting with dizziness to an emergency room, 31 percent had a "serious" cause (stroke, medication side effect, seizure, or arrhythmia). In a study of patients with dizziness over 70 years old presenting to a neurologist, 23 percent had brainstem or cerebellar ischemia (Sloane and Baloh, 1989). High quality medical care may therefore prevent serious disability in a few patients and help to improve symptoms in many.

SCREENING

Some of the underlying causes of dizziness may have an asymptomatic interval, but there is no evidence that diagnosing these conditions prior to the onset of dizziness would have any benefit.

DIAGNOSIS

Table 22.1 lays out the differential diagnostic considerations for dizziness. Prevalence statistics are taken from the cohort studies summarized in McGee (1995): 102 patients in a dizziness clinic, 100 patients in a primary care practice (Kroenke et al., 1992), 116 patients in a neurology clinic (Sloane and Baloh, 1989), and 123 patients in an emergency room (Herr et al., 1989). Less common disorders that were not reported in these studies but that should be considered in the differential diagnosis of dizziness are marked in Table 22.1 with an asterisk. Patients may also have more than one cause of dizziness simultaneously. A recent study of 117 men over age 50 presenting with dizziness to a general neurology clinic found that 49 percent had more than one contributing diagnosis (Davis, 1994). Patients with symptoms of more than one type of dizziness should therefore have history, physical examination, and laboratory testing appropriate for each type.

History

The history provides crucial information for the initial classification of a patient's dizziness into one of four categories: vertigo, disequilibrium, presyncope, or nonspecific lightheadedness. For this reason, every patient presenting with dizziness should have documentation of symptoms that support at least one of these categories.

Vertigo

Vertigo is an illusion of movement, either of the person's body or of the environment. Words commonly used to describe the sensation include spinning, tilting, and moving sideways. Any patient with a final diagnosis in the vertigo category should have some abnormal sensation of movement documented. The many potential causes of vertigo are best distinguished by sub-classifying vertigo according the duration of symptoms, and whether the vertigo is brought on by changes in position or occurs spontaneously. Association of vertigo with hearing loss or tinnitus also provides important diagnostic information. Excellent quality care would therefore include documentation of these factors in the patient chart (Indicator 1) (Ruckenstein, 1995). We next consider the causes of each important sub-syndrome of vertigo. Details of making this subclassification are elaborated in Table 22.1.

Recurrent positional vertigo

Benign positional vertigo (BPV) is caused by otolithic debris floating free in the posterior semicircular canal (Epley, 1995). Vertigo occurs in episodes lasting less than a minute, initiated by sudden head movements. Central vertigo (which may result from many causes, including posterior fossa infarction, tumor, multiple sclerosis (MS), and carcinomatous cerebellar degeneration) may also rarely cause vertigo triggered by head movements, but episodes tend to last more than one minute (McGee, 1995). Vertigo is an initial complaint in five percent of patients first presenting with MS (Ruckenstein, 1995). Differentiation between central and benign positional vertigo rests on the physical examination, as described in the next section.

Recurrent spontaneous vertigo

Posterior circulation transient ischemic attacks (TIAs) tend to cause spontaneous attacks of vertigo, with or without other neurologic symptoms, that last four to eight minutes (Grad and Baloh, 1989). A prior history of cerebrovascular disease or risk factors such as hypertension (HTN), diabetes mellitus (DM), and smoking may contribute to making this diagnosis (Indicator 2). Meniere's syndrome, or endolymphatic hydrops, causes acute-onset vertigo resolving gradually over hours to days and is often associated with unilateral hearing loss, tinnitus and a sensation of ear fullness.

Prolonged spontaneous vertigo

Vestibular neuritis (also incorrectly called labyrinthitis) causes abrupt onset of sustained vertigo lasting one to seven days. Acute, ongoing vertigo is also a "cardinal sign" of posterior circulation stroke, and vertigo is not always accompanied by other neurologic findings. In a case series of 153 patients with posterior circulation strokes, vertigo was present in 78 percent of cases (Fisher, 1967). In approximately one fourth of the cases with dizziness, it was the sole initial symptom, with other neurologic symptoms usually evolving over at most six weeks. Since the history may not differentiate vestibular neuritis from a posterior circulation vascular event in patients with acute persistent vertigo, the patient's risk factors for cerebrovascular disease are important to choosing further diagnostic testing. The chart should document some consideration of the patient's age, prior vascular disease, and history of HTN, DM, and smoking (Indicator 2)(Oas and Baloh, 1992; Ruckenstein 1995; Baloh et al., 1996). Case reports show that patients even in their 50s with significant vascular risk factors may have posterior circulation strokes heralded by episodes of isolated vertigo (Oas and Baloh, 1992).

Rare causes of vertigo may also be distinguished by history. Perilymphatic fistula is an abnormal communication between the middle and inner ear that may be caused by head trauma, ear surgery, cholesteatoma, otosyphilis, and anomalies of the temporal bone. It is suggested if vertigo is set off by changes in pressure, such as ascent in an airplane, valsalva, insufflation with an otoscope, or even loud noises (Ruckenstein, 1995; Baloh and Hamalgyi, 1996). A history of chronic otitis media may suggest cholesteatoma (Reilly, 1991). Significant ear pain with vertigo may suggest herpes zoster oticus (Reilly, 1991). Each of these conditions is rare enough, however, that requiring documentation of their consideration would probably not be productive as a quality indicator.

Disequilibrium

Disequilibrium is a sensation of unsteadiness, not localized to the head, that occurs when walking and that resolves at rest. The most common cause of disequilibrium is "multiple sensory deficits" in elderly patients, who may have reductions in vestibular, visual and proprioceptive function—all three of the balance-preserving senses. One characteristic of multiple sensory deficits is that symptoms will often resolve when the patient adds proprioceptive information by touching a wall or table (McGee, 1995). Risk factors for peripheral neuropathy and cerebellar degeneration should be elicited, including alcohol consumption, nutrition, diabetes mellitus, and family history (e.g., of porphyria or amyloidosis) (Indicator 3). Bilateral or gradual vestibular dysfunction usually causes disequilibrium rather than vertigo. Hearing loss would be associated with many causes of gradual vestibular dysfunction, such as acoustic neuroma, so hearing loss should be sought on history for disequilibrium as well as vertigo (Reilly, 1991).

Presyncope

Presyncope is the lightheadedness of a near-faint. This review does not cover patients with full loss of consciousness or syncope. Features of a patient's dizziness may suggest specific diagnoses, so the following features should be documented: sudden onset of presyncope is suspicious for arrhythmia (Reilly, 1991); exertional presyncope classically suggests aortic stenosis; presyncope with emotional stress or on urination suggests more benign, vasomotor syncope. Presyncope on standing, or orthostatic hypotension, has an enormous differential diagnosis (Reilly, 1991) (Indicator 4). Clinically evident causes, such as pregnancy, advanced Parkinsonism, and sepsis, are beyond the scope of this review. Medications

are a common cause of orthostasis, especially diuretics but also
vasodilators, tricyclic antidepressants, and many others. A careful
medication history is therefore necessary. Peripheral neuropathy is also a
common cause, most often from diabetes, but also potentially from rarer
causes including amyloidosis and porphyria (Reilly, 1991). Other uncommon
causes include hypoadrenalism and Shy-Drager syndrome.

Nonspecific dizziness

Many patients with dizziness have neither vertigo, disequilibrium, nor
presyncope. These patients often cannot describe their symptoms beyond
simply saying that they are "dizzy". Their history is distinguished mostly
by its vagueness and the lack of any features that would point to causes in
one of the other categories (Reilly, 1991). They may or may not have other
nonspecific symptoms, such as a feeling of floating, disconnectedness,
unreality, or fear of losing control. These patients tend to have a
psychiatric disorder such as anxiety or panic disorder (Reilly, 1991).
Among 16 patients in one study whose dizziness was considered to be due
primarily to a psychiatric disorder, six had a mood disorder, seven had
anxiety disorders including panic, nine had somatization disorder, and nine
had personality disorders (Kroenke et al., 1992). Many patients had more
than one diagnosis. A history of depressive symptoms (sadness, anhedonia,
sleep pattern, loss of appetite, concentration disturbance, and suicidal
ideation) and panic symptoms (diaphoresis, flushing, palpitations, chest
pressure, paresthesias, and nausea) should be sought.

Physical Examination

Provocation maneuvers are the focus of the physical examination for
dizziness but several routine elements of the exam should also be performed
in each patient with dizziness. The tympanic membranes and external canals
should be inspected with an otoscope for evidence of zoster, cholesteatoma,
or other destructive process (Indicator 5) (Reilly, 1991). The cranial
nerves should always document eye movements (for spontaneous and gaze-
evoked nystagmus), facial strength and sensation (for V and VII palsies
from cerebellopontine angle tumor), and some assessment of hearing. Eye
movements are particularly important for differentiating central from

peripheral causes of vertigo. Vertical nystagmus is always central in origin (Fisher, 1967). Spontaneous nystagmus from peripheral lesions should be unidirectional, increasing with gaze in the direction of the nystagmus and decreasing with gaze away. Central lesions, on the other hand, often cause nystagmus that changes direction with gaze in different directions (Baloh et al., 1996). Many generalists may be uncomfortable making this distinction, however. Patients with acute ongoing vertigo should therefore be referred to a neurologist or otolaryngologist unless the chart documents unidirectional nystagmus consistent with a peripheral lesion.

Five provocation tests may help to categorize the diagnosis: the Hallpike maneuver, gait observation, Romberg testing, orthostatic BP and pulse, and hyperventilation for three minutes. One author recommends that each of these tests should be performed on every dizzy patient, since more than one diagnosis may coexist (Reilly, 1991). Given the lack of evidence for this approach and the time constraints of modern practice it seems more reasonable to require a provocative maneuver only when some element of the patient's history points toward its potential usefulness.

The Hallpike maneuver (Dix and Hallpike, 1952), is also sometimes called (incorrectly) the Nylen-Baranay test after the authors who first described BPV (McGee, 1995). The procedure involves holding the patient's head in extension and rotation while moving the patient from a seated to a head-hanging supine position in less than two seconds. A positive test elicits vertigo and a practically pathognomonic torsional-vertical nystagmus, confirming the diagnosis of BPV (Indicator 6). A negative test does not rule out BPV, however, since spontaneous remissions and exacerbations are common. Inexperienced clinicians may have difficulty distinguishing BPV's torsional vertical nystagmus from the pure vertical or horizontal nystagmus that may be found on Hallpike testing in central vertigo (McGee, 1995; Robert Baloh, personal communication). Case reports also suggest that BPV may be distinguished from central positional vertigo by the latency, duration, and fatigability of nystagmus elicited by Hallpike testing (see Table 22.1) (McGee, 1995). Patients who have nystagmus induced by Hallpike maneuver that does not have a clearly torsional component should therefore be referred for neurologic consultation.

Gait observation and Romberg testing should be undertaken in patients with disequilibrium (Indicator 9). Particular attention should be paid for signs of ataxia, foot drop, Parkinsonism, veering, and ease of correction (Reilly, 1991). Visual acuity should be checked and eyes examined for cataracts (McGee, 1995) (Indicator 8).

Vital signs should be obtained in the supine, seated, and standing position for any patient suspected of having presyncopal episode (Reilly, 1991) (Indicator 7). A drop in BP of 10 mm systolic or rise in pulse rate more than 20 per minute indicates a positive test. A recent large cohort study showed that postural dizziness without significant changes in vital signs was even more strongly associated with future falls than true orthostatic hypotension (Ensrud et al., 1992). Postural dizziness should therefore be considered equivalent to postural hypotension. Some authors recommend asking the patient to hyperventilate for three minutes in an attempt to reproduce the patient's symptoms, with strict criteria for calling the test positive (Reilly, 1991). In prospective studies, however, the hyperventilation test has had relatively high false positive rates, though these studies may not have been as strict in interpreting the test results (Kroenke et al., 1992; McGee, 1995). In one prospective study the sensitivity was 100 percent but specificity only 79 percent for hyperventilation syndrome (Herr et al., 1989). Because the prevalence of hyperventilation syndrome was much lower than that of other diagnoses, the test had only a 19 percent positive predictive value. Its 100 percent negative predictive value would appear more useful, but since only five patients with hyperventilation syndrome were tested this statistic is also uncertain. Kroenke found a similarly poor specificity in a primary care practice (Kroenke et al., 1992). Given its inadequate specificity, this review will not recommend hyperventilation testing (Kroenke et al., 1992; McGee, 1995).

Other maneuvers, including Valsalva, carotid sinus stimulation, and the Quix test for past-pointing showed little benefit in one trial (Herr et al., 1989).

Laboratory And Radiologic Testing

Most patients with dizziness do not require laboratory or radiologic testing, the major exception being the need for neuroimaging in patients who may have posterior fossa tumors or strokes. Strokes are especially important to detect at initial presentation, since they can evolve to further deficits, brain swelling, and death. MRI should be the first imaging modality for disease in the posterior fossa, according to guidelines based on evidence of "moderate" quality (American College of Physicians, 1994). Patients with onset of vertigo associated with new neurological deficits such as dysarthria or numbness should definitely undergo MRI (Indicator 10). Imaging of patients who have spontaneous vertigo without other neurologic findings has more uncertain benefit. As noted above, the history and physical examination may not fully distinguish stroke from vestibular neuritis, but the prior probabilities of these disorders remain uncertain. A recent review (Froehling et al., 1994a) concluded that patients less than 70 years old with true vertigo and no other neurologic deficit may not need further testing, since a prospective study of ER patients with dizziness (Herr et al., 1989) found that only 12 percent of them had a 'serious' cause of dizziness (stroke, medication side effect, seizure, or arrhythmia). However, the authors later agreed with a correspondent who suggested that most physicians would not be comfortable accepting that they will miss 12 percent of serious causes in this setting (Froehling et al., 1994b). In deciding whether to obtain MRI, risk factors for cerebrovascular disease (HTN, diabetes, smoking, age > 65, and history of prior atherosclerotic vascular disease) should probably be considered, though evidence for the strength of risk factors in vertebrobasilar vascular disease is weak or nonexistent. A more conservative alternative to requiring MRI for patients with acute prolonged vertigo and any risk factors for cerebrovascular disease would instead require that such patients be referred to a neurologist for a more detailed neurologic assessment. MRI is not necessary for younger vertiginous patients without risk factors for cerebrovascular disease, especially with gaze-evoked nystagmus typical of a peripheral lesion.

CT scan of the head is recommended if normal pressure hydrocephalus (NPH) is suspected (American College of Physicians, 1994). Patients with a history of disequilibrium, gait imbalance, and new dementia or incontinence should therefore have a head CT. NPH is a rare disorder, however, so its detection is probably not warranted as a quality indicator.

Audiometry is the test of first choice for any patient with suspected acoustic neuroma (Ruckenstein, 1995). Acoustic neuroma causes imbalance far more often than vertigo, however, so our quality indicator requires audiometry for patients with a history of hearing loss with disequilibrium or vertigo (Indicator 11). Audiometry often shows a characteristic low-frequency hearing loss in Meniere's disease (Baloh et al., 1996). Audiometry may also aid in the diagnosis of vestibular neuritis, ototoxic medications, and spinocerebellar degeneration. This broad utility has led to the recommendation that it be used as a screening test for every patient with non-positional vertigo (Robert Baloh, personal communication). Because the operating characteristics of audiometry remain uncertain, however, no further quality indicators will be specified for audiometry.

Electronystagmogram (ENG) has been recommended for confirming vestibular damage in Meniere's disease and aminoglycoside ototoxicity (Ruckenstein, 1995; Baloh et al., 1996), but ENG testing has had problems with poor quality control (Robert Baloh, personal communication). Another author states that ENG usually only confirms diagnoses "obvious" from the history and physical (Reilly, 1991). This review makes no recommendations for quality indiators for ENG.

Electrocardiograms (ECGs) should be performed on patients with potential arrhythmias. Such patients would include those with sudden presyncope episodes with or without palpitations, and those with ongoing lightheadedness and tachycardia or bradycardia on examination (Indicator 12). Patients with episodic presyncope should also be considered for ambulatory ECG (Holter) or event monitoring. In one study of Holter monitoring, the test resulted in a management change in 29 percent of patients with dizziness and palpitations, and seven percent of patients with dizziness without palpitations (Kessler et al., 1995). A small randomized crossover trial in patients with palpitations found that Holter monitors detected no clinically significant arrhythmias while event monitors detected significant arrhythmias in 19 percent (Kinlay et al., 1996).

Hemoglobin and hematocrit (H&H) testing has been recommended for patients with orthostatic hypotension to identify occult anemia (Reilly, 1991). Several case series support the utility of the H&H in this setting (Davis, 1994; Herr et al., 1989; Madlon-Kay, 1985). Testing for the many less common causes of orthostatic hypotension, such as hypoadrenalism would also make sense if symptoms persist, but this review will not recommend further quality indicators.

TREATMENT

Ninety percent of patients with dizziness leave the physician's office with a prescription, often for meclizine, while four percent are referred to specialists (McGee, 1995). Only two small randomized placebo-controlled trials of meclizine are quoted in our review articles, one supporting the effectiveness of meclizine based on 31 patients with vertigo, and the other supporting meclizine combined with dimenhydrinate in 50 elderly patients with dizziness from a variety of causes (McGee, 1995). Animal studies, however, show that vestibular suppressant medications actually hinder recovery from a vestibular insult by suppressing the vestibular input from the uninjured side that is essential for recovery (Peppard, 1986). Meclizine therefore probably does more harm than good (Robert Baloh, personal communication), but given the uncertainty of evidence this review will not suggest quality indicators for or against meclizine.

For BPV, the canalith repositioning procedure, or Epley's maneuver, is safe and effective. This maneuver takes the patient through a series of head positions to return debris from the semicircular canal into the utricle where its movement ceases to cause vertigo. In the initial case series of 30 BPV patients treated with the procedure, 90 percent had immediate complete resolution of vertigo. The remaining ten percent had full resolution of positional vertigo, but only partial relief of vertigo overall. Though 30 percent later had one or more recurrences, 86 percent of these had complete resolution on retreatment (Epley, 1992). At another institution, 19 of 25 patients with BPV (76%) had complete resolution of symptoms from the canalith repositioning procedure (Welling and Barnes, 1994). Other recent randomized trials have yielded similar results (Lynn, et al. 1995; Li, 1995; Blakeley, 1994; Herdman, et al. 1993). Patients can also be given an instruction page teaching them to perform this maneuver on themselves should their symptoms recur (Baloh et al., 1996). The best treatment for BPV prior to Epley's maneuver consisted of head movement exercises that repeatedly precipitated symptoms with the intent of dispersing debris within the semicircular canal. This led to complete relief in 66 of 67 patients within three to 14 days (Brandt and Daroff, 1980). These exercises often induce nausea and vomiting, however, and must be performed several times a day to be effective. Thus patients outside of trials may fail to complete the course and continue to have vertigo (Baloh, personal communication). Given the simplicity of the canalith repositioning procedure and the marked differences in the time spent ill between the two treatments, this review recommends as a quality indicator the canalith repositioning procedure be used as the standard treatment for BPV (Indicator 13).

Treatment of Meniere's disease has been difficult to evaluate because the disease has a naturally remitting and relapsing course, though it usually progresses over ten to 20 years to severe permanent hearing loss (2/3 unilateral). Vertigo episodes stop when this "burned out" stage of Meniere's is reached (Baloh et al., 1996). Guidelines for treatment of Meniere's disease from the American Academy of Otolaryngology recommend sodium restriction to 1-2 g/day in combination with a diuretic such as hydrochlorothiazide (HCTZ) (Santos et al., 1993). A retrospective case series of 26 patients who reported compliance with this regimen found that hearing loss stabilized and vertigo improved during an average follow-up of six years (Santos et al., 1993). Better evidence for diuretic use comes from a randomized double-blind crossover trial in 30 patients that found modest improvement in episodes of vertigo and hearing loss when patients were on HCTZ rather than placebo (Klockhoff and Lindblom, 1967). Another retrospective series, however, emphasized salt restriction (Boles et al., 1975). Some experts recommend that salt restriction should be initiated first and diuretics added only if episodes of vertigo continue (Baloh et al., 1996). Given the incomplete evidence this review recommends that medical therapy for Meniere's disease include either salt restriction or diuretic therapy or both (Indicator 14). Surgery may be contemplated for the occasional patient with disabling, refractory vertigo. Endolymphatic shunt surgery was once widely performed, and is still recommended by some authors (Ruckenstein, 1995), but it has gradually fallen out of favor after two negative trials. Shunt surgery was no better than sham mastoidectomy in one trial (75 percent of patients in both groups had improved at 3 years), and had no better outcome than those who refused surgery in another trial (60 percent of patients in both groups had improved at two years) (McGee, 1995). A more logical surgery for debilitating, refractory Meniere's disease is simple ablation of vestibular function on the affected side so that the central nervous system can complete the process of compensation (Baloh et al., 1996). Options are either selective section of the vestibular nerve, or a chemical vestibulectomy created by infusing gentamycin into the middle ear. A six to 12 month trial of medical therapy would generally be reasonable before proceeding to surgery (Baloh, personal communication). Because there is no clear consensus on appropriate surgery for Meniere's disease, however, our indicators will not address this topic.

Patients with prolonged vertigo probably benefit from vestibular rehabilitation therapy (VRT), though evidence remains meager and no quality indicators are recommended (Baloh et al., 1996). A randomized trial of head turning/visual fixation exercises and gait exercises in 21 patients after acoustic neuroma resection found markedly better gait and balance after three days of VRT compared with less specific exercises (Herdman et al., 1995). This benefit may be generalizable to other acute peripheral lesions such as vestibular neuritis. VRT is less effective in patients whose vertigo is due to head trauma or bilateral ototoxicity, though in the latter case a controlled trial has shown that the benefit is still statistically significant (Shepard and Telian, 1995). Patients with central vertigo, (e.g. from stroke or multiple sclerosis) have more difficulty adapting to loss of vestibular function. Though VRT has not been systematically studied in this group (Shepard and Telian, 1995), they almost certainly benefit at least from gait training (Baloh et al., 1996).

Patients with multiple sensory deficits should have their deficits addressed wherever possible (McGee, 1995). Patients with visual impairment should therefore have referral for ophthalmologic evaluation (Indicator 16), and patients with significant gait disorder or proprioceptive loss should be referred to physical therapy for gait and balance training, and consideration of the use of a walker.

Most cases of orthostatic hypotension require treatment of the underlying cause, most commonly the discontinuance of offending medications. Other common causes of orthostatic hypotension, such as peripheral neuropathy due to diabetes, do not have specific treatments. Many cases of orthostatic hypotension also remain idiopathic. Treatment of these patients may initially be nonpharmacologic (e.g., avoiding dehydration, salt supplements, support stockings) and may progress to mineralocorticoid therapy (Reilly, 1991; see Tables 5-11 and 5-12 in this reference).

The treatment of more serious conditions, such as brainstem infarction or cardiac arrhythmia, would typically be carried out by a specialist and is beyond the scope of this review. Although many cases of anxiety and depression may be treated by a primary care physician, their treatment is also beyond the scope of this review (see Chapter 8 for indicators related to treatment of depression).

FOLLOW-UP

There are no specific recommendations in the literature for follow-up of patients with dizziness. Since many of the treatments outlined above require empiric adjustments it would make sense to schedule regular follow-up, but given the lack of evidence this review will not create quality indicators for follow-up.

Table 22.1

Differential Diagnostic Considerations for Dizziness

'*' indicates conditions that were not assigned a prevalence in existing cohort studies of patients presenting with dizziness.

Cause	Prevalence (%)	Key History	Key Physical Exam	Testing
Vertigo	38-46	Illusion of movement	Nystagmus	
Benign positional vertigo (BPV)	12-26	Vertigo in episodes lasting seconds, provoked by changes in position, like turning in bed, or reaching for a high shelf. (Syndrome: Recurrent positional vertigo)	Hallpike test: torsional- vertical nystagmus should have 2-20 sec. latency, adapt in less than 50 sec., and lessen with prompt repetition.	
Central vertigo (posterior circulation CVA, MS, cerebello-pontine angle tumor, and many more).	2-3	Acute disorders (e.g. CVA) cause sustained vertigo (syndrome: prolonged spontaneous vertigo). Slow-growing tumors cause imbalance, but minimal, if any, vertigo. 5% of MS initially presents with vertigo.	Usually direction-changing gaze-evoked nystagmus. Hallpike nystagmus is typically pure vertical or horizontal, has no latency, and does not fatigue; Acoustic neuroma always has at least some hearing loss; sometimes V, VII palsy.	MRI of posterior fossa; Audiometry. III

Cause	Prevalence (%)	Key History	Key Physical Exam	Testing
Vertebrobasilar TIA	5-7	Acute spontaneous episodes of vertigo lasting minutes (typically 4-8 min). (syndrome: Recurrent spontaneous vertigo) Associated neurologic symptoms (numbness, diplopia, etc.) frequent. Risk factors: age, HTN, DM, smoking, anticoagulation.	Exam is usually normal.	Vertebro-basilar MR angiography only helpful if dx uncertain, e.g., if good history but few risk factors.
Meniere's syndrome	3-8	Vertigo in spontaneous episodes, lasting hours, with hearing loss, tinnitus, unilateral ear fullness. (Syndrome: Recurrent spontaneous vertigo).	Spontaneous torsional horizontal nystagmus, only during an acute attack.	Audiometry: Low frequency loss is highly specific.
Vestibular neuritis (Labyrinthitis)	3-9	Acute sustained vertigo, lasting 1-7 days or longer, without hearing loss. Recent febrile illness in 25-50% (Syndrome: Prolonged spontaneous vertigo).	Spontaneous unidirectional torsional-horizontal nystagmus. Decreased caloric responses in the affected ear. Nystagmus suppressed by visual fixation.	Audiometry MRI not necessary.

Cause	Prevalence (%)	Key History	Key Physical Exam	Testing
Other, including:	7-10			
migraine	Next to BPV, most common cause.	Vertigo in spontaneous episodes, lasting hours, headache may be dissociated (Syndrome: Recurrent spontaneous vertigo). Up to 25% of migraines are associated with vertebrobasilar symptoms.	Usually normal.	Audiometry.
Ototoxic medications	*	Usually no vertigo with bilateral vestibular insult. Instead, dis-equilibrium and oscillopsia (vision unsteady with head movements).	Bilateral hearing decrement, except with aminoglycosides, which do not affect hearing.	Audiometry.
Cholesteatoma	*	Prolonged spontaneous vertigo. History of chronic otitis media. Otorrhea.	Visualization of the tympanic membrane Conductive hearing loss.	
Perilymphatic fistula	*	Vertigo set off by air pressure changes or straining. (Recurrent pressure-provoked vertigo) RFs: head trauma, otosyphilis, congenital temporal bone anomaly.	Nystagmus and vertigo from otoscope insufflation.	
Herpes zoster oticus	*	Prolonged spontaneous vertigo. Hearing loss. In full Ramsay Hunt syndrome, ear pain & facial paralysis.	Vesicles on the TM or canal ± facial paralysis.	
Disequilibrium		Unsteady walking.	Gait testing.	

Cause	Prevalence (%)	Key History	Key Physical Exam	Testing
Multiple sensory deficits	1-17	No dizziness at rest. Relieved when touching wall.	Gait testing with right-angle turns; Romberg. Visual acuity, fundoscopy for cataracts, macular degeneration.	
Ototoxic medications		Usually *no* vertigo with bilateral vestibular insult. Instead, dis-equilibrium and oscillopsia (vision unsteady with head movements).	Bilateral hearing decrement, except with aminoglyco-sides, which do not affect hearing.	Audiometry III.
Peripheral Neuropathy	up to 5	Risk factors: alcohol, DM, toxins, vitamin deficiency.	Romberg positive Sensory loss, decreased deep tendon reflexes.	
Cerebellar disease or spinocerebellar disease	*	Slow posterior fossa neoplasms cause imbalance rather than vertigo.	Ataxia, dysmetria, etc.	Audiometry if any hearing loss. CT or MRI.
Normal Pressure Hydrocephalus	*	Incontinence.	Wide-based gait, extensor plantar reflex.	
Presyncope	3-16	Impending faint.	Orthostatic vitals.	
Orthostatic hypotension (incl. meds, infection)	2-7	Dizziness occurs after assuming upright posture.	Upright drop in BP or dizzy symptoms. Rectal for occult blood.	CBC.
Arrhythmia	up to 5	Abrupt onset; ± palpitations.	If ongoing, tachycardia- or bradycardia	ECG;Holter / event monitor.

Cause	Prevalence (%)	Key History	Key Physical Exam	Testing
Vasomotor or "vasovagal"	*	History of prior similar episodes; +/- emotional stress.		
Other cardiac (AS, PE, etc.)	*	Exertional symptoms for AS Risk factors for PE.	Heart exam (murmur, rub).	
Situational (e.g. micturition)	1	History of events surrounding episode.		
Nonspecific lightheadedness		None of the above syndromes.		
Psychiatric (Anxiety, depression, panic, somatization)	5-16	Hard to describe. May feel floating, disembodied, head fullness. Life stress. Panic syndrome: palpitations, doom sensation, diaphoresis.	DSM criteria for depression or panic on mental status exam.	
Hyperventilation	1-23	Circumoral and acral paresthesias may be present. Other panic symptoms.	3 minute hyperventilation: positive predictive value = 20%	

381

REFERENCES

American College of Physicians. 1994. Magnetic resonance imaging of the brain and spine: a revised statement. *Archives of Internal Medicine* 120: 872-5.

Baloh RW, Fife TD, Furman JM, and Zee DS. 1996. *Neurotology, Part A. Continuum: Lifelong Learning in Neurology.* Minneapolis: American Academy of Neurology.

Baloh RW, and G. Halmagyi. 1996. *Disorders of the Vestibular System.* New York: Oxford University Press.

Bernard ME, Bachenberg TC, and Brey RH. 1996. Benign paroxysmal positional vertigo: the canalith repositioning procedure. *American Family Physician* 53: 2613-6, 2621.

Blakeley BW. 1994 April. A randomized, controlled assessment of the canalith repositioning maneuver. *Otolaryngology - Head and Neck Surgery* 110(4):391-6.

Boles R, Rice DH, Hybels R, and Work WP. July 1975. Conservative management of Meniere's disease: Furstenberg regimen revisited. *Annals of Otology, Rhinology and Laryngology* 84 ((4 Pt 1)): 513-7.

Brandt T, and Daroff RB. August 1980. Physical therapy for benign paroxysmal positional vertigo. *Archives of Otolaryngology* 106 (8): 484-5.

Davis LE. 1994. Dizziness in elderly men. *Journal of the American Geriatric Society* 42: 1184-8.

Dix M, and Hallpike C. 1952. The pathology, symptomatology, and diagnosis of certain common disorders of the vestibular system. *Proceedings of the Royal Society of London* 45: 341-54.

Ensrud KE, Nevitt MC, Yunis C, Hulley SB, et al. 1992. Postural hypotension and postural dizziness in elderly women. The study of osteoporotic fractures. The Study of Osteoporotic Fractures Research Group. *Archives of Internal Medicine* 152: 1058-64.

Epley J. 1992. The canalith repositioning procedure for treatment of benign paroxysmal positional vertigo. *Otolaryngoly - Head and Neck Surgery* 107: 399-404.

Epley J. 1995. Positional vertigo related to semicircular canalithiasis. *Otolaryngology - Head and Neck Surgery* 112: 154-61.

Fisher C. 1967. Vertigo in cerebrovascular disease. *Archives of Otolaryngology* 85: 529-34.

Froehling DA, Silverstein MD, Mohr DN, and Beatty CW. 1 1994. Does this dizzy patient have a serious form of vertigo? *Journal of the American Medical Association* 271: 385-8.

Grad A, and Baloh RW. 1989. Vertigo of vascular origin: clinical and electronystagmographic features in 84 cases. *Archives of Neurology* 46: 281-284.

Herdman SJ, Tusa RJ, Zee DS, et al. 1993 April. Single treatment approaches to benign paroxysmal positional vertigo. *Archives of Otolaryngology - Head and Neck Surgery* 119 (4):450-4.

Herdman SJ, Clenandiel RA, Mattox DE, et al. 1995. Vestibular adaptation exercises and recovery: acute stage after acoustic neuroma resection. *Otolaryngology - Head and Neck Surgery* 113: 77-87.

Herr RD, Zun L, and Mathews JJ. 1989. A directed approach to the dizzy patient. *Annals of Emergency Medicine* 18: 664-72.

Hoffman R, Einstadter D, and Kroenke K. 30 August 1996. Diagnosing Dizziness. From the Section of General Internal Medicine, Albuquerque VA Medical Center and the Dept. of Medicine, Univeristy of New Mexico School of Medicine; Sectional of General Internal Medicine, MetroHealth Medical Center and the Departement of Medicine, Case Western University; Division of General Internal Medicine and the Department of Medicine, Uniformed Services University of the Health Sciences.

Kent DL, Haynor DR, Longstreth WT, et al. 1994. The clinical efficacy of magnetic resonance imaging in neuroimaging [see comments]. *Archives of Internal Medicine* 120: 856-71.

Kessler DK, Kessler KM, and Myerburg RJ. 1995. Ambulatory electrocardiography. A cost per management decision analysis. *Archives of Internal Medicine* 155: 165-9.

Kinlay S, Leitch JW, Neil A, et al. 1996. Cardiac event recorders yield more diagnoses and are more cost-effective than 48-hour Holter monitoring in patients with palpitations. A controlled clinical trial. *Archives of Internal Medicine* 124: 16-20.

Klockhoff I, and Lindblom U. 1967. Meniere's disease and hydrochlorothiazide--A critical analysis of symptoms and therapeutic effects. *Acta Otolaryngology* 63: 347-65.

Kroenke K, Hoffman R, and Einstadter D. How Common are Various Causes of Dizziness? A critical review of the literature. *Regenstref Institute for Health Care, Albuquerque VA and Medical Center, MetroHealth*

Medical Center, and the Clinical Efficacy Assessment Program of the American College of Physicians

Kroenke K, and Hoffman R. 1997. A Rational Approach to the Dizzy Patient. *Journal of Clinical Outcomes Management* 4: 23-41.

Kroenke K, Lucas CA, Rosenberg ML, et al. 1992. Causes of persistent dizziness. A prospective study of 100 patients in ambulatory care. *Archives of Internal Medicine* 117: 898-904.

Kroenke K, Lucas C, Rosenberg ML, et al. 1994. One-year outcome for patients with a chief complaint of dizziness. *Journal of General Internal Medicine* 9: 684-9.

Lempert T, Gresty MA, and Bronstein AM. 1995. Benign positional vertigo: recognition and treatment. *British Medical Journal* 311: 489-91.

Li JC. 1995. Mastoid oscillation: a critical factor for success in canalith repositioning procedure. *Otolaryngology - Head and Neck Surgery* 112(6):670-5.

Lynn S, Pool A, Rose D, et al. 1995 Dec. Randomized trial of the canalith repositioning procedure. *Otolaryngology - Head and Neck Surgery* 113(6):712-20.

.Madlon-Kay DJ. 1985. Evaluation and outcome of the dizzy patient. *Journal of Family Practice* 21: 109-13.

McGee SR. 1995. Dizzy patients. Diagnosis and treatment [see comments]. *Western Journal of Medicine* 162: 37-42.

Oas JG, and Baloh RW. 1992. Vertigo and the anterior inferior cerebellar artery syndrome. *Neurology* 42: 2274-9.

Peppard SB. 1986. Effect of drug therapy on compensation from vestibular injury. *Laryngoscope* Aug, 96 (8): 878-98.

Reilly B. 1991. *Dizziness. In Practical Strategies in Outpatient Medicine.* Philadelphia: Saunders, pp. 162-236.

Ruckenstein MJ. 1995. A practical approach to dizziness. Questions to bring vertigo and other causes into focus. *Postgraduate Medicine* 97: 70-2, 75-8, 81.

Santos PM, Hall RA, Snyder JM, et al. 1993. Diuretic and diet effect on Meniere's disease evaluated by the Committee on Hearing and Equilibrium guidelines. *Otolaryngology - Head and Neck Surgery* 109: 680-689.

Shepard NT, and Telian SA. 1995. Programmatic vestibular rehabilitation. *Otolaryngology - Head and Neck Surgery* 112: 172-182.

Sloane P, and Baloh R. 1989. Persistent dizziness in geriatric patients. *Journal of the American Geriatric Society* 37: 1031-8.

Welling D, and Barnes D. 1994. Particle repositioning procedure for benign paroxysmal positional vertigo. *Laryngoscope* 104: 946-9.

RECOMMENDED QUALITY INDICATORS FOR VERTIGO AND DIZZINESS

The following indicators apply to men and women age 18 and older.

Indicator	Quality of Evidence	Literature	Benefits	Comments
Diagnosis				

1. Patients who present with vertigo[1] should have all of the following documented at the time of initial presentation with symptoms:
  a. the duration of episodes;
  b. presence or absence of precipitation by head movements;
  c. presence or absence of any association with hearing loss or tinnitus.
	III	Ruckenstein, 1995	Prevent morbidity leading from incorrect diagnosis.	Characteristics of vertigo are key to further diagnosis.

2. Patients who present with prolonged spontaneous vertigo[2] should have documentation of risk factors for cerebrovascular disease[3] at the time of presentation.	III	Baloh et al., 1996; Oas and Baloh, 1992; Ruckenstein, 1995	Prevent evolution of stroke, posterior fossa edema, and death.	Critical to choosing further testing and treatment, since exam may not fully differentiate neuritis from CVA.

3. Patients who present with disequilibrium[4] should have all of the following documented at the time of initial presentation:
  a. presence or absence of diabetes;
  b. presence or absence of alcohol consumption;
  c. use of ototoxic medications;
  d. recent poor oral intake.
	III	Reilly, 1991	Prevent disabling falls.	Sensory loss due to peripheral neuropathy may be correctable. Poor oral intake can cause orthostasis.

4. Patients who present with presyncope[4] should be asked about all of the following possible precipitants at the time of initial presentation:
  a. standing up;
  b. urination;
  c. exertion;
  d. emotional stress.
	III	Reilly, 1991	Reduce morbidity and death by identifying causes for presyncope.	History guides further testing.

386

Indicator	Quality of Evidence	Literature	Benefits	Comments
5. Patients who present with vertigo should have documented an examination of tympanic membranes at the time of presentation.	III	Ruckenstein, 1995	Decrease morbidity.	Examination can lead to diagnosis of cholesteatoma and herpes zoster oticus -which are rare, but easy to diagnose.
6. Patients who present with recurrent positional vertigo[5] should have documented the results of a Hallpike maneuver[6] at the time of presentation.	II-2	McGee, 1995; Baloh et al., 1996	Decrease morbidity.	Benign positional vertigo is immediately treatable. Central vertigo is usually serious and requires referral.
7. Patients who present with presyncope should have all of the following documented at the time of presentation: a. orthostatic vital signs; b. heart examination.	III	McGee, 1995	Decrease morbidity and mortality.	Orthostasis is a very common cause of presyncope, but one also needs to consider serious arrythmias.
8. Patients who present with disequilibrium should have documentation of visual acuity testing at the time of presentation.	III	Reilly, 1991; McGee, 1995	Prevent disabling falls.	Cataract extraction may cure some cases of disequilibrium.
9. Patients who present with disequilibrium should have documentation of the following components of a neurological examination at the time of presentation: a. cerebellar exam; b. gait observation; c. Romberg testing.	III	McGee, 1995	Prevent disabling falls.	Some sensory loss or disequilibrium may be correctable, especially through physical therapy.
10. Patients who present with vertigo and new neurological deficits should have MRI within 2 weeks of presentation.	III	American College of Physicians, 1994	Prevent evolution of CVA and decrease morbidity.	Patients with acute onset of deficits should be considered for emergent MRI.
11. Patients who present with disequilibrium and unilateral hearing loss[7] should have audiometry within 3 weeks of presentation.	III	Ruckenstein, 1995	Decrease morbidity from CPA tumor.	Documentation of hearing loss needed prior to surgery for acoustic neuroma.

387

	Indicator	Quality of Evidence	Literature	Benefits	Comments
12.	Patients who present with sudden presyncope[8] and HR < 55 on exam should have an ECG at the time of presentation.	III	Reilly, 1991	Prevent mortality and decrease morbidity.	
Treatment					
13.	Patients who present with torsional-vertical nystagmus on Hallpike testing[7] should have the canalith repositioning procedure within 1 week of presentation.	I, II-2	Bernard et al, 1996; Lempert et al, 1995; Lynn, 1995; Li, 1995; Blakeley, 1994	Decrease disability from symptoms of vertigo.	Canalith repositioning is 76–100% effective. The 30% who recur can be retreated.
14.	Patients who present with a diagnosis of Meniere's syndrome should be advised to follow a 1–2 gram sodium/day diet or be given a diuretic or both within one month of presentation.	I, II-2	Santos et al., 1993 Klockhoff & Lindblom, 1967	Decrease disability from symptoms of vertigo.	A small but randomized controlled trial supports HCTZ.
15.	Patients who present with recurrent spontaneous vertigo[9] and any risk factor for cerebrovascular disease[3] should start aspirin or ticlopidine at the time of presentation or be referred to a neurologist within 2 weeks of presentation.	II-2	Grad and Baloh, 1989	Prevent CVA.	Twelve of 42 Patients 28% with posterior circulation stroke had prior vertigo TIAs.
16.	Patients who present with disequilibrium and decreased visual acuity should be referred to an opthalmologist or optometrist within one month of presentation.	III	Reilly, 1991; McGee, 1995	Prevent disabling falls.	Cataract extraction may cure some cases of disequilibrium.

388

Definitions and Examples

1 Vertigo: an illusion of movement.

2 Prolonged spontaneous vertigo: Continuous vertigo, either ongoing or resolved only after several days.

3 High risk for stroke (CVD) includes one or more of the following risk factors:

   a. Prior stroke
   b. Diabetes mellitus
   c. Hypertension -- any of the following:

      • At least three measurements on different days with a mean SBP>140 mm Hg and/or a mean DBP>90 mm Hg documented in the medical record
      • A diagnosis of hypertension mentioned in the chart
      • Documentation of chronic antihypertensive therapy

   d. Age >65 years old
   e. Heart failure — any charted diagnosis of heart failure
   f. Clinical coronary heart disease (angina or myocardial infarction mentioned in the chart)
   g. Mitral stenosis
   h. Prosthetic heart valves
   i. Echo criteria:

      • Left atrial enlargement (>4.5 cm)
      • Impaired left ventricular function (ejection fraction <50% or LV dyskinesis, hypokinesis, or akinesis).

4 Presyncope: a sensation of impending faint.

5 Recurrent positional vertigo: Vertigo, recurring in episodes brought on by changes in head position, often lasting seconds.

6 Hallpike maneuver (also sometimes called the Nylen-Baranay test): The procedure involves holding the patient's head in extension and rotation while moving the patient from a seated to a head-hanging supine position in less than two seconds.

7 Hearing loss: any noticeable decrease in aural acuity.

8 Sudden presyncope: presyncope occurring in sudden, unprovoked episodes.

9 Recurrent spontaneous vertigo: Vertigo, recurring and abating spontaneously in episodes lasting minutes to hours.

389

APPENDIX A: PANEL RATING SUMMARY BY CONDITION

NOTE: This chapter was revised from Q1.
There were no new or revised indicators to
rate.

NOTE: This chapter was revised from Q1.
Only new or revised indicators were rated.

SCREENING

1. All patients should be screened for
problem drinking. This assessment of
pattern of alcohol use should include at
least one of the following:

- Use of a validated questionnaire (such
  as AUDIT, MAST, CAGE)
- Quantity (e.g., drinks per day)
- Binge drinking (e.g., more than 5 drinks
  in a day in the last month)

```
                           5 4                  5 2 2
             1 2 3 4 5 6 7 8 9   1 2 3 4 5 6 7 8 9   ( 1-  2)
               (7.0, 0.4, A)       (7.0, 0.7, A)
```

2. All patients hospitalized with the
following conditions should be screened for
problem drinking at least once during their
hospital stay.

a. trauma

```
                           4 3 2                3 3 3
             1 2 3 4 5 6 7 8 9   1 2 3 4 5 6 7 8 9   ( 3-  4)
               (8.0, 0.7, A)       (8.0, 0.7, A)
```

b. hepatitis

```
                           3 3 3                1 3 5
             1 2 3 4 5 6 7 8 9   1 2 3 4 5 6 7 8 9   ( 5-  6)
               (8.0, 0.7, A)       (9.0, 0.6, A)
```

c. pancreatitis

```
                           3 3 3                1 3 5
             1 2 3 4 5 6 7 8 9   1 2 3 4 5 6 7 8 9   ( 7-  8)
               (8.0, 0.7, A)       (9.0, 0.6, A)
```

3. The record should indicate assessment for
dependence, tolerance of psychoactive
effects, loss of control, and consequences
of use if the medical record indicates the
patient is a daily or binge drinker.

```
                         1   6 2              1 1   2 5
             1 2 3 4 5 6 7 8 9   1 2 3 4 5 6 7 8 9   ( 9- 10)
               (7.0, 0.4, A)       (8.0, 1.0, A)
```

Scales: 1 = low validity or feasibility; 9 = high validity or feasibility

NOTE: This chapter was revised from Q1.
There were no new or revised indicators to
rate.

DIAGNOSIS

1. Men age 50 and older who present for routine care should be asked at least once a year about recent symptoms of prostatism.

```
1     2 2 1 1 2           2   1 1 2 2 1
1 2 3 4 5 6 7 8 9   1 2 3 4 5 6 7 8 9   ( 1- 2)
    (5.0, 1.7, I)         (7.0, 1.7, I)
```

2. If the patient has recent symptoms of prostatism, the provider should document one of the following on the same visit:

- AUA symptom score
- How bothersome the patient considers the symptoms

```
      1 3 4 1             1 1 3 2 2
1 2 3 4 5 6 7 8 9   1 2 3 4 5 6 7 8 9   ( 3- 4)
    (8.0, 0.7, A)         (7.0, 1.0, A)
```

3. Patients with new recent symptoms of prostatism should have the presence of absence of at least one of the following conditions documented:

- Parkinson's disease
- Diabetes mellitus
- Stroke
- History of urethral instrumentation

```
      2 3 1 3             1 4 2   2
1 2 3 4 5 6 7 8 9   1 2 3 4 5 6 7 8 9   ( 5- 6)
    (4.0, 1.0, A)         (4.0, 1.0, I)
```

4. Patients with new recent symptoms of prostatism should be offered a digital rectal examination (DRE) within one month after the visit in which the symptoms are noted, if they have not had a DRE in the past year.

```
      2 1   1   3 1 1           2 1 2 3 1
1 2 3 4 5 6 7 8 9   1 2 3 4 5 6 7 8 9   ( 7- 8)
    (7.0, 2.1, D)         (7.0, 1.1, I)
```

5. If a patient has new recent symptoms of moderate prostatism the health care provider should offer at least one of the following within one month of the note of symptoms:

- Uroflowometry
- Post void residual
- Pressure flow study

```
      1 1 4 1 2           1   5 1 1 1
1 2 3 4 5 6 7 8 9   1 2 3 4 5 6 7 8 9   ( 9- 10)
    (4.0, 0.9, A)         (5.0, 0.9, I)
```

6. If a patient has new recent symptoms prostatism, the provider should order the following tests within one month of the note of symptoms, unless done in the past year:

a. Urine analysis

```
        5 2 2               3 2 4
1 2 3 4 5 6 7 8 9   1 2 3 4 5 6 7 8 9   ( 11- 12)
    (7.0, 0.7, A)         (8.0, 0.8, A)
```

b. Serum creatinine

```
        7 1 1               1 2 2 4
1 2 3 4 5 6 7 8 9   1 2 3 4 5 6 7 8 9   ( 13- 14)
    (7.0, 0.3, A)         (8.0, 0.9, A)
```

TREATMENT

7. Patients diagnosed with BPH who report recent symptoms of prostatism, and who are on anticholinergic or sympathomimetic medications, should have discontinuation or dose reduction of these medications offered or discussed within one month of the note of symptoms.

```
      1 5 3             1 1 1   3 1 2
1 2 3 4 5 6 7 8 9   1 2 3 4 5 6 7 8 9   ( 15- 16)
    (7.0, 0.4, A)         (7.0, 1.6, I)
```

Scales: 1 = low validity or feasibility; 9 = high validity or feasibility

TREATMENT, CONT.

8. Patients diagnosed with BPH who report symptoms of moderate prostatism should have treatment options offered or discussed within one month of the note of symptoms.

```
            1   3 5            1 1 2 3 2
1 2 3 4 5 6 7 8 9   1 2 3 4 5 6 7 8 9   ( 17- 18)
   (8.0, 0.7, A)      (8.0, 1.0, A)
```

9. Patients diagnosed with BPH should be offered surgical therapy within one month of either of the following conditions being noted:

a. Acute renal insufficiency with dilated upper tracts

```
            2 5 2              2 4 3
1 2 3 4 5 6 7 8 9   1 2 3 4 5 6 7 8 9   ( 19- 20)
   (8.0, 0.4, A)      (8.0, 0.6, A)
```

b. Persistant renal insufficiency after catheterization trial

```
        1   4 2 2            1 1 2 4 1
1 2 3 4 5 6 7 8 9   1 2 3 4 5 6 7 8 9   ( 21- 22)
   (7.0, 1.0, A)      (8.0, 0.9, A)
```

10. Patients diagnosed with BPH should be offered surgical therapy within two months of any of the following conditions being noted unless the patient is not a surgical candidate:

a. Continued complaints of moderate symptoms of prostatism after at least 2 months of alpha 1 adrenergic therapy

```
        1 1 4 3              2 3 3 1
1 2 3 4 5 6 7 8 9   1 2 3 4 5 6 7 8 9   ( 23- 24)
   (7.0, 0.7, A)      (7.0, 0.8, A)
```

b. More than one urinary tract infection in the past year

```
        2 3 2   2            1 1 4 2 1
1 2 3 4 5 6 7 8 9   1 2 3 4 5 6 7 8 9   ( 25- 26)
   (5.0, 1.1, A)      (7.0, 0.8, A)
```

c. Bladder stones

```
            2 3 3 1          1 1 3 3 1
1 2 3 4 5 6 7 8 9   1 2 3 4 5 6 7 8 9   ( 27- 28)
   (7.0, 0.8, A)      (7.0, 0.9, A)
```

FOLLOW-UP

11. Patients diagnosed with BPH who have received alpha 1 adrenergic or surgical therapy should have their symptoms reassessed 6 months after initiation of therapy.

```
        1 2 5 1            1   3 4 1
1 2 3 4 5 6 7 8 9   1 2 3 4 5 6 7 8 9   ( 29- 30)
   (8.0, 0.6, A)      (8.0, 0.8, A)
```

12. Patients with persistent moderate symptoms of prostatism 6 months after surgical therapy should be offered urodynamic evaluation.

```
        2 4 3              1 4 3 1
1 2 3 4 5 6 7 8 9   1 2 3 4 5 6 7 8 9   ( 31- 32)
   (7.0, 0.6, A)      (7.0, 0.7, A)
```

Scales: 1 = low validity or feasibility; 9 = high validity or feasibility

	Validity	Feasibility

SCREENING

1. All patients aged 55 and older should have documentation of their visual function every 3 years.

```
                3 2 1 3          1   1   3 3 1
        1 2 3 4 5 6 7 8 9   1 2 3 4 5 6 7 8 9   ( 1- 2)
          (6.0, 1.1, I)        (7.0, 1.2, A)
```

DIAGNOSIS

2. Patients who report difficulty with corrected visual function should receive a complete eye exam that includes all of the following within 3 months of the report:

a. visual acuity measurement
```
                2 2 4 1              1 2 3 3
        1 2 3 4 5 6 7 8 9   1 2 3 4 5 6 7 8 9   ( 3- 4)
          (8.0, 0.8, A)        (8.0, 0.8, A)
```

b. intraocular pressure measurement
```
                1 1 2 4 1            1 2 3 3
        1 2 3 4 5 6 7 8 9   1 2 3 4 5 6 7 8 9   ( 5- 6)
          (8.0, 0.9, A)        (8.0, 0.8, A)
```

c. pupil exam
```
                1 2 5 1              1 2 3 3
        1 2 3 4 5 6 7 8 9   1 2 3 4 5 6 7 8 9   ( 7- 8)
          (8.0, 0.6, A)        (8.0, 0.8, A)
```

d. motility exam
```
                1 2 4 2              1 2 3 3
        1 2 3 4 5 6 7 8 9   1 2 3 4 5 6 7 8 9   ( 9- 10)
          (8.0, 0.7, A)        (8.0, 0.8, A)
```

e. slit lamp exam
```
                1 1 2 4 1          2 1 1 3 2
        1 2 3 4 5 6 7 8 9   1 2 3 4 5 6 7 8 9   ( 11- 12)
          (8.0, 0.9, A)        (8.0, 1.2, I)
```

f. dilated fundus exam
```
                2 2 4 1            1 2 1 3 2
        1 2 3 4 5 6 7 8 9   1 2 3 4 5 6 7 8 9   ( 13- 14)
          (8.0, 0.8, A)        (8.0, 1.1, I)
```

3. Patients should be offered refraction in the affected eye within 4 months before surgery unless a prior refraction made no improvement in otherwise stable vision in the past two years.
```
              2   3 3 1          1   2 4 2
        1 2 3 4 5 6 7 8 9   1 2 3 4 5 6 7 8 9   ( 15- 16)
          (7.0, 1.0, A)        (8.0, 0.8, A)
```

TREATMENT

4. Patients with cataracts should be offered surgery if any of the following situations are present:

a. phacomorphic glaucoma
```
                  4 4 1                2 6 1
        1 2 3 4 5 6 7 8 9   1 2 3 4 5 6 7 8 9   ( 17- 18)
          (8.0, 0.6, A)        (8.0, 0.3, A)
```

b. phacolytic glaucoma
```
                  4 4 1                2 6 1
        1 2 3 4 5 6 7 8 9   1 2 3 4 5 6 7 8 9   ( 19- 20)
          (8.0, 0.6, A)        (8.0, 0.3, A)
```

c. lens-related uveitis
```
                  4 4 1                2 6 1
        1 2 3 4 5 6 7 8 9   1 2 3 4 5 6 7 8 9   ( 21- 22)
          (8.0, 0.6, A)        (8.0, 0.3, A)
```

d. disrupted anterior lens capsule in otherwise phakic eye
```
                  4 4 1                2 6 1
        1 2 3 4 5 6 7 8 9   1 2 3 4 5 6 7 8 9   ( 23- 24)
          (8.0, 0.6, A)        (8.0, 0.3, A)
```

e. cataract prevents adequate monitoring or treatment of glaucoma or diabetes
```
                  5 4                  3 6
        1 2 3 4 5 6 7 8 9   1 2 3 4 5 6 7 8 9   ( 25- 26)
          (7.0, 0.4, A)        (8.0, 0.3, A)
```

Scales: 1 = low validity or feasibility; 9 = high validity or feasibility

TREATMENT, CONT.

5. In the absence of a medical indication for
cataract surgery, the ophthalmologist should
offer cataract surgery only when both of the
following conditions are met:

- the patient's visual functioning is
  impaired
- there is either a normal fundus exam or a
  statement that the surgeon believes the
  patient's visual function would improve
  after the surgery.
- a lens opacity exists.

```
          1   1   3 3 1           1   4 3 1
1 2 3 4 5 6 7 8 9   1 2 3 4 5 6 7 8 9   ( 27- 28)
   (7.0, 1.2, A)       (7.0, 0.8, A)
```

FOLLOW-UP

7. Within 90 days of surgery, the surgeon
should do at least one of the following:

- examine the patient
- refer the patient for further care
- document inability to contact patient

```
1 1 1 2     1 1 2         1     1 3 2 2
1 2 3 4 5 6 7 8 9   1 2 3 4 5 6 7 8 9   ( 29- 30)
   (4.0, 2.6, D)       (7.0, 1.2, A)
```

8. Within 48 hours of surgery, an
optometrist or ophthalmologist should offer
patients who have undergone cataract
extraction a complete anterior segment eye
examination, including all of the following:

a. visual acuity measurement

```
              3 3 3               1 3 5
1 2 3 4 5 6 7 8 9   1 2 3 4 5 6 7 8 9   ( 31- 32)
   (8.0, 0.7, A)       (9.0, 0.6, A)
```

b. intraocular pressure measurement

```
              3 3 3               1 3 5
1 2 3 4 5 6 7 8 9   1 2 3 4 5 6 7 8 9   ( 33- 34)
   (8.0, 0.7, A)       (9.0, 0.6, A)
```

c. slit lamp exam

```
              3 3 3               1 3 5
1 2 3 4 5 6 7 8 9   1 2 3 4 5 6 7 8 9   ( 35- 36)
   (8.0, 0.7, A)       (9.0, 0.6, A)
```

9. Patients who have undergone cataract
extraction should have their visual
functioning assessed within 90 days of
surgery.

```
            4 4 1             1 2 4 2
1 2 3 4 5 6 7 8 9   1 2 3 4 5 6 7 8 9   ( 37- 38)
   (8.0, 0.6, A)       (8.0, 0.7, A)
```

Scales: 1 = low validity or feasibility; 9 = high validity or feasibility

TREATMENT

1. Patients who are diagnosed with a
complication of gallstones should receive a
cholecystectomy within one month of the
complication, unless the medical record
states that they are not a surgical
candidate.

```
                 2 5 2                     2 3 4
1 2 3 4 5 6 7 8 9   1 2 3 4 5 6 7 8 9   (  1-  2)
   (8.0, 0.4, A)        (8.0, 0.7, A)
```

2. If a patient undergoes cholecystectomy
for gallstones, one of the following should
be documented within the 6 months prior to
surgery:

- biliary pain
- complications from gallstone

```
               1   3 3 2                   2 3 4
1 2 3 4 5 6 7 8 9   1 2 3 4 5 6 7 8 9   (  3-  4)
   (8.0, 0.9, A)        (8.0, 0.7, A)
```

3. Patients who are diagnosed with biliary
pain should be offered cholecystectomy within
6 months of the symptoms, unless the medical
record states that they are not a surgical
candidate.

```
               6 2 1                     3 4 2
1 2 3 4 5 6 7 8 9   1 2 3 4 5 6 7 8 9   (  5-  6)
   (7.0, 0.4, A)        (8.0, 0.6, A)
```

Scales: 1 = low validity or feasibility; 9 = high validity or feasibility

Validity   Feasibility

DIAGNOSIS

1. If a patient has new symptoms of
cognitive impairment, all of the following
information should be documented within 3
months:

a. Have the patient's cognitive abilities
declined from a previous level?

```
1        2 1 4 1              2 1 1 3 2
1 2 3 4 5 6 7 8 9   1 2 3 4 5 6 7 8 9  ( 1- 2)
   (8.0, 1.3, I)       (8.0, 1.2, I)
```

b. Do the patient's symptoms of cognitive
impairment interfere with daily
functioning?

```
1        1 2 3 2              2 1 1 3 2
1 2 3 4 5 6 7 8 9   1 2 3 4 5 6 7 8 9  ( 3- 4)
   (8.0, 1.3, A)       (8.0, 1.2, I)
```

c. Medications being taken (both
prescription and non-prescription)

```
         1 5 3                1 2 2 4
1 2 3 4 5 6 7 8 9   1 2 3 4 5 6 7 8 9  ( 5- 6)
   (8.0, 0.4, A)       (8.0, 0.9, A)
```

d. The use of alcohol or other substances
that may affect cognition

```
         2 4 3              1 1 1 2 4
1 2 3 4 5 6 7 8 9   1 2 3 4 5 6 7 8 9  ( 7- 8)
   (8.0, 0.6, A)       (8.0, 1.1, A)
```

e. The presence or absence of delirium

```
       2 1 1 3 2            1 2   2   2 2
1 2 3 4 5 6 7 8 9   1 2 3 4 5 6 7 8 9  ( 9- 10)
   (8.0, 1.2, I)       (6.0, 1.9, I)
```

f. The presence or absence of depression

```
         2 5 2              2 3 1 2 1
1 2 3 4 5 6 7 8 9   1 2 3 4 5 6 7 8 9  ( 11- 12)
   (8.0, 0.4, A)       (6.0, 1.1, I)
```

2. All of the following information should
be documented within 3 months of onset for
patients with a new diagnosis of dementia:

a. The onset of symptoms

```
         1 2 5 1              1 2 1 3 2
1 2 3 4 5 6 7 8 9   1 2 3 4 5 6 7 8 9  ( 13- 14)
   (8.0, 0.6, A)       (8.0, 1.1, I)
```

b. The nature of progression

```
         3 1 4 1            1 1 2   3 2
1 2 3 4 5 6 7 8 9   1 2 3 4 5 6 7 8 9  ( 15- 16)
   (8.0, 0.9, I)       (8.0, 1.4, I)
```

3. "O" If a patient has any new symptoms of
cognitive impairment, the health care
provider should perform a mental status
examination within 3 months.

```
     1 1 2 2 1 1 1            2 2 2 2 1
1 2 3 4 5 6 7 8 9   1 2 3 4 5 6 7 8 9  ( 17- 18)
   (6.0, 1.4, I)       (7.0, 1.1, I)
```

3. "X" If a patient has any new symptoms of
of cognitive impairment, the health care
provider should perform a neurological
examination within 3 months.

```
         2 3 3 1              1 2 1 3 2
1 2 3 4 5 6 7 8 9   1 2 3 4 5 6 7 8 9  ( 19- 20)
   (7.0, 0.8, A)       (8.0, 1.1, I)
```

4. If a patient has a new diagnosis of
dementia, the following blood tests should
be offered within 3 months:

a. CBC

```
       3   4 1 1              1   4 4
1 2 3 4 5 6 7 8 9   1 2 3 4 5 6 7 8 9  ( 21- 22)
   (7.0, 1.0, I)       (8.0, 0.7, A)
```

b. Chemistry panel (electrolytes, BUN,
creatinine, bicarbonate, chloride, glucose,
calcium)

```
         2 4 2 1              1   4 4
1 2 3 4 5 6 7 8 9   1 2 3 4 5 6 7 8 9  ( 23- 24)
   (7.0, 0.7, A)       (8.0, 0.7, A)
```

c. TSH

```
         2 3 3 1              1   4 4
1 2 3 4 5 6 7 8 9   1 2 3 4 5 6 7 8 9  ( 25- 26)
   (7.0, 0.8, A)       (8.0, 0.7, A)
```

Scales: 1 = low validity or feasibility; 9 = high validity or feasibility

DIAGNOSIS, CONT.

5. If a patient has a new diagnosis of
dementia, a head CT or MRI should be offered
within 30 days if one or more of the
following criteria is met:

b. head trauma within 2 weeks preceding
the onset of symptoms of cognitive
impairment

```
              1   6 2              1 2 4 1 1
1 2 3 4 5 6 7 8 9    1 2 3 4 5 6 7 8 9   ( 27- 28)
   (7.0, 0.4, A)        (7.0, 0.8, I)
```

c. onset of seizures in the past 2 years

```
   1      3 3 1 1           2 1    3 2 1
1 2 3 4 5 6 7 8 9    1 2 3 4 5 6 7 8 9   ( 29- 30)
   (6.0, 1.1, I)        (7.0, 1.3, I)
```

d. gait disorder in the past 2 years

```
   1   1 3 1 2 1           2 3    1 2 1
1 2 3 4 5 6 7 8 9    1 2 3 4 5 6 7 8 9   ( 31- 32)
   (5.0, 1.3, I)        (5.0, 1.6, I)
```

e. focal neurologic findings

```
   1        1 4 3          1   5 2 1
1 2 3 4 5 6 7 8 9    1 2 3 4 5 6 7 8 9   ( 33- 34)
   (7.0, 1.0, A)        (7.0, 0.7, A)
```

f. new headache that persists despite at
least 4 weeks of medical treatment

```
   1     1 1 4 2           2 2    2 1 2
1 2 3 4 5 6 7 8 9    1 2 3 4 5 6 7 8 9   ( 35- 36)
   (7.0, 1.1, I)        (7.0, 1.7, I)
```

TREATMENT

6. Patients with a diagnosis of dementia and
who are having behavioral problems should be
offered at least one of the following
interventions:

- counseling the caregivers about
  non-pharmacological measures to control
  symptoms
- providing pharmacological means to
  control symptoms
- referral to specialists who may assist
  with symptoms

```
      1 1 3 4              2 2 1 3 1
1 2 3 4 5 6 7 8 9    1 2 3 4 5 6 7 8 9   ( 37- 38)
   (7.0, 0.8, A)        (7.0, 1.2, I)
```

7. Caregivers of demented persons should be
asked about their need for support services
within 3 months of the diagnosis.

```
         6 1 2        1   3 1 1 1 2
1 2 3 4 5 6 7 8 9    1 2 3 4 5 6 7 8 9   ( 39- 40)
   (7.0, 0.6, A)        (6.0, 1.7, I)
```

8. For patients diagnosed with dementia, the
presence or absence of all of the following
risk factors for vascular etiology should be
documented:

a. hypertension

```
   4 3 2                   2 2 1 2 2
1 2 3 4 5 6 7 8 9    1 2 3 4 5 6 7 8 9   ( 41- 42)
   (5.0, 0.7, A)        (7.0, 1.3, I)
```

b. smoking

```
   4 3 2                   2 3    2 2
1 2 3 4 5 6 7 8 9    1 2 3 4 5 6 7 8 9   ( 43- 44)
   (5.0, 0.7, A)        (6.0, 1.3, I)
```

c. hypercholesterolemia

```
   4 3 2                   2 2 1 2 2
1 2 3 4 5 6 7 8 9    1 2 3 4 5 6 7 8 9   ( 45- 46)
   (5.0, 0.7, A)        (7.0, 1.3, I)
```

9. Patients with vascular or multi-infarct
dementia should be offered aspirin, unless
active peptic ulcer disease or aspirin
intolerance is noted.

```
   1 2 4 2                 2 3 1 1 2
1 2 3 4 5 6 7 8 9    1 2 3 4 5 6 7 8 9   ( 47- 48)
   (5.0, 0.7, A)        (6.0, 1.2, I)
```

Scales: 1 = low validity or feasibility; 9 = high validity or feasibility

	Validity	Feasibility

TREATMENT, CONT.

10. Persons with dementia should not be
taking long-acting sedatives unless there is
explicit justification in the medical record.

```
                                    4 4 1              1 1 4 3
                          1 2 3 4 5 6 7 8 9   1 2 3 4 5 6 7 8 9   ( 49- 50)
                             (8.0, 0.6, A)        (8.0, 0.7, A)
```

FOLLOW-UP

11. Patients with symptoms of cognitive
impairment who do not receive a diagnosis of
dementia should have documented that the
provider inquired again about those symptoms
within 12 months of first presentation.

```
                                    3 5 1             1 3 2 1 2
                          1 2 3 4 5 6 7 8 9   1 2 3 4 5 6 7 8 9   ( 51- 52)
                             (7.0, 0.4, I)        (6.0, 1.1, I)
```

Scales: 1 = low validity or feasibility; 9 = high validity or feasibility

Note: This chapter was revised from Q1.
Only new or revised indicators were rated.

FOLLOW-UP

11. Patients with major depression who have
medical record documentation of improvement
of symptoms within 6 weeks of starting
antidepressant treatment should be continued
on and antidepressant for at least 4
additional months.

                                                    3 4 2   1   2 3 3
                                    1 2 3 4 5 6 7 8 9   1 2 3 4 5 6 7 8 9   (1- 2)
                                       (8.0, 0.6, A)   (8.0, 0.9, A)

NOTE: This chapter was revised from Q1.
Only new or revised indicators were rated.

DIAGNOSIS

1. Patients < 75 years old with more than
one fasting blood sugar >126 or postprandial
blood sugar >200 should have diagnosis of
diabetes noted in progress notes or problem   1   3 5   2 6 1
list.   1 2 3 4 5 6 7 8 9 1 2 3 4 5 6 7 8 9 (1- 2)
                                               (8.0, 0.7, A)   (8.0, 0.3, A)

2. Patients with the diagnosis of Type 1
diabetes should have all of the following:

  c. Total serum cholesterol and HDL   1 4 3 1   1   1 2 3 2
  cholesterol tests documented   1 2 3 4 5 6 7 8 9 1 2 3 4 5 6 7 8 9 (3- 4)
                                               (7.0, 0.7, A)   (8.0, 1.1, A)

3. Patients with the diagnosis of Type 2
diabetes should have all of the following:

  c. Total serum cholesterol and HDL   1 5 3   1   1 2 3 2
  cholesterol tests documented   1 2 3 4 5 6 7 8 9 1 2 3 4 5 6 7 8 9 (5- 6)
                                               (7.0, 0.4, A)   (8.0, 1.1, A)

8. Diabetics with proteinuria should be
offered an ACE inhibitor within 3 months of
the notation of proteinuria unless   6 3   3 4 2
contraindicated.   1 2 3 4 5 6 7 8 9 1 2 3 4 5 6 7 8 9 (7- 8)
                                               (7.0, 0.3, A)   (8.0, 0.6, A)

1. Women with intact uteri should not use
unopposed oral or transdermal estrogen
unless both of the following are true:

  - The patient has been tried on cyclic or
    continuous estrogen plus progestin
    regimen
  - Endometrial sampling is performed at   1 3 4 1   2 3 4
    least every 2 years   1 2 3 4 5 6 7 8 9 1 2 3 4 5 6 7 8 9 (1- 2)
                                     (8.0, 0.7, A)   (8.0, 0.7, A)

2. Women with a new diagnosis of menopause   2 4 3   2 1 2 2 2
should receive counseling about the risks and 1 2 3 4 5 6 7 8 9 1 2 3 4 5 6 7 8 9 (3- 4)
benefits of HRT within one year of diagnosis.   (8.0, 0.6, A)   (6.0, 1.7, I)

3. Post-menopausal women being initiated on
HRT should receive counseling about the risks
and benefits of HRT within 1 year prior to   3 5 1   3 2 4
initiation.   1 2 3 4 5 6 7 8 9 1 2 3 4 5 6 7 8 9 (5- 6)
                                     (8.0, 0.4, A)   (7.0, 0.8, I)

Scales: 1 = low validity or feasibility; 9 = high validity or feasibility

NOTE: This chapter was revised from Q1.
There were no new or revised indicators to
rate.

DIAGNOSIS

1. Patients with symptoms or signs of hip
fracture should offered one of the following
imaging studies of the affected hip within 1
day unless documented not to be a surgical
candidate:

- a radiograph
- a technetium-99m bone scan
- an MRI

```
                     2 3 4          1     1 3 4
         1 2 3 4 5 6 7 8 9  1 2 3 4 5 6 7 8 9  ( 1- 2)
           (8.0, 0.7, A)      (8.0, 1.0, A)
```

2. Patients who have had surgical repair of
a hip fracture should have been offered a
complete medical evaluation preoperatively,
including all of the following:

a. medical history

```
         1     1   2 2 3               2 3 4
         1 2 3 4 5 6 7 8 9  1 2 3 4 5 6 7 8 9  ( 3- 4)
           (8.0, 1.6, A)      (8.0, 0.7, A)
```

b. physical examination

```
         1     1   2 2 3               2 3 4
         1 2 3 4 5 6 7 8 9  1 2 3 4 5 6 7 8 9  ( 5- 6)
           (8.0, 1.6, A)      (8.0, 0.7, A)
```

c. laboratory evaluation for patients
    >= age 50

```
         1       1 1 1 2 3            1 2 2 4
         1 2 3 4 5 6 7 8 9  1 2 3 4 5 6 7 8 9  ( 7- 8)
           (8.0, 1.7, I)      (8.0, 0.9, A)
```

d. electrocardiogram for patients >= age 50

```
         1       1 1 1 2 3            1 2 2 4
         1 2 3 4 5 6 7 8 9  1 2 3 4 5 6 7 8 9  ( 9- 10)
           (8.0, 1.7, I)      (8.0, 0.9, A)
```

TREATMENT

3. Patients who have had surgical repair of
a hip fracture should have received
antibiotics prophylactically on the **same** day
that surgery was performed.

```
           1 2 3 1 2                1 2 2 4
         1 2 3 4 5 6 7 8 9  1 2 3 4 5 6 7 8 9  ( 11- 12)
           (7.0, 1.0, I)      (8.0, 0.9, A)
```

4. Patients who have a surgically repaired
hip fracture should begin rehabilitation on
post-operative day one.

```
           3 3 1 2                3 1 3 2
         1 2 3 4 5 6 7 8 9  1 2 3 4 5 6 7 8 9  ( 13- 14)
           (6.0, 0.9, I)      (8.0, 1.0, I)
```

5. Persons with hip fractures should be
given prophylactic antithrombotics on
admission to the hospital.

```
           1 2 5 1                  2 4 3
         1 2 3 4 5 6 7 8 9  1 2 3 4 5 6 7 8 9  ( 15- 16)
           (8.0, 0.6, A)      (8.0, 0.6, A)
```

6. Patients hospitalized with hip fracture
who are at risk for developing pressure sores
should have both of the following done while
hospitalized:

a. Be repositioned every 2 hours

```
           3 3 1 2            1     3 1 4
         1 2 3 4 5 6 7 8 9  1 2 3 4 5 6 7 8 9  ( 17- 18)
           (7.0, 0.9, I)      (7.0, 1.1, I)
```

b. Be provided a pressure-reducing mattress

```
         1 2 1 2 2 1                3   3 3
         1 2 3 4 5 6 7 8 9  1 2 3 4 5 6 7 8 9  ( 19- 20)
           (6.0, 1.3, I)      (7.0, 1.0, I)
```

Scales: 1 = low validity or feasibility; 9 = high validity or feasibility

| | Validity | Feasibility |

FOLLOW-UP

7.   Patients who have had a hip fracture should have documented within 2 months (before or after) the presence or absence of at least one modifiable risk factors for hip fracture.

```
                    1    3 5              1 4 4
          1 2 3 4 5 6 7 8 9  1 2 3 4 5 6 7 8 9  ( 21- 22)
             (8.0, 0.7, A)      (7.0, 0.6, A)
```

8.   Patients over 65 who report falling should be assessed for at least two modifiable risk factors for hip fracture within 3 months of the report.

```
                    1 6 2              1   3 3 2
          1 2 3 4 5 6 7 8 9  1 2 3 4 5 6 7 8 9  ( 23- 24)
             (7.0, 0.3, A)      (7.0, 0.9, I)
```

Scales: 1 = low validity or feasibility; 9 = high validity or feasibility

Validity   Feasibility

1. If a woman undergoes a hysterectomy with
the indication of fibroid uterus at least one
of the following should be recorded in the
medical record:

- The uterus is significantly enlarged
  and the patient is concerned about the
  fibroids
- Excessive menstrual bleeding
- Pelvic discomfort
- Bladder pressure with urinary frequency

```
                    1 6 2              1 2 3 2 1
          1 2 3 4 5 6 7 8 9   1 2 3 4 5 6 7 8 9  ( 1- 2)
            (7.0, 0.3, A)        (7.0, 0.9, I)
```

2. If a pre- or peri-menopausal woman
undergoes a hysterectomy with the indication
of abnormal uterine bleeding, then the
medical record should indicate that at least
one month of medical therapy was offered in
the six months prior to the hysterectomy
without relief of symptoms.

```
                    5 2 2              4 3 2
          1 2 3 4 5 6 7 8 9   1 2 3 4 5 6 7 8 9  ( 3- 4)
            (7.0, 0.7, A)        (8.0, 0.7, A)
```

3. Women who have a hysterectomy for
post-menopausal bleeding should have been
offered a biopsy of the endometrium within
six months prior to the procedure.

```
                    4 3 2              2 3 2 2
          1 2 3 4 5 6 7 8 9   1 2 3 4 5 6 7 8 9  ( 5- 6)
            (8.0, 0.7, A)        (7.0, 0.9, A)
```

4. Women with post-menopausal bleeding
should be offered an office endometrial
biopsy within three months of presentation.

```
                    7 1 1              3 2 2 2
          1 2 3 4 5 6 7 8 9   1 2 3 4 5 6 7 8 9  ( 7- 8)
            (7.0, 0.3, A)        (7.0, 1.0, I)
```

Scales: 1 = low validity or feasibility; 9 = high validity or feasibility

Validity   Feasibility

DIAGNOSIS

1. For a patient < age 65 diagnosed with inguinal hernia, the medical record should document the time duration since the patient first noticed symptoms of hernia.

```
    1   4 2 2                    3 2 1   2 1
1 2 3 4 5 6 7 8 9   1 2 3 4 5 6 7 8 9   ( 1- 2)
  (4.0, 0.9, A)        (5.0, 1.6, I)
```

TREATMENT

2. A patient diagnosed with a strangulated inguinal hernia should receive emergency groin exploration within 24 hours of presentation.

```
          1 5 3                    2 2 5
1 2 3 4 5 6 7 8 9   1 2 3 4 5 6 7 8 9   ( 3- 4)
  (8.0, 0.4, A)        (9.0, 0.7, A)
```

3. For a patient diagnosed with symptomatic inguinal hernia, the medical record should document that elective herniorrhaphy was discussed.

```
            7 2              1   4 2 2
1 2 3 4 5 6 7 8 9   1 2 3 4 5 6 7 8 9   ( 5- 6)
  (7.0, 0.2, A)        (7.0, 0.9, A)
```

4. Patients with a newly documented inguinal hernia should, at the same visit, receive education on the symptoms that would necessitate emergency surgery.

```
          1 6 2            1 3   1 3 1
1 2 3 4 5 6 7 8 9   1 2 3 4 5 6 7 8 9   ( 7- 8)
  (7.0, 0.3, A)        (6.0, 1.6, I)
```

Scales: 1 = low validity or feasibility; 9 = high validity or feasibility

NOTE: This chapter was revised from Q1.
There were no new or revised indicators to
rate.

SHOULDER: DIAGNOSIS

1. Patients presenting with new onset
shoulder pain should have a history obtained
at the time of presentation that includes at
least 4 of the following:

- duration of pain
- location of pain
- activity at time the pain began
- activities that worsen the pain
- past history of injury
- past history of surgery
- therapeutic interventions attempted
  (e.g., NSAIDs, rest, physical therapy)
- involvement of other joints

```
         1 1   2 3   2              2 3 1 2 1
1 2 3 4 5 6 7 8 9   1 2 3 4 5 6 7 8 9  ( 1- 2)
   (6.0, 1.4, I)        (6.0, 1.1, I)
```

2. Patients who present with new onset
shoulder pain should have a physical
examination performed at time of presentation
that includes at least 3 of the following:

- range of passive motion testing
- range of active motion testing
- the drop arm test
- testing for presence of impingement sign
- palpation to localize the site of pain
- cervical spine examination

```
      1   1 2 2 1 2              1 4 2 2
1 2 3 4 5 6 7 8 9   1 2 3 4 5 6 7 8 9  ( 3- 4)
   (6.0, 1.4, I)        (6.0, 0.8, I)
```

SHOULDER: TREATMENT

3. Patients diagnosed with impingement
syndrome should be offered at least 1 of the
following within 2 weeks:

- NSAIDs, including aspirin
- steroid injection
- avoidance of inciting activities
- physical therapy
- instructions for a home exercise program

```
      1   1   1 4 2              1 1 4 3
1 2 3 4 5 6 7 8 9   1 2 3 4 5 6 7 8 9  ( 5- 6)
   (7.0, 1.2, I)        (7.0, 0.7, A)
```

6. Patients diagnosed with adhesive
capsulitis should receive education regarding
shoulder exercises at the time of diagnosis.

```
      1 1 3   2 2              3 2 2 2
1 2 3 4 5 6 7 8 9   1 2 3 4 5 6 7 8 9  ( 7- 8)
   (4.0, 1.4, I)        (5.0, 1.0, A)
```

KNEE: DIAGNOSIS

7. Patients presenting with new onset knee
pain should have a history taken at time of
initial presentation that includes at least 3
of the following:

- duration
- activity at time of onset
- exacerbating and relieving factors
- ability to ambulate
- history of prior trauma, surgery, or knee
  problems

```
      1 1 1 3   1 2              3 2 1 3
1 2 3 4 5 6 7 8 9   1 2 3 4 5 6 7 8 9  ( 9- 10)
   (5.0, 1.6, I)        (6.0, 1.1, I)
```

Scales: 1 = low validity or feasibility; 9 = high validity or feasibility

KNEE: DIAGNOSIS, CONT.

8. Patients presenting with new onset knee pain after injury to their knee should undergo at least 2 of the following maneuvers during physical examination within one month of initial presentation:

- Lachman's test
- anterior drawer test
- posterior drawer test
- posterior sag test
- joint line palpation
- McMurray's test
- valgus stress
- varus stress

```
         1    2 1 1 4                    1 1 4 3
       1 2 3 4 5 6 7 8 9    1 2 3 4 5 6 7 8 9   ( 11- 12)
         (7.0, 1.6, I)         (7.0, 0.7, A)
```

9. Patients presenting with new onset knee effusion should have a history taken at time of initial presentation that includes:

a. duration of swelling

```
         1    1 2 3 2                      2 3 4
       1 2 3 4 5 6 7 8 9    1 2 3 4 5 6 7 8 9   ( 13- 14)
         (7.0, 1.2, I)         (7.0, 0.7, A)
```

b. history of trauma and injury

```
         1    1 2 3 2                      2 3 4
       1 2 3 4 5 6 7 8 9    1 2 3 4 5 6 7 8 9   ( 15- 16)
         (7.0, 1.2, I)         (7.0, 0.7, A)
```

c. presence of pain

```
         1    3 1 2 2                    1 2 3 3
       1 2 3 4 5 6 7 8 9    1 2 3 4 5 6 7 8 9   ( 17- 18)
         (6.0, 1.4, I)         (7.0, 0.8, I)
```

d. history of crystalline-induced arthropathies

```
         1      2 4 2                    1 2 2 4
       1 2 3 4 5 6 7 8 9    1 2 3 4 5 6 7 8 9   ( 19- 20)
         (7.0, 1.0, I)         (7.0, 0.9, I)
```

e. presence or absence of fever

```
         1        5 3                      1 3 5
       1 2 3 4 5 6 7 8 9    1 2 3 4 5 6 7 8 9   ( 21- 22)
         (7.0, 0.9, A)         (8.0, 0.6, A)
```

10. Patients presenting with new onset knee effusion who do not have a history of recent trauma should undergo arthrocentesis at time of presentation.

```
         1 1 4 3                        1 3 4 1
       1 2 3 4 5 6 7 8 9    1 2 3 4 5 6 7 8 9   ( 23- 24)
         (5.0, 0.7, A)         (7.0, 0.7, I)
```

11. Patients who undergo an arthrocentesis for new onset knee effusion should have the fluid analyzed for all of the following:

a. cell count

```
              5 4                          4 3 2
       1 2 3 4 5 6 7 8 9    1 2 3 4 5 6 7 8 9   ( 25- 26)
         (7.0, 0.4, A)         (8.0, 0.7, A)
```

b. culture

```
           1 4 1 1 2                     1 3 3 2
       1 2 3 4 5 6 7 8 9    1 2 3 4 5 6 7 8 9   ( 27- 28)
         (5.0, 1.1, I)         (8.0, 0.8, A)
```

c. Gram stain

```
                4 4 1                    1 3 3 2
       1 2 3 4 5 6 7 8 9    1 2 3 4 5 6 7 8 9   ( 29- 30)
         (8.0, 0.6, A)         (8.0, 0.8, A)
```

d. crystals

```
              5 4                        1 3 3 2
       1 2 3 4 5 6 7 8 9    1 2 3 4 5 6 7 8 9   ( 31- 32)
         (7.0, 0.4, A)         (8.0, 0.8, A)
```

Scales: 1 = low validity or feasibility; 9 = high validity or feasibility

KNEE: TREATMENT

12. Patients diagnosed with an ACL rupture
should have surgical options discussed within
2 weeks of the rupture unless documented not
to be a surgical candidate.

```
                2   5 2                    2 2 3 2
1 2 3 4 5 6 7 8 9  1 2 3 4 5 6 7 8 9  ( 33- 34)
  (7.0, 0.7, A)        (8.0, 0.9, A)
```

13. Patients newly diagnosed with
patellofemoral syndrome should receive the
following at time of diagnosis:

a. prescription or recommendation for
NSAIDs, unless contraindicated

```
                2 2 3   2              1 2 2 4
1 2 3 4 5 6 7 8 9  1 2 3 4 5 6 7 8 9  ( 35- 36)
  (6.0, 1.1, A)        (7.0, 0.9, I)
```

b. education on quadriceps-strengthening
exercises

```
                1 3 3   2                2 1   2 4
1 2 3 4 5 6 7 8 9  1 2 3 4 5 6 7 8 9  ( 37- 38)
  (6.0, 1.0, A)        (7.0, 1.3, I)
```

14. Patients diagnosed with a septic joint
should be treated with intravenous
antibiotics.

```
                  3 2 4                    3 1 5
1 2 3 4 5 6 7 8 9  1 2 3 4 5 6 7 8 9  ( 39- 40)
  (8.0, 0.8, A)        (9.0, 0.8, A)
```

15. Patients who report having at least 6
months of knee pain that limits function,
despite regular use of NSAIDS and/or
intrarticular steroid joint injection, should
have the following offered or discussed
within 1 month of the report of continued
pain:

- physical therapy (if not already tried)
- surgery/arthroscopy

```
              1   2 5 1                3 1 4 1
1 2 3 4 5 6 7 8 9  1 2 3 4 5 6 7 8 9  ( 41- 42)
  (7.0, 0.7, I)        (7.0, 0.9, I)
```

Scales: 1 = low validity or feasibility; 9 = high validity or feasibility

DIAGNOSIS

1. Providers caring for patients with
symptoms of OA should document at least one
of the following at least once in 2 years:

  - the location of symptoms
  - the presence or absence of limitations
    in daily activities
  - the use and effectiveness of treatment   1   2 1 3 2   1 1 3 1 2 1
    modalities   1 2 3 4 5 6 7 8 9 1 2 3 4 5 6 7 8 9 (1- 2)
                                              (7.0, 1.2, I)   (6.0, 1.2, I)

2. Providers caring for patients with
incident symptoms of OA should document at
least one of the following within 3 months
of symptom documentation:

  - the presence or absence of a history of
    any systemic or inflammatory disease that
    may mimic OA
  - the presence of absence of any current
    symptoms of systemic or inflammatory
    disease that may mimic OA
  - the presence or absence of a history of   1   3 2 1 2   1 2 2 1 2 1
    joint trauma or surgery   1 2 3 4 5 6 7 8 9 1 2 3 4 5 6 7 8 9 (3- 4)
                                              (6.0, 1.2, I)   (6.0, 1.3, I)

3. Providers caring for patients with
incident symptoms of OA should document at
least one of the following within 3 months
of symptom documentation:

  - the presence or absence of effusion
  - the presence or absence of bony
    enlargement
  - the presence or absence of tenderness
  - the presence or absence of limitations   1 1 1 2 2 2   1   2 2 3 1
    in range of motion   1 2 3 4 5 6 7 8 9 1 2 3 4 5 6 7 8 9 (5- 6)
                                              (6.0, 1.3, I)   (6.0, 1.1, I)

4. Patients with incident symptoms of hip OA
should be offered an anteroposterior film of   1 2 2 3 1   2 3 3   1
the affected hip.   1 2 3 4 5 6 7 8 9 1 2 3 4 5 6 7 8 9 (7- 8)
                                              (4.0, 1.0, I)   (5.0, 0.9, A)

TREATMENT

5. Patients with a new diagnosis of OA who
wish to take medication for joint symptoms   3 5 1   1 3 4 1
should be offered a trial of acetaminophen. 1 2 3 4 5 6 7 8 9 1 2 3 4 5 6 7 8 9 (9- 10)
                                              (8.0, 0.4, A)   (8.0, 0.7, A)

Scales: 1 = low validity or feasibility; 9 = high validity or feasibility

TREATMENT, CONT.

6. Providers caring for patients with
symptoms of hip or knee OA should recommend
the following at least once in 2 years:

a. exercise programs for persons with hip
or knee OA

                                                     2 5 2   1 1 3 2 2
1 2 3 4 5 6 7 8 9   1 2 3 4 5 6 7 8 9   (11- 12)
                                                  (7.0, 0.4, A)   (6.0, 1.0, I)

b. weight loss among persons with knee OA
and a BMI >= 25

                                                   2 1   4 1 1   4 4 1
1 2 3 4 5 6 7 8 9   1 2 3 4 5 6 7 8 9   (13- 14)
                                                  (5.0, 1.2, I)   (6.0, 0.6, A)

FOLLOW-UP

7. Patients receiving care for symptoms of
OA should be seen in follow-up at least every
6 months.

                                                 1   2 2 2 2   2 3 2 2
1 2 3 4 5 6 7 8 9   1 2 3 4 5 6 7 8 9   (15- 16)
                                                  (4.0, 1.2, I)   (6.0, 0.9, I)

Scales: 1 = low validity or feasibility; 9 = high validity or feasibility

DYSPEPSIA DIAGNOSIS

1. Patients presenting with a new episode of
dyspepsia should have the presence or absence
of NSAID use noted in the medical record on
the date of presentation.

```
                    4 4 1                  3 3 3
        1 2 3 4 5 6 7 8 9  1 2 3 4 5 6 7 8 9  ( 1- 2)
          (8.0, 0.6, A)       (8.0, 0.7, A)
```

DYSPEPSIA TREATMENT: NON NSAID-ASSOCIATED
DYSPEPSIA

2. Dyspepsia patients whose persistent and
bothersome symptoms have not improved after
8 weeks of empiric antiulcer treatment and
who were not using NSAIDs within the
previous month should have at least one of
the following within one month:

- endoscopy
- H. pylori test
- upper GI series

```
            1 1   6 1              1 2 1 4 1
1 2 3 4 5 6 7 8 9  1 2 3 4 5 6 7 8 9  ( 3- 4)
  (7.0, 0.7, A)       (8.0, 1.0, I)
```

3. Patients with new dyspepsia who have any
of the following "alarm" indicators on the
date of presentation should have endoscopy
performed within 1 month, unless endoscopy
has been performed in the previous 6 months:

a. new anemia
```
            1   6 2                5 3 1
1 2 3 4 5 6 7 8 9  1 2 3 4 5 6 7 8 9  ( 5- 6)
  (7.0, 0.4, A)       (7.0, 0.6, A)
```

b. early satiety
```
            1 7 1                  2 3 4
1 2 3 4 5 6 7 8 9  1 2 3 4 5 6 7 8 9  ( 7- 8)
  (7.0, 0.2, A)       (7.0, 0.7, A)
```

c. significant unintentional weight loss
(exceeding 15 pounds in the past 3 months)
```
            1 7 1                  6 3
1 2 3 4 5 6 7 8 9  1 2 3 4 5 6 7 8 9  ( 9- 10)
  (7.0, 0.2, A)       (7.0, 0.3, A)
```

d. guaiac-positive stool if not on NSAIDs
```
            1 6 2                  5 3 1
1 2 3 4 5 6 7 8 9  1 2 3 4 5 6 7 8 9  ( 11- 12)
  (7.0, 0.3, A)       (7.0, 0.6, A)
```

e. dysphagia
```
              8 1                  2 4 3
1 2 3 4 5 6 7 8 9  1 2 3 4 5 6 7 8 9  ( 13- 14)
  (7.0, 0.1, A)       (7.0, 0.6, A)
```

f. over age 60 if not on NSAIDs
```
        1   1 4 1 2              1 1 3 4
1 2 3 4 5 6 7 8 9  1 2 3 4 5 6 7 8 9  ( 15- 16)
  (5.0, 1.0, I)       (6.0, 0.8, I)
```

4. Patients who are prescribed H. pylori
eradication antibiotic treatment within 3
months after presentation for a new episode
of dyspepsia should have one of the following
noted in the medical record before start of
antibiotic treatment:

- prior positive test for H. pylori
- both a history of documented duodenal
  ulcer and absence of NSAID use.

```
            3 2   4              1 2 2 4
1 2 3 4 5 6 7 8 9  1 2 3 4 5 6 7 8 9  ( 17- 18)
  (6.0, 1.2, I)       (7.0, 0.9, I)
```

Scales: 1 = low validity or feasibility; 9 = high validity or feasibility

PEPTIC ULCER DISEASE: SECONDARY AND TERTIARY
PREVENTION

5.   For patients with documented PUD who
have been noted to use NSAIDs or aspirin
within 2 months before diagnosis, the
medical record should indicate one of the
following at the time of diagnosis:

- a reason why NSAIDs or aspirin will be
  continued
- advice to the patient to discontinue
  NSAIDs or aspirin

```
                       6 2 1                    6 2 1
           1 2 3 4 5 6 7 8 9   1 2 3 4 5 6 7 8 9   ( 19- 20)
             (7.0, 0.4, A)       (7.0, 0.4, A)
```

PEPTIC ULCER DISEASE: TREATMENT OF
UNCOMPLICATED PUD

6.   Patients in whom peptic ulceration is
confirmed on endoscopy should have antiulcer
treatment for a minimum of 4 weeks.

```
                     3 4 2                    1 1 5 2
         1 2 3 4 5 6 7 8 9   1 2 3 4 5 6 7 8 9   ( 21- 22)
           (8.0, 0.6, A)       (8.0, 0.6, A)
```

7.   Patients with endoscopically confirmed
gastric ulcer should have H. pylori testing
within 3 months before or 1 month after
endoscopy, unless the medical record, in the
same time period, documents a past positive
H. pylori test for which no H. pylori
eradication treatment was given.

```
                   1 1 3 2 2                  3 2 2 2
         1 2 3 4 5 6 7 8 9   1 2 3 4 5 6 7 8 9   ( 23- 24)
           (7.0, 1.0, A)       (7.0, 1.0, I)
```

8.   Eradication therapy for H. pylori should
be offered within 1 month when all of the
following conditions are met:

- documentation of history of positive
  H. pylori test at any time in the past
- documentation of endoscopically
  confirmed ulceration of the duodenum at
  any time in the past
- no previous H. pylori eradication
  therapy

```
                   1 6 1 1                  1   5 2 1
         1 2 3 4 5 6 7 8 9   1 2 3 4 5 6 7 8 9   ( 25- 26)
           (7.0, 0.4, A)       (7.0, 0.7, A)
```

PEPTIC ULCER DISEASE: TREATMENT

9. Patients with a gastric ulcer confirmed by
endoscopy should have at least one of the
following:

- a minimum of 3 biopsies during endoscopy
- follow-up endoscopy within 3 months

```
                   1 4 4                      2 7
         1 2 3 4 5 6 7 8 9   1 2 3 4 5 6 7 8 9   ( 27- 28)
           (7.0, 0.6, A)       (8.0, 0.2, A)
```

10.   Patients with endoscopically documented
gastric ulcer who have follow-up endoscopy
within 6 months should have one of the
following at the follow-up endoscopy:

- complete healing of the gastric ulcer
  noted
- a minimum of 3 biopsies of the ulcer

```
                   2 2 5                      1 8
         1 2 3 4 5 6 7 8 9   1 2 3 4 5 6 7 8 9   ( 29- 30)
           (8.0, 0.7, A)       (8.0, 0.1, A)
```

Scales: 1 = low validity or feasibility; 9 = high validity or feasibility

PEPTIC ULCER DISEASE: TREATMENT OF
COMPLICATED PUD

11. Patients with endoscopically documented
PUD should be offered endoscopic treatment or
surgery within the next 24 hours if either of
the following are documented in the endoscopy
note:

a. continued oozing, bleeding, or spurting
of blood

> 1 4 2 2   3 4 2
> 1 2 3 4 5 6 7 8 9   1 2 3 4 5 6 7 8 9   (31- 32)
> (7.0, 0.8, A)   (8.0, 0.6, A)

b. a visible vessel (or "pigmented
protuberance")

> 1 4 2 2   1 2 4 2
> 1 2 3 4 5 6 7 8 9   1 2 3 4 5 6 7 8 9   (33- 34)
> (7.0, 0.8, A)   (8.0, 0.7, A)

12. Patients with a documented PUD
complication who have had a positive
H. pylori test (by biopsy, breath test, or
positive serology not previously treated)
within 3 months after the complication
should be started on an H. pylori eradication
regimen within 1 month of the positive test.

> 4 4 1   1 1 6 1
> 1 2 3 4 5 6 7 8 9   1 2 3 4 5 6 7 8 9   (35- 36)
> (8.0, 0.6, A)   (8.0, 0.4, A)

PEPTIC ULCER DISEASE: FOLLOW-UP

13. Patients with endoscopically confirmed
PUD whose symptoms of dyspepsia or documented
ulcers recur within 6 months after
eradication therapy for H. pylori should
receive confirmatory testing for successful
H. pylori cure by endoscopic biopsy or urease
breath test within 1 month of symptom
recurrence.

> 1 6 2   2 7
> 1 2 3 4 5 6 7 8 9   1 2 3 4 5 6 7 8 9   (37- 38)
> (7.0, 0.3, A)   (8.0, 0.2, A)

14. Patients with a history of PUD
complications in the past year should have
results of H. pylori testing documented in
the medical record in the same time period.

> 1 5 3   1   7 1
> 1 2 3 4 5 6 7 8 9   1 2 3 4 5 6 7 8 9   (39- 40)
> (7.0, 0.4, A)   (8.0, 0.3, A)

Scales: 1 = low validity or feasibility; 9 = high validity or feasibility

NOTE: This chapter was revised from Q1.
Only new or revised indicators were rated.

IMMUNIZATIONS

2. There should be documentation in the
medical record that patients over the age of
50 were offered a tetanus/diphtheria booster
after their 50th birthday or in the last 10
years.

```
              1   6 2              2 1 4 2
    1 2 3 4 5 6 7 8 9    1 2 3 4 5 6 7 8 9   ( 1-  2)
      (7.0, 0.4, A)        (8.0, 0.8, A)
```

3. Patients receiving medical attention for
any wound should receive Td injection under
either of the following conditions:

    a. For clean minor wounds, if the last Td
    booster was greater than 10 years

```
                3 6                  3 3 3
    1 2 3 4 5 6 7 8 9    1 2 3 4 5 6 7 8 9   ( 3-  4)
      (8.0, 0.3, A)        (8.0, 0.7, A)
```

    b. For other/dirty wounds, if the last Td
    booster was greater than 5 years

```
                2 7                  3 3 3
    1 2 3 4 5 6 7 8 9    1 2 3 4 5 6 7 8 9   ( 5-  6)
      (8.0, 0.2, A)        (8.0, 0.7, A)
```

4. All patients aged 65 and over should have
been offered influenza vaccine annually or
have documentation that they received it
elsewhere.

```
              3 4 2                2 2 3 2
    1 2 3 4 5 6 7 8 9    1 2 3 4 5 6 7 8 9   ( 7-  8)
      (8.0, 0.6, A)        (8.0, 0.9, A)
```

5. All patients under age 65 with any of the
following conditions should have been offered
influenza vaccination annually:

    a. Living in a nursing home

```
              2 3 4              1 2 2 4
    1 2 3 4 5 6 7 8 9    1 2 3 4 5 6 7 8 9   ( 9- 10)
      (8.0, 0.7, A)        (8.0, 0.9, A)
```

    b. Chronic obstructive pulmonary disease

```
              2 4 3                4 3 2
    1 2 3 4 5 6 7 8 9    1 2 3 4 5 6 7 8 9   ( 11- 12)
      (8.0, 0.6, A)        (8.0, 0.7, A)
```

    c. Asthma

```
              3 3 3              2 2 3 2
    1 2 3 4 5 6 7 8 9    1 2 3 4 5 6 7 8 9   ( 13- 14)
      (8.0, 0.7, A)        (8.0, 0.9, A)
```

    d. Chronic cardiovascular disorders

```
              3 3 3              3 1 3 2
    1 2 3 4 5 6 7 8 9    1 2 3 4 5 6 7 8 9   ( 15- 16)
      (8.0, 0.7, A)        (8.0, 1.0, I)
```

    e. Renal failure

```
              3 3 3              2 2 3 2
    1 2 3 4 5 6 7 8 9    1 2 3 4 5 6 7 8 9   ( 17- 18)
      (8.0, 0.7, A)        (8.0, 0.9, A)
```

    f. Immunosuppression

```
              2 4 3              2 1 4 2
    1 2 3 4 5 6 7 8 9    1 2 3 4 5 6 7 8 9   ( 19- 20)
      (8.0, 0.6, A)        (8.0, 0.8, A)
```

    g. Diabetes mellitus

```
              3 3 3              2 2 3 2
    1 2 3 4 5 6 7 8 9    1 2 3 4 5 6 7 8 9   ( 21- 22)
      (8.0, 0.7, A)        (8.0, 0.9, A)
```

    h. Hemoglobinopathies (e.g. sickle cell)

```
              3 3 3              2 2 3 2
    1 2 3 4 5 6 7 8 9    1 2 3 4 5 6 7 8 9   ( 23- 24)
      (8.0, 0.7, A)        (8.0, 0.9, A)
```

Scales: 1 = low validity or feasibility; 9 = high validity or feasibility

Validity   Feasibility

IMMUNIZATIONS, CONT.

6. There should be documentation that all patients in the following groups and otherwise presenting for care were offered pneumococcal vaccine at least once:

a. Patients aged 65 and older
```
                4 3 2                    2 2 3 2
    1 2 3 4 5 6 7 8 9   1 2 3 4 5 6 7 8 9    ( 25- 26)
       (8.0, 0.7, A)       (8.0, 0.9, A)
```

b. Chronic cardiac or pulmonary disease
```
                4 3 2                    2 2 3 2
    1 2 3 4 5 6 7 8 9   1 2 3 4 5 6 7 8 9    ( 27- 28)
       (8.0, 0.7, A)       (8.0, 0.9, A)
```

c. Diabetes mellitus
```
                4 3 2                    2 2 3 2
    1 2 3 4 5 6 7 8 9   1 2 3 4 5 6 7 8 9    ( 29- 30)
       (8.0, 0.7, A)       (8.0, 0.9, A)
```

d. Anatomic asplenia
```
                4 3 2                    2 2 3 2
    1 2 3 4 5 6 7 8 9   1 2 3 4 5 6 7 8 9    ( 31- 32)
       (8.0, 0.7, A)       (8.0, 0.9, A)
```

e. Persons over age 50 who are institutionalized
```
                4 3 2                    2 1 4 2
    1 2 3 4 5 6 7 8 9   1 2 3 4 5 6 7 8 9    ( 33- 34)
       (8.0, 0.7, A)       (8.0, 0.8, A)
```

f. Other immunocompromising conditions
```
    2   1   1   1 3 1   2         1 1 1 3 1
    1 2 3 4 5 6 7 8 9   1 2 3 4 5 6 7 8 9    ( 35- 36)
       (7.0, 2.6, D)       (7.0, 2.2, I)
```

7. There should be documentation that all patients identified as being in the following high risk groups were offered hepatitis B vaccination within one year after identification of the risk, unless the patient has serologic evidence of immunity:

a. Hemodialysis patients
```
                3 3 3                    3 3 3
    1 2 3 4 5 6 7 8 9   1 2 3 4 5 6 7 8 9    ( 37- 38)
       (8.0, 0.7, A)       (8.0, 0.7, A)
```

b. Sexually active homosexual men
```
              1 3 3 2                  2 1   4 2
    1 2 3 4 5 6 7 8 9   1 2 3 4 5 6 7 8 9    ( 39- 40)
       (8.0, 0.8, A)       (8.0, 1.1, I)
```

c. Household and sexual contacts of HBV carriers
```
                3 4 2              1   2 1 3 2
    1 2 3 4 5 6 7 8 9   1 2 3 4 5 6 7 8 9    ( 41- 42)
       (8.0, 0.6, A)       (8.0, 1.2, I)
```

d. Intravenous drug users
```
                4 3 2                1 1 1 1 3 2
    1 2 3 4 5 6 7 8 9   1 2 3 4 5 6 7 8 9    ( 43- 44)
       (8.0, 0.7, A)       (8.0, 1.3, I)
```

e. Persons with occupational risk
```
                4 3 2                    2 2 3 2
    1 2 3 4 5 6 7 8 9   1 2 3 4 5 6 7 8 9    ( 45- 46)
       (8.0, 0.7, A)       (8.0, 0.9, A)
```

f. Persons who have a history of sexual activity with multiple sexual partners in the past 6 months.
```
              1 3 4 1              1 2 2   3 1
    1 2 3 4 5 6 7 8 9   1 2 3 4 5 6 7 8 9    ( 47- 48)
       (8.0, 0.7, A)       (6.0, 1.4, I)
```

g. Persons who have recently acquired another sexually transmitted disease.
```
              1 3 4 1                    3 2 3 1
    1 2 3 4 5 6 7 8 9   1 2 3 4 5 6 7 8 9    ( 49- 50)
       (8.0, 0.7, A)       (7.0, 0.9, I)
```

8. All persons otherwise presenting for care in the following high risk groups should have documentation of measles immunization status:

a. College students
```
                2 6 1                1 2 1 4 1
    1 2 3 4 5 6 7 8 9   1 2 3 4 5 6 7 8 9    ( 51- 52)
       (8.0, 0.3, A)       (8.0, 1.0, I)
```

b. Health-care workers
```
                2 6 1                1 2 1 4 1
    1 2 3 4 5 6 7 8 9   1 2 3 4 5 6 7 8 9    ( 53- 54)
       (8.0, 0.3, A)       (8.0, 1.0, I)
```

Scales: 1 = low validity or feasibility; 9 = high validity or feasibility

SCREENING

9. There should be documentation of PPD reactivity status for all patients otherwise presenting for care who are identified as being in the following risk groups in the year following identification of the risk:

a. Foreign born persons from countries of high TB prevalence (Asia, Africa, Latin America) who have been in the US less than 5 years

```
            5 2 2               1   2   4 2
1 2 3 4 5 6 7 8 9   1 2 3 4 5 6 7 8 9   ( 55- 56)
  (7.0, 0.7, A)        (8.0, 1.1, I)
```

b. Injection drug users

```
            5 2 2               3 1   3 2
1 2 3 4 5 6 7 8 9   1 2 3 4 5 6 7 8 9   ( 57- 58)
  (7.0, 0.7, A)        (8.0, 1.4, I)
```

c. Persons with immunosuppression

```
            5 2 2                 2 3 3 1
1 2 3 4 5 6 7 8 9   1 2 3 4 5 6 7 8 9   ( 59- 60)
  (7.0, 0.7, A)        (7.0, 0.8, A)
```

d. Residents of long-term care facilities such as nursing homes

```
              3 4 2               1 2 3 3
1 2 3 4 5 6 7 8 9   1 2 3 4 5 6 7 8 9   ( 61- 62)
  (8.0, 0.6, A)        (8.0, 0.8, A)
```

e. Homeless persons

```
            5 2 2               3 2   3 1
1 2 3 4 5 6 7 8 9   1 2 3 4 5 6 7 8 9   ( 63- 64)
  (7.0, 0.7, A)        (5.0, 1.8, I)
```

f. Health care workers

```
              3 4 2                 2   5 2
1 2 3 4 5 6 7 8 9   1 2 3 4 5 6 7 8 9   ( 65- 66)
  (8.0, 0.6, A)        (8.0, 0.7, A)
```

12. Persons identified as having a newly positive or reactive PPD should have a chest radiograph performed within 1 month.

```
              1 5 3               1 4 4
1 2 3 4 5 6 7 8 9   1 2 3 4 5 6 7 8 9   ( 67- 68)
  (8.0, 0.4, A)        (8.0, 0.6, A)
```

13. Persons in the following risk groups who are identified as having TB infection (not disease) should be offered INH preventive therapy unless they have clear contraindications:

a. Patients with diabetes mellitus

```
            5 2 2                 4 3 2
1 2 3 4 5 6 7 8 9   1 2 3 4 5 6 7 8 9   ( 69- 70)
  (7.0, 0.7, A)        (8.0, 0.7, A)
```

b. Patients with chronic renal failure

```
            5 2 2                 4 3 2
1 2 3 4 5 6 7 8 9   1 2 3 4 5 6 7 8 9   ( 71- 72)
  (7.0, 0.7, A)        (8.0, 0.7, A)
```

c. Recent exposure to a case of active TB

```
          4 3 2             1     2 4 2
1 2 3 4 5 6 7 8 9   1 2 3 4 5 6 7 8 9   ( 73- 74)
  (8.0, 0.7, A)        (8.0, 0.9, A)
```

d. Recent conversion of PPD (documented negative test in the previous 2 years)

```
          4 3 2                 2 5 2
1 2 3 4 5 6 7 8 9   1 2 3 4 5 6 7 8 9   ( 75- 76)
  (8.0, 0.7, A)        (8.0, 0.4, A)
```

e. Immunocompromised or chronic high dose corticosteroids

```
            3 4 2                 3 4 2
1 2 3 4 5 6 7 8 9   1 2 3 4 5 6 7 8 9   ( 77- 78)
  (8.0, 0.6, A)        (8.0, 0.6, A)
```

f. Injection drug users

```
            5 2 2               3   2 2 2
1 2 3 4 5 6 7 8 9   1 2 3 4 5 6 7 8 9   ( 79- 80)
  (7.0, 0.7, A)        (7.0, 1.3, I)
```

g. Foreign born persons from high prevalence countries less than 35 years of age.

```
            5 2 2                 3 2 2 2
1 2 3 4 5 6 7 8 9   1 2 3 4 5 6 7 8 9   ( 81- 82)
  (7.0, 0.7, A)        (7.0, 1.0, I)
```

14. If the initial PPD test on nursing home patients is negative, retesting (two-step testing) should be performed within 2 weeks.

```
          2 2 3 2               2 5 2
1 2 3 4 5 6 7 8 9   1 2 3 4 5 6 7 8 9   ( 83- 84)
  (8.0, 0.9, A)        (8.0, 0.4, A)
```

Scales: 1 = low validity or feasibility; 9 = high validity or feasibility

SCREENING, CONT.

15. Patients age 65 and older noted to have
a hearing problem or complaint without
reversible cause or that persists despite
treatment for reversible cause should have
formal evaluation for amplification offered
or discussed.

```
                              2 4 2 1             1 1 3 4
                1 2 3 4 5 6 7 8 9   1 2 3 4 5 6 7 8 9   ( 85- 86)
                   (7.0, 0.7, A)       (7.0, 0.8, A)
```

COUNSELING

22. Patients with the following current HIV
risk factors should have HIV testing offered
or discussed at the visit in which the risk
factor is noted:

a. Having had sex with more that 2 male
partners in the past 6 months

```
                                  6 3               2 5 2
                1 2 3 4 5 6 7 8 9   1 2 3 4 5 6 7 8 9   ( 87- 88)
                   (7.0, 0.3, A)       (7.0, 0.4, A)
                                  6 3               2 5 2
```

b. Injection drug use

```
                1 2 3 4 5 6 7 8 9   1 2 3 4 5 6 7 8 9   ( 89- 90)
                   (7.0, 0.3, A)       (7.0, 0.4, A)
                                  6 3         1     2 4 2
```

c. Exchanging sex for money or drugs

```
                1 2 3 4 5 6 7 8 9   1 2 3 4 5 6 7 8 9   ( 91- 92)
                   (7.0, 0.3, A)       (7.0, 0.9, I)
```

d. Present sex partners are HIV-infected
or injection drug users

```
                                  6 3         1     2 4 2
                1 2 3 4 5 6 7 8 9   1 2 3 4 5 6 7 8 9   ( 93- 94)
                   (7.0, 0.3, A)       (7.0, 0.9, I)
```

23. There should be documentation that
patients' level of physical activity was
assessed on at least one occasion.

```
                2     3 2   1 1       1 2 1 3     2
                1 2 3 4 5 6 7 8 9   1 2 3 4 5 6 7 8 9   ( 95- 96)
                   (5.0, 1.4, I)       (6.0, 1.3, I)
```

24. Patients with the following past HIV risk
factors should have HIV testing offered or
discussed at the visit in which the
past risk factor is noted (unless HIV status
has been documented since the termination of
the risk factor).

a. Past injection drug use

```
                               5 4                6 3
                1 2 3 4 5 6 7 8 9   1 2 3 4 5 6 7 8 9   ( 97- 98)
                   (7.0, 0.4, A)       (7.0, 0.3, A)
```

b. Having had sex with more than two
male partners in a six month period

```
                               5 4                6 3
                1 2 3 4 5 6 7 8 9   1 2 3 4 5 6 7 8 9   ( 99-100)
                   (7.0, 0.4, A)       (7.0, 0.3, A)
```

c. Exchanged sex for money or drugs in
the past

```
                               5 4         1      5 3
                1 2 3 4 5 6 7 8 9   1 2 3 4 5 6 7 8 9   (101-102)
                   (7.0, 0.4, A)       (7.0, 0.8, A)
```

d. Past sex partners were HIV-infected
or injection drug users

```
                               5 4         1      5 3
                1 2 3 4 5 6 7 8 9   1 2 3 4 5 6 7 8 9   (103-104)
                   (7.0, 0.4, A)       (7.0, 0.8, A)
```

e. History of transfusion between 1978
and 1985

```
                               5 4                6 3
                1 2 3 4 5 6 7 8 9   1 2 3 4 5 6 7 8 9   (105-106)
                   (7.0, 0.4, A)       (7.0, 0.3, A)
```

25. Patients over age 65 should be asked
about hearing difficulties at least every 2
years.

```
                    1 2   2 4         1 1      4 3
                1 2 3 4 5 6 7 8 9   1 2 3 4 5 6 7 8 9   (107-108)
                   (7.0, 1.2, I)       (7.0, 1.1, A)
```

Scales: 1 = low validity or feasibility; 9 = high validity or feasibility

NOTE: This chapter was revised from Q1.
Only new or revised indicators were rated.

URETHRITIS - DIAGNOSIS

9. If a sexually active male patient
presents with penile discharge he should be
tested for both chlamydia and gonorrhea at
the time of presentation.

                                        1 1 6 1   1 1 6 1
                           1 2 3 4 5 6 7 8 9 1 2 3 4 5 6 7 8 9 (1- 2)
                             (8.0, 0.4, A)   (8.0, 0.4, A)

GENITAL ULCERS - DIAGNOSIS

16. If a patient presents with the new onset
of genital ulcers then all of the following
should be offered at the time of
presentation:

    a. Cultures or DFA for HSV

                                        3 5 1   1 7 1
                           1 2 3 4 5 6 7 8 9 1 2 3 4 5 6 7 8 9 (3- 4)
                             (8.0, 0.4, A)   (8.0, 0.2, A)

    c. Blood test for syphilis

                                        2 6 1   1 7 1
                           1 2 3 4 5 6 7 8 9 1 2 3 4 5 6 7 8 9 (5- 6)
                             (8.0, 0.3, A)   (8.0, 0.2, A)

Scales: 1 = low validity or feasibility; 9 = high validity or feasibility

Note: This chapter was revised from Q1.
Only new or revised indicators were rated.

DIAGNOSIS

3. Patients who present with dysuria and are
started on antimicrobial treatment for
urinary tract infection should have had a
urinalysis or dipstick evaluation on the day
of presentation.

```
 1 1 1   3 1 1 1                    1   2 6
 1 2 3 4 5 6 7 8 9   1 2 3 4 5 6 7 8 9  ( 1- 2)
   (5.0,  1.7,  I)       (8.0,  0.6,  A)
```

Scales: 1 = low validity or feasibility; 9 = high validity or feasibility

DIAGNOSIS

1. Patients who present with vertigo should have all of the following documented at the time of initial presentation with symptoms:

a. the duration of episodes

```
              1           6 2                    2    4 2 1
              1 2 3 4 5 6 7 8 9   1 2 3 4 5 6 7 8 9   ( 1- 2)
                (7.0, 0.9, A)        (7.0, 0.9, A)
```

b. presence or absence of precipitation by head movements

```
              1           6 2                 1 1    4 2 1
              1 2 3 4 5 6 7 8 9   1 2 3 4 5 6 7 8 9   ( 3- 4)
                (7.0, 0.9, A)        (7.0, 1.0, A)
```

c. presence or absence of any association with hearing loss or tinnitus

```
              1      2 1 4 1                    2    5 2
              1 2 3 4 5 6 7 8 9   1 2 3 4 5 6 7 8 9   ( 5- 6)
                (7.0, 1.3, I)        (7.0, 0.7, A)
```

2. Patients who present with prolonged spontaneous vertigo should have documentation of risk factors for cerebrovascular disease at the time of presentation.

```
              3   1 3 2                  2   1 1 4    1
              1 2 3 4 5 6 7 8 9   1 2 3 4 5 6 7 8 9   ( 7- 8)
                (4.0, 1.3, I)        (5.0, 1.4, I)
```

3. Patients who present with disequilibrium should have all of the following documented at the time of initial presentation:

a. presence or absence of diabetes

```
              3      3 2 1                 2      3 2 2
              1 2 3 4 5 6 7 8 9   1 2 3 4 5 6 7 8 9   ( 9- 10)
                (4.0, 1.4, I)        (4.0, 1.3, A)
```

b. presence or absence of alcohol consumption

```
              3      3 2 1                 2      3 2 2
              1 2 3 4 5 6 7 8 9   1 2 3 4 5 6 7 8 9   ( 11- 12)
                (4.0, 1.4, I)        (4.0, 1.3, A)
```

c. use of ototoxic medications

```
              3      1 3 2                 2      2 3 1 1
              1 2 3 4 5 6 7 8 9   1 2 3 4 5 6 7 8 9   ( 13- 14)
                (5.0, 1.7, I)        (5.0, 1.4, I)
```

d. recent poor oral intake

```
              3   1 3 1 1                2   1 3 2 1
              1 2 3 4 5 6 7 8 9   1 2 3 4 5 6 7 8 9   ( 15- 16)
                (4.0, 1.4, I)        (4.0, 1.2, I)
```

4. Patients who present with presyncope should be asked about all of the following possible precipitants at the time of initial presentation:

a. standing up

```
              2 1   3 2 1                 2      1 4 1 1
              1 2 3 4 5 6 7 8 9   1 2 3 4 5 6 7 8 9   ( 17- 18)
                (5.0, 1.6, I)        (5.0, 1.3, I)
```

b. urination

```
              2   1 1 4 1                 2   1 1 2 3
              1 2 3 4 5 6 7 8 9   1 2 3 4 5 6 7 8 9   ( 19- 20)
                (5.0, 1.3, I)        (5.0, 1.6, I)
```

c. exertion

```
              2   1 1 4 1                 2   1 1 2 2 1
              1 2 3 4 5 6 7 8 9   1 2 3 4 5 6 7 8 9   ( 21- 22)
                (5.0, 1.3, I)        (5.0, 1.7, I)
```

d. emotional stress

```
              2 1 1 1 3 1               2 1   1 3 2
              1 2 3 4 5 6 7 8 9   1 2 3 4 5 6 7 8 9   ( 23- 24)
                (4.0, 1.6, I)        (5.0, 1.6, I)
```

5. Patients who present with vertigo should have documented an examination of tympanic membranes at the time of presentation.

```
              2 1 1 2 2 1               2      1 2 2 1 1
              1 2 3 4 5 6 7 8 9   1 2 3 4 5 6 7 8 9   ( 25- 26)
                (4.0, 1.4, I)        (5.0, 1.8, I)
```

6. Patients who present with recurrent positional vertigo should have documented the results of a Hallpike maneuver at the time of presentation.

```
              2   1 1 2 2 1             2   1   4   2
              1 2 3 4 5 6 7 8 9   1 2 3 4 5 6 7 8 9   ( 27- 28)
                (5.0, 1.7, I)        (5.0, 1.6, I)
```

Scales: 1 = low validity or feasibility; 9 = high validity or feasibility

Validity   Feasibility

DIAGNOSIS, CONT.

7. Patients who present with presyncope
should have all of the following documented
at the time of presentation:

```
                              6 2 1                 5 3 1
  a. orthostatic vital signs
                    1 2 3 4 5 6 7 8 9   1 2 3 4 5 6 7 8 9   ( 29- 30)
                      (7.0, 0.4, A)       (7.0, 0.6, A)
                                7 2                   6 3
  b. heart examination
                    1 2 3 4 5 6 7 8 9   1 2 3 4 5 6 7 8 9   ( 31- 32)
                      (7.0, 0.2, A)       (7.0, 0.3, A)
```

8. Patients who present with disequilibrium
should have documentation of visual acuity
testing at the time of presentation.

```
                    2   3 2 2           2     1 4   1 1
                    1 2 3 4 5 6 7 8 9   1 2 3 4 5 6 7 8 9   ( 33- 34)
                      (3.0, 1.1, I)       (5.0, 1.6, I)
```

9. Patients who present with disequilibrium
should have documentation of the following
components of a neurological examination at
the time of presentation:

```
                    1   1 1 3 2 1       1     1 5   2
  a. cerebellar exam
                    1 2 3 4 5 6 7 8 9   1 2 3 4 5 6 7 8 9   ( 35- 36)
                      (5.0, 1.2, I)       (5.0, 1.0, I)
                    1   1 1 3 2 1       1     1 5 1 1
  b. gait observation
                    1 2 3 4 5 6 7 8 9   1 2 3 4 5 6 7 8 9   ( 37- 38)
                      (5.0, 1.2, I)       (5.0, 0.9, A)
                    1   1 2 3 1 1       1     1 5 1 1
  c. Romberg testing
                    1 2 3 4 5 6 7 8 9   1 2 3 4 5 6 7 8 9   ( 39- 40)
                      (5.0, 1.2, I)       (5.0, 0.9, A)
```

10. Patients who present with vertigo and
new neurological deficits should have MRI
within 2 weeks of presentation.

```
                    4     2 1   1 1     3     1 1 1 1 2
                    1 2 3 4 5 6 7 8 9   1 2 3 4 5 6 7 8 9   ( 41- 42)
                      (4.0, 2.2, I)       (5.0, 2.4, D)
```

11. Patients who present with disequilibrium
and unilateral hearing loss should have
audiometry within 3 weeks of presentation.

```
                    2 1     2 2 2       2 1   1 1 2 2
                    1 2 3 4 5 6 7 8 9   1 2 3 4 5 6 7 8 9   ( 43- 44)
                      (5.0, 1.9, I)       (5.0, 2.0, I)
```

12. Patients who present with sudden
presyncope and HR < 55 on exam should have an
ECG at the time of presentation.

```
                    2 1     2 3   1     2 1     2 3 1
                    1 2 3 4 5 6 7 8 9   1 2 3 4 5 6 7 8 9   ( 45- 46)
                      (5.0, 1.9, I)       (5.0, 1.8, I)
```

TREATMENT

13. Patients who present with
torsional-vertical nystagmus on Hallpike
testing should have the canalith
repositioning procedure within 1 week of
presentation.

```
                    2   4 1 2           2   3 1 1 2
                    1 2 3 4 5 6 7 8 9   1 2 3 4 5 6 7 8 9   ( 47- 48)
                      (3.0, 1.0, I)       (3.0, 1.4, I)
```

14. Patients who present with a diagnosis of
Meniere's syndrome and have bothersome
symptoms should be advised to follow a
1-2 gram sodium/day diet or be given a
diuretic or both within one month of
presentation.

```
                    2   1 2 2 2         2     2 2 2 1
                    1 2 3 4 5 6 7 8 9   1 2 3 4 5 6 7 8 9   ( 49- 50)
                      (4.0, 1.4, I)       (5.0, 1.6, I)
```

15. Patients who present with recurrent
spontaneous vertigo and any risk factor for
cerebrovascular disease should start aspirin
or ticlopidine at the time of presentation or
be referred to a neurologist within 2 weeks
of presentation.

```
                    2 1 1 2 1 1 1       2 1 1 2 1 2
                    1 2 3 4 5 6 7 8 9   1 2 3 4 5 6 7 8 9   ( 51- 52)
                      (4.0, 1.7, I)       (4.0, 1.6, I)
```

Scales: 1 = low validity or feasibility; 9 = high validity or feasibility

TREATMENT, CONT.

16. Patients who present with disequilibrium
and decreased visual acuity should be
referred to an opthalmologist or optometrist   2   2 1 2   2   2   1   4   2
within one month of presentation.   1 2 3 4 5 6 7 8 9 1 2 3 4 5 6 7 8 9 (53- 54)
                                                   (4.0, 1.8, I)   (5.0, 1.6, I)

APPENDIX B: CROSSWALK TABLE OF ORIGINAL AND FINAL INDICATORS

Chapter 1 - Acne

	Indicator Proposed by Staff		Indicator Voted on by Panel	Comments/Disposition
	Diagnosis			
1.	For patients presenting with a chief complaint of acne, the following history should be documented in their chart: a. location of lesions (back, face, neck, chest), b. previous treatments, and c. medications and drug use.	1. a. b. c.	For patients presenting with a chief complaint of acne, the following history should be documented in their chart: a. location of lesions (back, face, neck, chest), b. previous treatments, and c. medications and drug use.	INCLUDED BASED ON Q1 PANEL RATING
	Treatment			
2.	If oral antibiotics are prescribed, papules and/or pustules must be present.	2.	If oral antibiotics are prescribed, papules and/or pustules must be present.	INCLUDED BASED ON Q1 PANEL RATING
3.	If isotretinoin is prescribed, there must be documentation of cysts and/or nodules.	3.	If isotretinoin is prescribed, there must be documentation of cysts and/or nodules.	INCLUDED BASED ON Q1 PANEL RATING
	Follow-up			
4.	If isotretinoin is prescribed, monthly liver function tests should be performed, for three months.	4.	If isotretinoin is prescribed, monthly liver function tests should be performed, for three months.	INCLUDED BASED ON Q1 PANEL RATING

430

Chapter 2- Alcohol Dependence

	Indicator Proposed by Staff		Indicator Voted on by Panel	Comments/Disposition
	Screening			
1.	All new patients or those receiving a routine history and physical should be screened for problem drinking. This assessment of pattern of alcohol use should include at least one of the following: • Quantity (e.g., drinks per day); • Binge drinking (e.g., more than 5 drinks in a day in the last month).	1.	All new patients or those receiving a routine history and physical should be screened for problem drinking. This assessment of pattern of alcohol use should include at least one of the following: • Use of a validated screening questionnaire (such as AUDIT, MAST or CAGE) • Quantity (e.g., drinks per day); • Binge drinking (e.g., more than 5 drinks in a day in the last month).	MODIFIED: Panelists felt that screening once is sufficient and that use of a validated screening tool would be sufficient even in the absence of other documentation. ACCEPTED AS MODIFIED
2.	All patients hospitalized with the following conditions should be screened for problem drinking at least once during their hospital stay. a. trauma; b. hepatitis; c. pancreatitis; d. gastrointestinal bleeding.	2.	All patients hospitalized with the following conditions should be screened for problem drinking at least once during their hospital stay. a. trauma; b. hepatitis; c. pancreatitis. d. gastrointestinal bleeding	"a-c" ACCEPTED "d" DROPPED PRIOR TO PANEL. Overlaps with discussion of gastrointestinal bleeding in Chapter 18.
	Diagnosis			
3.	The record should indicate more detailed screening for dependence, tolerance of psychoactive effects, loss of control, and consequences of use with a validated screening questionnaire (examples include but are not confined to the CAGE, MAST, HSS, AUDIT, SAAST, and SMAST), if the medical record indicates the patient is a regular or binge drinker.	3.	The record should indicate more detailed screening assessment for dependence, tolerance of psychoactive effects, loss of control, and consequences of use with a validated screening questionnaire (examples include but are not confined to the CAGE, MAST, HSS, AUDIT, SAAST, and SMAST), if the medical record indicates the patient is a regular daily or binge drinker.	MODIFIED: Panelists clarified indicator language. Pre-panel comments indicated that the use of validated screening questionnaires should be sufficient to pass the indicator, but should not be required. ACCEPTED AS MODIFIED
	Treatment			
4.	Regular or binge drinkers should be advised to decrease their drinking.	4.	Regular or binge drinkers should be advised to decrease their drinking.	INCLUDED BASED ON Q1 PANEL RATING

	Indicator Proposed by Staff		Indicator Voted on by Panel	Comments/Disposition
5.	Patients diagnosed with alcohol dependence should be referred for further treatment to at least one of the following: • inpatient rehabilitation program; • outpatient rehabilitation program; • mutual help group (e.g., AA); • substance abuse counseling; • aversion therapy.	5.	Patients diagnosed with alcohol dependence should be referred for further treatment to at least one of the following: • inpatient rehabilitation program; • outpatient rehabilitation program; • mutual help group (e.g., AA); • substance abuse counseling; • aversion therapy.	INCLUDED BASED ON Q1 PANEL RATING
Follow-up				
6.	Providers should reassess the alcohol intake of patients who report regular or binge drinking at the next routine health visit.	6.	Providers should reassess the alcohol intake of patients who report regular or binge drinking at the next routine health visit.	INCLUDED BASED ON Q1 PANEL RATING

432

Chapter 3 - Allergic Rhinitis

	Indicator Proposed by Staff		Indicator Voted on by Panel	Comments/Disposition
	Diagnosis			
1.	If a diagnosis of allergic rhinitis is made, the search for a specific allergen by history should be documented in the chart (for initial history).	1.	If a diagnosis of allergic rhinitis is made, the search for a specific allergen by history should be documented in the chart (for initial history).	INCLUDED BASED ON Q1 PANEL RATING
2.	If a diagnosis of allergic rhinitis is made, history should include whether the patient uses any topical nasal decongestants.	2.	If a diagnosis of allergic rhinitis is made, history should include whether the patient uses any topical nasal decongestants.	INCLUDED BASED ON Q1 PANEL RATING
	Treatment			
3.	Treatment for allergic rhinitis should include at least one of the following: • allergen avoidance counseling; • antihistamines; • nasal steroids; • nasal cromolyn.	3.	Treatment for allergic rhinitis should include at least one of the following: • allergen avoidance counseling; • antihistamines; • nasal steroids; • nasal cromolyn.	INCLUDED BASED ON Q1 PANEL RATING
4.	If topical nasal decongestants are prescribed for patients with allergic rhinitis, duration of treatment should be for no longer than 4 days.	4.	If topical nasal decongestants are prescribed for patients with allergic rhinitis, duration of treatment should be for no longer than 4 days.	INCLUDED BASED ON Q1 PANEL RATING

Chapter 4 - Benign Prostatic Hyperplasia (BPH)

	Indicator Proposed by Staff		Indicator Voted on by Panel	Comments/Disposition
	Diagnosis			
1.	Men age 50 and older who present for routine care should be asked at least once a year about recent symptoms of prostatism.	--	Men age 50 and older who present for routine care should be asked at least once a year about recent symptoms of prostatism.	**DROPPED due to low validity score.** Panelists felt that the evidence of benefit is lacking.
2.	If the patient has recent symptoms of prostatism, the provider should document one of the following on the same visit: • AUA symptom score; • How bothersome the patient considers the symptoms.	1.	If the patient has recent symptoms of prostatism, the provider should document one of the following on the same visit: • AUA symptom score; • How bothersome the patient considers the symptoms.	**ACCEPTED**
3.	Patients with new recent symptoms of prostatism[1] should have the presence or absence of at least one of the following conditions documented: • Parkinson's disease; • Diabetes mellitus; • Stroke; • History of urethral instrumentation.	--	Patients with new recent symptoms of prostatism should have the presence or absence of at least one of the following conditions documented: • Parkinson's disease; • Diabetes mellitus; • Stroke; • History of urethral instrumentation.	**DROPPED due to low validity score.** Documentation could legitimately vary depending on the severity of symptoms and the nature of the patient-physician relationship.
4.	Patients with new recent symptoms of prostatism should be offered a digital rectal examination (DRE) on the same visit that the symptoms are noted, if they have not had a DRE in the past year.	--	Patients with new recent symptoms of prostatism should be offered a digital rectal examination (DRE) ~~on the same visit that~~ **within one month after the visit in which** the symptoms are noted, if they have not had a DRE in the past year.	**DROPPED due to disagreement on validity.** A DRE may not be warranted in all cases due to its questionable sensitivity.
5.	If a patient has new recent symptoms of moderate prostatism the health care provider should offer at least one of the following within one month of the note of symptoms: • Uroflowometry; • Post void residual; • Pressure flow study.	--	If a patient has new recent symptoms of moderate prostatism the health care provider should offer at least one of the following within one month of the note of symptoms: • Uroflowometry; • Post void residual; • Pressure flow study.	**DROPPED due to low validity score.** Panelists felt these tests were linked to improved outcomes only in a subset of cases.

434

#	Indicator Proposed by Staff	#	Indicator Voted on by Panel	Comments/Disposition
6.	If a patient has new recent symptoms of prostatism, the provider should order the following tests within one month of the note of symptoms, unless done in the past year: a. Urine analysis; b. Serum creatinine.	2. a. b.	If a patient has new recent symptoms of prostatism, the provider should order the following tests within one month of the note of symptoms, unless done in the past year: a. Urine analysis; b. Serum creatinine.	ACCEPTED
	Treatment			
7.	Patients diagnosed with BPH who report recent symptoms of prostatism, and who are on anticholinergic or sympathomimetic medications, should be offered discontinuation of these medications within one month of the note of symptoms.	3.	Patients diagnosed with BPH who report recent symptoms of prostatism, and who are on anticholinergic or sympathomimetic medications, should be offered ~~have~~ discontinuation **or dose reduction** of these medications **offered or discussed** within one month of the note of symptoms.	MODIFIED: Panelists wanted to broaden the indicator to encompass standard of care. ACCEPTED AS MODIFIED
8.	Patients diagnosed with BPH who report symptoms of moderate prostatism should be offered alpha 1 adrenergic therapy within one month of the note of symptoms.	4.	Patients diagnosed with BPH who report symptoms of moderate prostatism should be offered ~~alpha 1 adrenergic therapy~~ **have treatment options discussed or offered** within one month of the note of symptoms.	MODIFIED: Panelists wanted to broaden the indicator to encompass standard of care. ACCEPTED AS MODIFIED
9.	Patients diagnosed with BPH should be offered surgical therapy within one month of either of the following conditions being noted: a. Acute renal insufficiency with dilated upper tracts; b. Persistent renal insufficiency after catheterization trial.	5. a. b.	Patients diagnosed with BPH should be offered surgical therapy within one month of either of the following conditions being noted: a. Acute renal insufficiency with dilated upper tracts; b. Persistent renal insufficiency after catheterization trial.	ACCEPTED
10.	Patients diagnosed with BPH should be offered surgical therapy within two months of any of the following conditions being noted: a. Continued complaints of moderate symptoms of prostatism after 6 months of alpha 1 adrenergic therapy, b. More than one urinary tract infection in the past year, c. Bladder stones.	6. a. -- b.	Patients diagnosed with BPH should be offered surgical therapy within two months of any of the following conditions being noted **unless the patient is not a surgical candidate:** a. Continued complaints of moderate symptoms of prostatism after ~~6 months~~ **at least 2 months** of alpha 1 adrenergic therapy, b. More than one urinary tract infection in the past year, c. Bladder stones.	MODIFIED **"a" ACCEPTED AS MODIFIED.** Panelists felt that a 2 month trial is adequate. **"b" DROPPED due to low validity score.** There is no clear medical evidence to support surgery. **"c" ACCEPTED**

		Indicator Proposed by Staff			Indicator Voted on by Panel	Comments/Disposition
		Follow-up				
11.		Patients diagnosed with BPH who have received alpha 1 adrenergic or surgical therapy should have their symptoms reassessed 6 months after initiation of therapy.	7.		Patients diagnosed with BPH who have received alpha 1 adrenergic or surgical therapy should have their symptoms reassessed 6 months after initiation of therapy.	**ACCEPTED**
12.		Patients with persistent recent symptoms of prostatism[1] 6 months after appropriate surgical therapy should be offered urodynamic evaluation.	8.		Patients with persistent ~~recent~~ **moderate** symptoms of prostatism 6 months after ~~appropriate~~ surgical therapy should be offered urodynamic evaluation.	MODIFIED: "Recent" conflicts with "persistent", the term "moderate" is more accurate. It is difficult to identify "appropriate" surgical therapy. **ACCEPTED AS MODIFIED**

Chapter 5 - Cataracts

		Indicator Voted on by Panel	Comments/Disposition
Screening			
1. Patients aged 55 and older presenting for non-urgent care should be offered a complete eye exam by an annually if they are having difficulty with visual function.	--	All patients aged 55 and older presenting for non-urgent care should be asked annually if they are having difficulty with visual function should have documentation of their visual function every 3 years.	**DROPPED due to low validity score.** Evidence of benefit is lacking. Also, patients will present for care if they experience visual difficulties.
Diagnosis			
2. Patients who report difficulty with visual function should be offered a complete eye exam by an optometrist or ophthalmologist. This examination should be performed at least annually and should include all of the following: a. visual acuity measurement; b. intraocular pressure measurement; c. pupil exam; d. motility exam; e. slit lamp exam; f. dilated fundus exam.	1. a. b. c. d. e. f.	Patients who report difficulty with **corrected** visual function should be offered receive a complete eye exam by an optometrist or ophthalmologist. This examination should be performed at least annually and should that includes all of the following **within 3 months of the report:** a. visual acuity measurement; b. intraocular pressure measurement; c. pupil exam; d. motility exam; e. slit lamp exam; f. dilated fundus exam.	MODIFIED: Panelists felt that specific actions were more important than specialist referrals. A time frame was specified. **ACCEPTED AS MODIFIED**
3. Patients should be offered refraction in the operative eye within 4 months before surgery unless a prior refraction made no improvement in otherwise stable vision in the past two years.	2.	Patients should be offered refraction in the operative **affected** eye within 4 months before surgery unless a prior refraction made no improvement in otherwise stable vision in the past two years.	MODIFIED: Terminology was clarified. **ACCEPTED AS MODIFIED**

437

Indicator Proposed by Staff		Indicator Voted on by Panel		Comments/Disposition
Treatment				
4. Patients with cataracts should be offered surgery if any of the following situations are present: a. phacomorphic glaucoma; b. phacolytic glaucoma; c. lens-related uveitis; d. disrupted anterior lens capsule in otherwise phakic eye; e. cataract prevents adequate monitoring or treatment of glaucoma or diabetes.	3.	Patients with cataracts should be offered surgery if any of the following situations are present: a. phacomorphic glaucoma; b. phacolytic glaucoma; c. lens-related uveitis; d. disrupted anterior lens capsule in otherwise phakic eye; e. cataract prevents adequate monitoring or treatment of glaucoma or diabetes.		ACCEPTED
5. In the absence of a medical indication for cataract surgery the ophthalmologist should offer cataract surgery only when both of the following conditions are met: • the patient's visual functioning is impaired; • there is either a normal fundus exam or a statement that the surgeon believes the patient's visual function would improve after the surgery.	4.	In the absence of a medical indication for cataract surgery the ophthalmologist should offer cataract surgery only when both of the following conditions are met: • the patient's visual functioning is impaired; • there is either a normal fundus exam or a statement that the surgeon believes the patient's visual function would improve after the surgery; • a lens opacity exists.		MODIFIED: A lens opacity is also a requirement for the diagnosis and surgical correction of cataracts. ACCEPTED AS MODIFIED
6. YAG capsulotomy should not be offered unless one condition from each of the following categories is met: • presence of opacity or impairment of the patient's visual function; • there is either a normal fundus exam or a statement that the surgeon believes the patient's visual function would improve after the surgery.	--	YAG capsulotomy should not be offered unless one condition from each of the following categories is met: • presence of opacity or impairment of the patient's visual function; • there is either a normal fundus exam or a statement that the surgeon believes the patient's visual function would improve after the surgery.		DROPPED PRIOR TO PANEL. Panelists had multiple criticisms, including awkward wording, ambiguous eligibility, and unclear benefit.

		Indicator Proposed by Staff		Indicator Voted on by Panel	Comments/Disposition
		Follow-up			
7.		Within 90 days of surgery, the surgeon should do at least one of the following: • examine the patient; • refer the patient for further care; • document inability to contact patient.	--	Within 90 days of surgery, the surgeon should do at least one of the following: • examine the patient; • refer the patient for further care; • document inability to contact patient.	**DROPPED due to low validity score.** This indicator overlaps with #8 and #9. There is no evidence of benefit.
8.		Within 48 hours of surgery, an optometrist or ophthalmologist should offer patients who have undergone cataract extraction a complete anterior segment eye examination, including all cf the following: a. visual acuity measurement; b. intraocular pressure measurement; c. slit lamp exam.	5. a. b. c.	Within 48 hours of surgery, an optometrist or ophthalmologist should offer patients who have undergone cataract extraction a complete anterior segment eye examination, including all of the following: a. visual acuity measurement; b. intraocular pressure measurement; c. slit lamp exam.	ACCEPTED
9.		Patients who have undergone cataract extraction should have their visual functioning assessed within 90 days of surgery.	6.	Patients who have undergone cataract extraction should have their visual functioning assessed within 90 days of surgery.	ACCEPTED

Chapter 6 - Cholelithiasis

	Indicator Proposed by Staff		Indicator Voted on by Panel	Comments/Disposition
	Treatment			
1.	Patients who are diagnosed with a complication of gallstones should receive a cholecystectomy within one month of the complication, unless the medical record states that they are not a surgical candidate.	1.	Patients who are diagnosed with a complication of gallstones should receive a cholecystectomy within one month of the complication, unless the medical record states that they are not a surgical candidate.	ACCEPTED
2.	If a patient undergoes cholecystectomy for gallstones, one of the following should be documented within the 6 months prior to surgery: • biliary pain; • complications from gallstone.	2.	If a patient undergoes cholecystectomy for gallstones, one of the following should be documented within the 6 months prior to surgery: • biliary pain; • complications from gallstone.	ACCEPTED
3.	Patients who are diagnosed with biliary pain should be offered cholecystectomy within 6 months of the symptoms, unless the medical record states that they are not a surgical candidate.	3.	Patients who are diagnosed with biliary pain should be offered cholecystectomy within 6 months of the symptoms, unless the medical record states that they are not a surgical candidate.	ACCEPTED

Chapter 7 - Dementia

		Indicator Proposed by Staff		Indicator Voted on by Panel	Comments/Disposition
		Treatment			
1.		If a patient has any symptoms of cognitive impairment, all of the following information should be documented:	1.	If a patient has ~~any~~ **new** symptoms of cognitive impairment, all of the following information should be documented **within 3 months:**	MODIFIED: Panelists wanted to clarify the intent and provide a time frame for action. Incident cases easier to operationalize.
	a.	Have the patient's cognitive abilities declined from a previous level?	a.	Have the patient's cognitive abilities declined from a previous level?	ACCEPTED AS MODIFIED
	b.	Do the patient's symptoms of cognitive impairment interfere with daily functioning?	b.	Do the patient's symptoms of cognitive impairment interfere with daily functioning?	
	c.	Medications being taken (both prescription and non-prescription);	c.	Medications being taken (both prescription and non-prescription);	
	d.	The use of alcohol or other substances that may affect cognition;	d.	The use of alcohol or other substances that may affect cognition;	
	e.	The presence or absence of delirium;	e.	The presence or absence of delirium;	
	f.	The presence or absence of depression.	f.	The presence or absence of depression.	
2.		All of the following information should be documented for patients with a diagnosis of dementia:	2.	All of the following information should be documented **within 3 months of onset** for patients with a **new** diagnosis of dementia:	MODIFIED: Panelists simplified and clarified the intent of the indicator.
	a.	The chronicity of symptoms (e.g. noted one week ago vs. 2 years ago, abrupt vs gradual);	a.	The ~~chronicity~~ **onset** of symptoms (~~e.g. noted one week ago vs. 2 years ago, abrupt vs. gradual~~);	ACCEPTED AS MODIFIED
	b.	The nature of progression (e.g., worsening, fluctuating, stable).	b.	The nature of progression (~~e.g., worsening, fluctuating, stable~~).	
3.		If a patient has any new symptoms of cognitive impairment, the health care provider should offer a neurological examination (including a mental status examination).	--	If a patient has any new symptoms of cognitive impairment, the health care provider should offer **perform** a ~~neurological examination (including a mental status examination)~~ **within 3 months.**	DROPPED due to low validity score. Panelists did not feel that a mental status examination should be specifically required.

441

	Indicator Proposed by Staff		Indicator Voted on by Panel	Comments/Disposition
		3. (3)	If a patient has any new symptoms of cognitive impairment, the health care provider should ~~offer~~ **perform** a neurological examination **within 3 months**. ~~(including a mental status examination)~~.	MODIFIED: Panelists wanted to consider the indicator without the mental status exam requirement. They also specified the time frame. Panelists felt that the term "offer" is not really appropriate for a demented person. **PANEL ACCEPTED INDICATOR AS MODIFIED TO NOT REQUIRE THE METAL STATUS EXAM**
4.	If patient has any new symptoms of cognitive impairment, the following blood tests should be offered within 30 days: a. CBC (if not ordered in last month), b. Chemistry panel (electrolytes, BUN, creatinine, bicarbonate, chloride, glucose, calcium) if not ordered in last 2 weeks; c. TSH if not ordered in last 6 months.	4. a. b. c.	If a patient has ~~any~~ **a new symptoms diagnosis** of ~~cognitive impairment~~ **dementia**, the following blood tests should be offered within ~~30 days~~ **3 months:** a. CBC ~~(if not ordered in last month)~~; b. Chemistry panel (electrolytes, BUN, creatinine, bicarbonate, chloride, glucose, calcium) ~~if not ordered in last 2 weeks~~; c. TSH ~~if not ordered in last 6 months~~.	MODIFIED: Panelists felt that there was no consensus on requiring these tests for patients without a known cause of the dementia. **ACCEPTED AS MODIFIED**
5.	If a patient has any new symptoms of cognitive impairment, a head CT or MRI should be offered within 30 days if one or more of the following criteria is met: a. onset of dementia in the past 2 years; b. head trauma in the past 2 years; c. onset of seizures in the past 2 years; d. gait disorder in the past 2 years; e. dementia with focal neurologic findings; f. dementia and headache.	5. -- a. -- -- b. c.	If a patient has ~~any~~ **a new symptoms diagnosis** of ~~cognitive impairment~~ **dementia**, a head CT or MRI should be offered within 30 days if one or more of the following criteria is met: ~~a. onset of dementia in the past 2 years~~; ~~b. head trauma in the past 2 years~~ **within 2 weeks preceding the onset of symptoms of cognitive impairment;** ~~c. onset of seizures in the past 2 years~~; ~~d. gait disorder in the past 2 years~~; e. dementia with focal neurologic findings; f. ~~dementia and~~ **new headache that persists despite at least 4 weeks of medical treatment.**	MODIFIED: Panelists felt that symptoms may not always warrant a CT or MRI. **"a" DROPPED PRIOR TO PANEL.** Panelists felt that reparable etiologies were unlikely to be revealed with a two year delay. **"b" ACCEPTED AS MODIFIED.** Two years is too long to get a reliable patient self-report. **"c" DROPPED due to low validity score.** CT/MRI is not likely to reveal anything treatable. **"d" DROPPED due to low validity score** **"e" ACCEPTED AS MODIFIED** **"f" ACCEPTED AS MODIFIED.** Panelists wanted to exclude patients with easily treated headaches.

442

	Indicator Proposed by Staff		Indicator Voted on by Panel	Comments/Disposition
	Treatment			
6.	Patients with a diagnosis of dementia and who are having behavioral problems should be offered at least one of the following interventions: • counseling the caregivers about non-pharmacological measures to control symptoms; • providing pharmacological means to control symptoms; • referral to specialists who may assist with symptoms.	6.	Patients with a diagnosis of dementia and who are having behavioral problems should be offered at least one of the following interventions: • counseling the caregivers about non-pharmacological measures to control symptoms; • providing pharmacological means to control symptoms; • referral to specialists who may assist with symptoms.	ACCEPTED
7.	Caregivers of demented persons should be asked about their need for support services.	7.	Caregivers of demented persons should be asked about their need for support services **within 3 months of the diagnosis.**	MODIFIED: Time frame was made explicit. **ACCEPTED AS MODIFIED**

8.	For patients diagnosed with dementia, the presence or absence of all of the following risk factors for vascular etiology should be documented:
	
	  a. hypertension;
	  b. smoking;
	  c. hypercholesterolemia.
		--	For patients diagnosed with dementia, the presence or absence of all of the following risk factors for vascular etiology should be documented:
			
			  a. hypertension;
			  b. smoking;
			  c. hypercholesterolemia.
				DROPPED due to low validity scores. Evidence of benefit is lacking.

9.	Patients with vascular or multi-infarct dementia should be offered aspirin, unless active peptic ulcer disease or aspirin intolerance is noted.	--	Patients with vascular or multi-infarct dementia should be offered aspirin, unless active peptic ulcer disease or aspirin intolerance is noted.	**DROPPED due to low validity score.** Evidence of benefit is not convincing.
10.	Persons with dementia should not be taking long-acting sedatives.	8.	Persons with dementia should not be taking long-acting sedatives **unless there is explicit justification in the medical record.**	MODIFIED: Panelists pointed out that there are possible exceptions. **ACCEPTED AS MODIFIED**
	Follow-up			
11.	Patients with symptoms of cognitive impairment who do not receive a diagnosis of dementia should have documented that the provider inquired again about those symptoms within 12 months of first presentation.	9.	Patients with symptoms of cognitive impairment who do not receive a diagnosis of dementia should have documented that the provider inquired again about those symptoms within 12 months of first presentation.	ACCEPTED

443

Chapter 8 - Depression

	Indicator Proposed by Staff		Indicator Voted on by Panel	Comments/Disposition
	Screening		**Screening**	
1.	Clinicians should ask about the presence or absence of depression or depressive symptoms in any person with any of the following risk factors for depression:	1.	Clinicians should ask about the presence or absence of depression or depressive symptoms in any person with any of the following risk factors for depression:	INCLUDED BASED ON Q1 PANEL RATING
	a. history of depression,	a.	a. history of depression,	
	b. death in family in past six months, or	b.	b. death in family in past six months, or	
	c. alcohol or other drug abuse.	c.	c. alcohol or other drug abuse.	
	Diagnosis		**Diagnosis**	
2.	If the diagnosis of depression is made, specific co-morbidities should be elicited and documented in the chart:	2.	If the diagnosis of depression is made, specific co-morbidities should be elicited and documented in the chart:	INCLUDED BASED ON Q1 PANEL RATING
	a. presence or absence of alcohol or other drug abuse;	a.	a. presence or absence of alcohol or other drug abuse;	
	b. medication use; and	b.	b. medication use; and	
	c. general medical disorder(s).	c.	c. general medical disorder(s).	
	Treatment		**Treatment**	
3.	Once diagnosis of major depression has been made, treatment with anti-depressant medication and/or psychotherapy should begin within 2 weeks.	3.	Once diagnosis of major depression has been made, treatment with anti-depressant medication and/or psychotherapy should begin within 2 weeks.	INCLUDED BASED ON Q1 PANEL RATING
4.	Presence or absence of suicidal ideation should be documented during the first or second diagnostic visit.	4.	Presence or absence of suicidal ideation should be documented during the first or second diagnostic visit.	INCLUDED BASED ON Q1 PANEL RATING
5.	Persons who have suicidality should be asked if they have specific plans to carry out suicide.	5.	Persons who have suicidality should be asked if they have specific plans to carry out suicide.	INCLUDED BASED ON Q1 PANEL RATING
6.	Persons who have suicidality and have any of the following risk factors should be hospitalized:	6.	Persons who have suicidality and have any of the following risk factors should be hospitalized:	INCLUDED BASED ON Q1 PANEL RATING
	a. psychosis;	a.	a. psychosis;	
	b. current alcohol or drug abuse or dependency;	b.	b. current alcohol or drug abuse or dependency;	
	c. specific plans to carry out suicide (e.g., obtaining a weapon, putting affairs in order, making a suicide note).	c.	c. specific plans to carry out suicide (e.g., obtaining a weapon, putting affairs in order, making a suicide note).	

	Indicator Proposed by Staff		Indicator Voted on by Panel	Comments/Disposition
7.	Antidepressants should be prescribed at appropriate dosages.	7.	Antidepressants should be prescribed at appropriate dosages.	INCLUDED BASED ON Q1 PANEL RATING
8.	Anti-anxiety agents should not be prescribed as a sole agent for the treatment of depression.	8.	Anti-anxiety agents should not be prescribed as a sole agent for the treatment of depression.	INCLUDED BASED ON Q1 PANEL RATING
	Follow-up			
9.	Medication treatment visits or telephone contacts should occur at least once in the 2 weeks following initial diagnosis.	9.	Medication treatment visits or telephone contacts should occur at least once in the 2 weeks following initial diagnosis.	INCLUDED BASED ON Q1 PANEL RATING
10.	Persons hospitalized for depression should have follow-up with a mental health specialist or their primary care doctor within two weeks of discharge.	10.	Persons hospitalized for depression should have follow-up with a mental health specialist or their primary care doctor within two weeks of discharge.	INCLUDED BASED ON Q1 PANEL RATING
11.	Patients with major depression who have medical record documentation of improvement of symptoms within 8 weeks of starting medication treatment should be continued on medication treatment for at least 2 additional months.	11.	Patients with major depression who have medical record documentation of improvement of symptoms within ~~8~~ 6 weeks of starting **antidepressant** ~~medication~~ treatment should be continued on **an antidepressant** ~~medication~~ treatment for at least ~~2~~ 4 additional months.	MODIFIED: Panelists wanted time frames to be consistent with AHCPR guidelines. ACCEPTED AS MODIFIED

445

	Indicator Proposed by Staff		Indicator Voted on by Panel	Comments/Disposition
12.	At least one of the following should occur if there is no or inadequate response to therapy for depression at 8 weeks: • Referral to psychotherapist, if not already seeing one; • Change or increase in dose of medication, if on medication; • Addition of medication, if only using psychotherapy, or • Change in diagnosis documented in chart	12.	At least one of the following should occur if there is no or inadequate response to therapy for depression at 8 weeks: • Referral to psychotherapist, if not already seeing one; • Change or increase in dose of medication, if on medication; • Addition of medication, if only using psychotherapy, or • Change in diagnosis documented in chart	INCLUDED BASED ON Q1 PANEL RATING
13.	At each visit during which depression is discussed, degree of response/remission and side effects of medication should be assessed and documented during the first year of treatment.	13.	At each visit during which depression is discussed, degree of response/remission and side effects of medication should be assessed and documented during the first year of treatment.	INCLUDED BASED ON Q1 PANEL RATING

Chapter 9 - Diabetes Mellitus

		Indicator Proposed by Staff		Indicator Voted on by Panel	Comments/Disposition
		Diagnosis			
1.		Patients with fasting blood sugar >126 or postprandial blood sugar >200 should have a diagnosis of diabetes noted in progress notes or problem list.	1.	Patients < 75 years old with more than one fasting blood sugar >126 or postprandial blood sugar >200 should have a diagnosis of diabetes noted in progress notes or problem list.	**ACCEPTED AS MODIFIED** MODIFIED: Panelists felt that the sensitivity of glucose to age required modification of this indicator. Guidelines universally recommend repeat measures of blood sugar.
2.		Patients with the diagnosis of Type 1 diabetes should have all of the following:	2.	Patients with the diagnosis of Type 1 diabetes should have all of the following:	**"a, b, d, e, f" INCLUDED BASED ON Q1 PANEL RATING**
	a.	Glycosylated hemoglobin or fructosamine every 6 months.	a.	Glycosylated hemoglobin or fructosamine every 6 months.	
	b.	Eye and visual exam (annual).	b.	Eye and visual exam (annual).	**"c" ACCEPTED AS MODIFIED** - panelists felt that annual requirement was too strict.
	c.	Total serum cholesterol and HDL cholesterol tests (annual).	c.	Total serum cholesterol and HDL cholesterol tests (~~annual~~) **documented**.	
	d.	Measurement of urine protein (annual).	d.	Measurement of urine protein (annual) documented.	
	e.	Examination of feet at least twice a year.	e.	Examination of feet at least twice a year.	
	f.	Measurement of blood pressure at every visit.	f.	Measurement of blood pressure at every visit.	
3.		Patients with the diagnosis of Type 2 diabetes should have all of the following:	2.	Patients with the diagnosis of Type 2 diabetes should have all of the following:	**"a, b, d, e, f" INCLUDED BASED ON Q1 PANEL RATING**
	a.	Glycosylated hemoglobin or fructosamine every 6 months;	a.	Glycosylated hemoglobin or fructosamine every 6 months;	**"c" ACCEPTED AS MODIFIED.** Panelists felt that the annual requirement was too strict.
	b.	Eye and visual exam (annual);	b.	Eye and visual exam (annual);	
	c.	Total serum cholesterol and HDL cholesterol tests (annual);	c.	Total serum cholesterol and HDL cholesterol tests (~~annual~~) **documented**;	
	d.	Measurement of urine protein (annual);	d.	Measurement of urine protein (annual);	
	e.	Examination of feet at least twice a year;	e.	Examination of feet at least twice a year;	
	f.	Measurement of blood pressure at every visit.	f.	Measurement of blood pressure at every visit.	
4.		Types 1 & 2 patients taking insulin should monitor their glucose at home unless documented to be unable or unwilling.	4.	Types 1 & 2 patients taking insulin should monitor their glucose at home unless documented to be unable or unwilling.	**INCLUDED BASED ON Q1 PANEL RATING**

447

	Indicator Proposed by Staff		Indicator Voted on by Panel	Comments/Disposition
	Treatment		*Treatment*	
5.	Newly diagnosed diabetics should receive dietary and exercise counseling.	5.	Newly diagnosed diabetics should receive dietary and exercise counseling.	INCLUDED BASED ON Q1 PANEL RATING
6.	Type 2 diabetics who have failed dietary therapy should receive oral hypoglycemic therapy.	6.	Type 2 diabetics who have failed dietary therapy should receive oral hypoglycemic therapy.	INCLUDED BASED ON Q1 PANEL RATING
7.	Type 2 diabetics who have failed oral hypoglycemics should be offered insulin.	7.	Type 2 diabetics who have failed oral hypoglycemics should be offered insulin.	INCLUDED BASED ON Q1 PANEL RATING
8.	Hypertensive diabetics with proteinuria should be offered an ACE inhibitor or a calcium channel blocker within 3 months of the notation of proteinuria.	8.	~~Hypertensive~~ Diabetics with proteinuria should be offered an ACE inhibitor ~~or a calcium channel blocker~~ within 3 months of the notation of proteinuria **unless contraindicated**.	MODIFIED: RCT evidence supports applicability to all diabetics. Calcium channel blockers are not a substitute for an ACE inhibitor. **ACCEPTED AS MODIFIED**
	Follow-up		*Follow-up*	
9.	All patients with diabetes should have a follow-up visit at least every 6 months.	9.	All patients with diabetes should have a follow-up visit at least every 6 months.	INCLUDED BASED ON Q1 PANEL RATING

448

Chapter 10 - Hormone Replacement Therapy

	Indicator Proposed by Staff		Indicator Voted on by Panel	Comments/Disposition
1.	Women with intact uteri should not use unopposed estrogen unless both of the following are true: • The patient has been tried on cyclic or continuous estrogen plus progestin regimen; • Endometrial sampling is performed yearly.	1.	Women with intact uteri should not use unopposed **oral or transdermal** estrogen unless both of the following are true: • The patient has been tried on cyclic or continuous estrogen plus progestin regimen; • Endometrial sampling is performed yearly— **at least every 2 years.**	MODIFIED: Panelists felt that endometrial sampling did not have to occur every year for every patient. **ACCEPTED AS MODIFIED**
2.	Women with a new diagnosis of menopause[1] should receive counseling about the risks and benefits of HRT.	2.	Women with a new diagnosis of menopause should receive counseling about the risks and benefits of HRT **within one year of diagnosis.**	MODIFIED: Time frame was made explicit **ACCEPTED AS MODIFIED**
		3.	**Post-menopausal women being initiated on HRT should receive counseling about the risks and benefits of HRT within 1 year prior to initiation.**	**PROPOSED and ACCEPTED by Q2 panel.** Panelists felt that patient education was important for patients prescribed HRT.

Chapter 11 - Headache

	Indicator Proposed by Staff		Indicator Voted on by Panel	Comments/Disposition
	Diagnosis			
1.	Patients with new onset headache should be asked about all of the following:	1.	Patients with new onset headache should be asked about all of the following:	INCLUDED BASED ON Q1 PANEL RATING
	a. location of the pain;	a.	a. location of the pain;	
	b. associated symptoms;	b.	b. associated symptoms;	
	c. temporal profile;	c.	c. temporal profile;	
	d. severity;	d.	d. severity;	
	e. family history; and	e.	e. family history; and	
	f. aggravating or alleviating factors.	f.	f. aggravating or alleviating factors.	
2.	Patients with new onset headache should have an examination evaluating all of the following:	2.	Patients with new onset headache should have an examination evaluating all of the following:	INCLUDED BASED ON Q1 PANEL RATING
	a. cranial nerves;	a.	a. cranial nerves;	
	b. fundi;	b.	b. fundi;	
	c. deep tendon reflexes; and	c.	c. deep tendon reflexes; and	
	d. blood pressure.	d.	d. blood pressure.	
3.	CT or MRI scanning is indicated in patients with new onset headache and any of the following circumstances:	3.	CT or MRI scanning is indicated in patients with new onset headache and any of the following circumstances:	INCLUDED BASED ON Q1 PANEL RATING
	a. abnormal neurological examination; or	a.	a. abnormal neurological examination; or	
	b. severe headache.	b.	b. severe headache.	
4.	Skull x-rays should not be part of an evaluation for headache.	4.	Skull x-rays should not be part of an evaluation for headache.	INCLUDED BASED ON Q1 PANEL RATING
	Treatment			
5.	Patients with acute mild migraine or tension headache should have tried aspirin, Tylenol, or other nonsteroidal anti-inflammatory agents before being offered any other medication.	5.	Patients with acute mild migraine or tension headache should have tried aspirin, Tylenol, or other nonsteroidal anti-inflammatory agents before being offered any other medication.	INCLUDED BASED ON Q1 PANEL RATING

450

	Indicator Proposed by Staff		Indicator Voted on by Panel	Comments/Disposition
6.	For patients with acute moderate or severe migraine headache, one of the following should have been tried before any other agent is offered: • ketorolac; • sumatriptan; • dihydroergotamine; • ergotamine; • chlorpromazine; or • metoclopramide.	6.	For patients with acute moderate or severe migraine headache, one of the following should have been tried before any other agent is offered: • ketorolac; • sumatriptan; • dihydroergotamine; • ergotamine; • chlorpromazine; or • metoclopramide.	INCLUDED BASED ON Q1 PANEL RATING
7.	Recurrent moderate or severe tension headaches should be treated with a trial of tricyclic antidepressant agents, if there are no medical contraindications to use.	7.	Recurrent moderate or severe tension headaches should be treated with a trial of tricyclic antidepressant agents, if there are no medical contraindications to use.	INCLUDED BASED ON Q1 PANEL RATING
8.	If a patient has more than 2 moderate to severe migraine headaches each month, then prophylactic treatment with one of the following agents should be offered: • beta blockers; • calcium channel blockers; • tricyclic antidepressants; • naproxen; • aspirin; • fluoxitene; • valproate; or • cyproheptadine.	8.	If a patient has more than 2 moderate to severe migraine headaches each month, then prophylactic treatment with one of the following agents should be offered: • beta blockers; • calcium channel blockers; • tricyclic antidepressants; • naproxen; • aspirin; • fluoxitene; • valproate; or • cyproheptadine.	INCLUDED BASED ON Q1 PANEL RATING
9.	Sumatriptan and ergotamine should not be concurrently administered.	9.	Sumatriptan and ergotamine should not be concurrently administered.	INCLUDED BASED ON Q1 PANEL RATING
10.	Opioid agonists and barbiturates should not be first-line therapy for migraine or tension headaches.	10.	Opioid agonists and barbiturates should not be first-line therapy for migraine or tension headaches.	INCLUDED BASED ON Q1 PANEL RATING
11.	Sumatriptan and ergotamine should not be given in patients with a history of: uncontrolled hypertension, atypical chest pain, or ischemic heart disease or angina.	11.	Sumatriptan and ergotamine should not be given in patients with a history of: uncontrolled hypertension, atypical chest pain, or ischemic heart disease or angina.	INCLUDED BASED ON Q1 PANEL RATING

451

Chapter 12 - Hip Fracture

	Indicator Proposed by Staff		Indicator Voted on by Panel	Comments/Disposition
	Diagnosis			
1.	Patients with symptoms or signs of hip fracture should be offered one of the following imaging studies of the affected hip within 1 day: • a radiograph; • a technetium-99m bone scan; • an MRI.	1.	Patients with symptoms or signs of hip fracture should be offered one of the following imaging studies of the affected hip within 1 day **unless documented not to be a surgical candidate:** • a radiograph; • a technetium-99m bone scan; • an MRI.	MODIFIED: Panelists felt that without a surgical option these tests were not useful. **ACCEPTED AS MODIFIED**
2.	Patients who have had surgical repair of a hip fracture should have been offered a complete medical evaluation preoperatively, including all of the following: a. medical history; b. physical examination; c. laboratory evaluation; d. electrocardiogram.	2. a. b. c. d.	Patients who have had surgical repair of a hip fracture should have been offered a complete medical evaluation preoperatively, including all of the following: a. medical history; b. physical examination; c. laboratory evaluation **for patients >= 50 years;** d. electrocardiogram **for patients >= 50 years.**	MODIFIED: Panelists felt that lab and ECG were indicated only for older patients. There was no consensus on use in the total population. **ACCEPTED AS MODIFIED**
	Treatment			
3.	Patients who have had surgical repair of a hip fracture should have received antibiotics prophylactically on the same day that surgery was performed.	3.	Patients who have had surgical repair of a hip fracture should have received antibiotics prophylactically on the same day that surgery was performed.	ACCEPTED
4.	Patients who have a surgically repaired hip fracture should begin rehabilitation on post-operative day one.	--	Patients who have a surgically repaired hip fracture should begin rehabilitation on post-operative day one.	**DROPPED due to low validity score.** The benefit is mainly reduced cost rather than improved functional outcome. May be difficult to define "rehabilitation".
5.	Persons with hip fractures should be given prophylactic thromboembolics on admission to the hospital.	4.	Persons with hip fractures should be given prophylactic ~~thromboembolics~~ **antithrombotics** on admission to the hospital.	MODIFIED: Clarified. **ACCEPTED AS MODIFIED**

	Indicator Proposed by Staff		Indicator Voted on by Panel	Comments/Disposition
6.	Patients hospitalized with hip fracture who are at risk for developing pressure sores should have both of the following done while hospitalized: a. Be repositioned every 2 hours; b. Be provided a pressure-reducing mattress.	5. a. --	Patients hospitalized with hip fracture who are at risk for developing pressure sores should have both of the following done while hospitalized: a. Be repositioned every 2 hours; b. Be provided a pressure-reducing mattress.	**"a" ACCEPTED** **"b" DROPPED due to low validity score.** May not be able to identify type of mattress from medical record, and some are not adequate.
Follow-up				
7.	Patients who have had a hip fracture should have documented within 2 months (before or after) the presence or absence of modifiable risk factors for subsequent hip fracture.	6.	Patients who have had a hip fracture should have documented within 2 months (before or after) the presence or absence of **at least one** modifiable risk factors for subsequent hip fracture.	MODIFIED: Panelists wanted to be specific on risk factors. **ACCEPTED AS MODIFIED**
		7. (8)	**Patients over 65 who report falling should be assessed for at least two modifiable risk factors within 3 months of the report.**	**PROPOSED AND ACCEPTED BY Q2 PANEL.** Panelists wanted to emphasize secondary prevention of falls.

453

Chapter 13 - Hysterectomy

	Indicator Proposed by Staff		Indicator Voted on by Panel	Comments/Disposition
1.	If a woman undergoes a hysterectomy with the indication of fibroid uterus at least one of the following should be recorded in the medical record: • The uterus is palpable abdominally and the patient is concerned about the fibroids; • Excessive menstrual bleeding; • Anemia; • Pelvic discomfort; or • Bladder pressure with urinary frequency.	1.	If a woman undergoes a hysterectomy with the indication of fibroid uterus at least one of the following should be recorded in the medical record: • The uterus is ~~palpable abdominally~~ and the **significantly enlarged** and the patient is concerned about the fibroids; • Excessive menstrual bleeding; • ~~Anemia;~~ • Pelvic discomfort; or • Bladder pressure with urinary frequency.	MODIFIED: Palpability can vary. Anemia dropped to make consistent with ACOG guidelines. **ACCEPTED AS MODIFIED**
2.	If a pre- or peri-menopausal woman undergoes a hysterectomy with the indication of abnormal uterine bleeding, then the medical record should indicate that at least one month of medical therapy was given in the six months prior to the hysterectomy without relief of symptoms.	2.	If a pre- or peri-menopausal woman undergoes a hysterectomy with the indication of abnormal uterine bleeding, then the medical record should indicate that at least one month of medical therapy was ~~given~~ **offered** in the six months prior to the hysterectomy without relief of symptoms.	MODIFIED: Panelists wanted to allow for patient choice and be consistent with other indicators. **ACCEPTED AS MODIFIED**
3.	Women who have a hysterectomy for post-menopausal bleeding should have had a biopsy of the endometrium within six months prior to the procedure.	3.	Women who have a hysterectomy for post-menopausal bleeding should have ~~had~~ **been offered** a biopsy of the endometrium within six months prior to the procedure.	MODIFIED: Panelists wanted to allow for patient choice and be consistent with other indicators. **ACCEPTED AS MODIFIED**
4.	Women with post-menopausal bleeding should be offered an office endometrial biopsy within one month of presentation.	4.	Women with post-menopausal bleeding should be offered an office endometrial biopsy within ~~one~~ **three** months of presentation.	MODIFIED: Panelists felt time frame was too short. **ACCEPTED AS MODIFIED**

454

Chapter 14 - Inguinal Hernia

	Indicator Proposed by Staff		Indicator Voted on by Panel	Comments/Disposition
	Diagnosis			
1.	For a patient < age 65 diagnosed with inguinal hernia, the medical record should document the time duration since the patient first noticed symptoms of hernia.	--	For a patient < age 65 diagnosed with inguinal hernia, the medical record should document the time duration since the patient first noticed symptoms of hernia.	**DROPPED due to low validity score.** Since patient recall is very flawed many providers may choose not to ask, or may not document if they did.
	Treatment			
2.	A patient diagnosed with a strangulated or incarcerated inguinal hernia should have emergency groin exploration within 24 hours of presentation.	1.	A patient diagnosed with a strangulated or incarcerated inguinal hernia should have **receive** emergency groin exploration within 24 hours of presentation.	MODIFIED: Panelists felt that an incarcerated hernia was not always emergent. **ACCEPTED AS MODIFIED**
3.	For a patient < age 65 diagnosed with inguinal hernia appearing within the prior 2 years, the medical record should document that elective herniorrhaphy was offered.	2.	For a patient < age 65 diagnosed with **symptomatic** inguinal hernia appearing within the prior 2 years, the medical record should document that elective herniorrhaphy was offered discussed.	MODIFIED: Panelists did not want to overly encourage surgery. Also, the quality of life benefits are unclear. The age cut-off is not applicable to symptomatic patients. **ACCEPTED AS MODIFIED**
		3. (4)	Patients with a newly documented inguinal hernia should, at the same visit, receive education on the symptoms that would necessitate emergency surgery.	PROPOSED AND ACCEPTED BY Q2 PANEL. Panelists felt that patient education was important.

Chapter 15 - Low Back Pain (Acute)

	Indicator Proposed by Staff		Indicator Voted on by Panel	Comments/Disposition
	Diagnosis			
1.	Patients presenting with acute low back pain should receive a focused medical history and physical examination. The history should include questions about "red flags" in at least one of the following areas: • Spine fracture: trauma, prolonged use of steroids; • Cancer: history of cancer, unexplained weight loss, immunosuppression; • Infection: fever, IV drug use; • "Red flags" for cauda equina syndrome (CES) or rapidly progressing neurologic deficit are: acute onset of urinary retention or overflow incontinence, loss of anal sphincter tone or fecal incontinence, saddle anesthesia, and global progressive motor weakness in the lower limbs.	1.	Patients presenting with acute low back pain should receive a focused medical history and physical examination. The history should include questions about "red flags" in at least one of the following areas: • Spine fracture: trauma, prolonged use of steroids; • Cancer: history of cancer, unexplained weight loss, immunosuppression; • Infection: fever, IV drug use; • "Red flags" for cauda equina syndrome (CES) or rapidly progressing neurologic deficit are: acute onset of urinary retention or overflow incontinence, loss of anal sphincter tone or fecal incontinence, saddle anesthesia, and global progressive motor weakness in the lower limbs.	INCLUDED BASED ON Q1 PANEL RATING
2.	For patients presenting with acute low back pain, the physical examination should include neurologic screening and straight leg raising.	2.	For patients presenting with acute low back pain, the physical examination should include neurologic screening and straight leg raising.	INCLUDED BASED ON Q1 PANEL RATING
	Treatment			
3.	Patients should NOT be taking any of the following medications for treatment of acute low back pain: a. Phenylbutazone; b. Dexamethasone; c. Other oral steroids; d. Colchicine; e. Anti-depressants.	3.	Patients should NOT be taking any of the following medications for treatment of acute low back pain: a. Phenylbutazone; b. Dexamethasone; c. Other oral steroids; d. Colchicine; e. Anti-depressants.	INCLUDED BASED ON Q1 PANEL RATING
4.	Patients should NOT be prescribed the following physical treatments for acute low back pain: a. Transcutaneous electrical nerve stimulation (TENS); b. Lumbar corsets and support belts; c. Spinal traction.	4.	Patients should NOT be prescribed the following physical treatments for acute low back pain: a. Transcutaneous electrical nerve stimulation (TENS); b. Lumbar corsets and support belts; c. Spinal traction.	INCLUDED BASED ON Q1 PANEL RATING
5.	Prolonged bed rest (> 4 days) should NOT be recommended for patients with acute low back pain.	5.	Prolonged bed rest (> 4 days) should NOT be recommended for patients with acute low back pain.	INCLUDED BASED ON Q1 PANEL RATING

Chapter 16 - Orthopedic Conditions

		Indicator Proposed by Staff		Indicator Voted on by Panel	Comments/Disposition
		Shoulder: *Diagnosis*			
1.		Patients presenting with new onset shoulder pain should have a history obtained at the time of presentation that includes at least 4 of the following: • duration of pain; • location of pain; • activity at time the pain began; • activities that worsen the pain; • past history of injury; • past history of surgery; • therapeutic interventions attempted (e.g., NSAIDs, rest, physical therapy); • involvement of other joints.	--	Patients presenting with new onset shoulder pain should have a history obtained at the time of presentation that includes at least 4 of the following: • duration of pain; • location of pain; • activity at time the pain began; • activities that worsen the pain; • past history of injury; • past history of surgery; • therapeutic interventions attempted (e.g., NSAIDs, rest, physical therapy); • involvement of other joints.	**DROPPED due to low validity score.** Panelists felt it was not reasonable to expect this level of documentation.
2.		Patients who present with new onset shoulder pain should have a physical examination performed at time of presentation that includes at least 3 of the following: • range of passive motion testing; • range of active motion testing; • the drop arm test; • testing for presence of impingement sign; • palpation to localize the site of pain; • cervical spine examination.	--	Patients who present with new onset shoulder pain should have a physical examination performed at time of presentation that includes at least 3 of the following: • range of passive motion testing; • range of active motion testing; • the drop arm test; • testing for presence of impingement sign; • palpation to localize the site of pain; • cervical spine examination.	**DROPPED due to low validity score.** Panelists felt it was not reasonable to expect this level of documentation.

457

	Indicator Proposed by Staff		Indicator Voted on by Panel	Comments/Disposition
	Shoulder: *Treatment*			
3.	Patients diagnosed with impingement syndrome should be offered at least 1 of the following: • NSAIDs at time of presentation; • intra-articular steroid injection within 1 week of presentation.	1.	Patients diagnosed with impingement syndrome should be offered at least 1 of the following **within 2 weeks:** • NSAIDs, at time of presentation including aspirin; • intra-articular steroid injection within 1 week of presentation; • **avoidance of inciting activities;** • **physical therapy;** • **instructions for a home exercise program.**	MODIFIED: Panelists specified a single time frame to simplify the indicator. They also included treatments from indicator #4. **ACCEPTED AS MODIFIED**
4.	Patients diagnosed with impingement syndrome should be offered 1 of the following within 2 weeks of diagnosis: • physical therapy referral; • instructions for a home exercise program.	--	~~Patients diagnosed with impingement syndrome should be offered 1 of the following within 2 weeks of diagnosis: • physical therapy referral; • instructions for a home exercise program.~~	DROPPED BY PANEL - The panel merged #4 with #3, and did not rate #4.
5.	Patients diagnosed with a medium or large rotator cuff tear who have not seen an orthopedist within 2 weeks before diagnosis, should be offered referral to an orthopedist at the time of diagnosis.	--	~~Patients diagnosed with a medium or large rotator cuff tear who have not seen an orthopedist within 2 weeks before diagnosis, should be offered referral to an orthopedist at the time of diagnosis.~~	DROPPED PRIOR TO PANEL. It is difficult to identify "medium or large" tears from the medical record. It may also be difficult to identify orthopedists.
6.	Patients diagnosed with adhesive capsulitis should receive education regarding shoulder exercises at time of diagnosis.	--	Patients diagnosed with adhesive capsulitis should receive education regarding shoulder exercises at time of diagnosis.	DROPPED due to low validity score. Evidence of benefit is lacking.

Indicator Proposed by Staff		Indicator Voted on by Panel		Comments/Disposition
Knee: *Diagnosis*				
7.	Patients presenting with new onset knee pain should have a history taken at time of initial presentation that includes at least 3 of the following: • duration; • activity at time of onset; • exacerbating and relieving factors; • ability to ambulate; • history of prior trauma, surgery, or knee problems.	1.	Patients presenting with new onset knee pain should have a history taken at time of initial presentation that includes at least 3 of the following: • duration; • activity at time of onset; • exacerbating and relieving factors; • ability to ambulate; • history of prior trauma, surgery, or knee problems.	**DROPPED due to low validity score**
8.	Patients presenting with new onset knee pain after injury to their knee should undergo at least 2 of the following maneuvers during physical examination: • Lachman's test; • anterior drawer test; • posterior drawer test; • posterior sag test; • joint line palpation; • McMurray's test; • valgus stress; • varus stress.	2.	Patients presenting with new onset knee pain after injury to their knee should undergo at least 2 of the following maneuvers during physical examination **within one month of initial presentation**: • Lachman's test; • anterior drawer test; • posterior drawer test; • posterior sag test; • joint line palpation; • McMurray's test; • valgus stress; • varus stress.	MODIFIED: Panelists wanted to extend time frame for tests. ACCEPTED AS MODIFIED
9.	Patients presenting with new onset knee effusion should have a history taken at time of initial presentation that includes: a. duration of swelling; b. history of trauma and injury; c. presence of pain; d. history of crystalline-induced arthropathies	3. a. b. c. d.	Patients presenting with new onset knee effusion should have a history taken at time of initial presentation that includes: a. duration of swelling; b. history of trauma and injury; c. presence of pain; d. history of crystalline-induced arthropathies; **e. presence or absence of fever.**	"a, b, d" ACCEPTED "c" DROPPED due to low validity score. Evidence of correlation with outcome is lacking. "e" PROPOSED AND ACCEPTED BY Q2 PANEL. Panelists felt that fever was important for diagnosis of a septic joint.

#	Indicator Proposed by Staff		Indicator Voted on by Panel	Comments/Disposition
10.	Patients presenting with new onset knee effusion who do not have a history of recent trauma should undergo arthrocentesis at time of presentation.	--	Patients presenting with new onset knee effusion who do not have a history of recent trauma should undergo arthrocentesis at time of presentation.	**DROPPED due to low validity score This may not be appropriate for all patients.**
11.	Patients who undergo an arthrocentesis for new onset knee effusion should have the fluid analyzed for all of the following: a. cell count; b. culture; c. microscopic evaluation.	4. a. -- b. c.	Patients who undergo an arthrocentesis for new onset knee effusion should have the fluid analyzed for all of the following: a. cell count; b. culture; c. ~~microscopic evaluation~~ Gram stain d. crystals.	MODIFIED: The microscopic evaluation was specified. "a" ACCEPTED "b" DROPPED due to low validity score "c" ACCEPTED AS MODIFIED "d" ADDED PRIOR TO PANEL AND ACCEPTED

Knee: *Treatment*

#	Indicator Proposed by Staff		Indicator Voted on by Panel	Comments/Disposition
12.	Patients diagnosed with an ACL rupture who have not seen an orthopedist within 2 weeks before diagnosis should be offered referral to an orthopedist at time of diagnosis.	5.	Patients diagnosed with an ACL rupture who ~~have not seen an orthopedist within 2 weeks before diagnosis should be offered referral to an orthopedist at time of diagnosis.~~ should have surgical options discussed within 2 weeks of the rupture unless documented not to be a surgical candidate.	MODIFIED: Panelists felt the focus should be on an intervention rather than on specialist referral. ACCEPTED AS MODIFIED
13.	Patients newly diagnosed with patellofemoral syndrome should receive the following at time of diagnosis: a. prescription or recommendation for NSAIDs, unless contraindicated; b. education on quadriceps-strengthening exercises.	--	Patients newly diagnosed with patellofemoral syndrome should receive the following at time of diagnosis: a. prescription or recommendation for NSAIDs, unless contraindicated; b. education on quadriceps-strengthening exercises.	DROPPED due to low validity score
14.	Patients diagnosed with a septic joint should be treated with intravenous antibiotics.	6.	Patients diagnosed with a septic joint should be treated with intravenous antibiotics.	ACCEPTED
		7. (15)	Patients who report having at least 6 months of knee pain that limits function, despite regular use of NSAIDs and/or intraarticular steroid joint injection, should have the following offered or discussed within 1 month of the report of continued pain: • physical therapy (if not already tried); • surgery/arthroscopy.	PROPOSED AND ACCEPTED BY Q2 PANEL. Panelists felt that indicators should address process of treatment.

460

Chapter 17 - Osteoarthritis

	Indicator Proposed by Staff		Indicator Voted on by Panel	Comments/Disposition
	Diagnosis			
1.	Providers caring for patients with symptoms of OA should document all of the following for at least once in 2 years: a. the location of symptoms; b. the presence or absence of limitations in daily activities; c. the presence or absence of a history or symptoms of systemic or inflammatory disease; d. the use and effectiveness of treatment modalities.	1.	Providers caring for patients with symptoms of OA should document all **at least one of the** following at least once in 2 years: • the location of symptoms; • the presence or absence of limitations in daily activities; • ~~the presence or absence of a history or symptoms of systemic or inflammatory disease;~~ • the use and effectiveness of treatment modalities.	MODIFIED: Panelists wanted to make the indicator more flexible. Option "c" was considered duplicative and dropped pre-panel. **ACCEPTED AS MODIFIED**
2.	Providers caring for patients with incident symptoms of OA should document at least one of the following: • the presence or absence of a history of any systemic or inflammatory disease that may mimic OA; • the presence of absence of any current symptoms of systemic or inflammatory disease that may mimic OA; • the presence or absence of a history of joint trauma or surgery.	--	Providers caring for patients with incident symptoms of OA should document at least one of the following **within 3 months of symptom documentation**: • the presence or absence of a history of any systemic or inflammatory disease that may mimic OA; • the presence of absence of any current symptoms of systemic or inflammatory disease that may mimic OA; • the presence or absence of a history of joint trauma or surgery.	DROPPED due to low validity score
3.	Providers caring for patients with symptoms of OA should document the following for any one affected joint at least once in 2 years: a. the presence or absence of effusion; b. the presence or absence of bony enlargement; c. the presence or absence of tenderness; d. the presence or absence of limitations in range of motion.	--	Providers caring for patients with incident symptoms of OA should document **at least one of the following within 3 months of symptom documentation:** ~~for any one affected joint at least once in 2 years:~~ • the presence or absence of effusion; • the presence or absence of bony enlargement; • the presence or absence of tenderness; • the presence or absence of limitations in range of motion.	**DROPPED due to low validity score.** Panelists felt that the link to improved outcomes is weak. Evaluation of function was felt to be more important than the physical exam.

	Indicator Proposed by Staff		Indicator Voted on by Panel	Comments/Disposition
4.	Patients with incident symptoms of hip OA should be offered an anteroposterior film of the affected hip.	--	Patients with incident symptoms of hip OA should be offered an anteroposterior film of the affected hip.	**DROPPED due to low validity score.** Panelists felt it would be reasonable not to do this the first time the patient complains of pain.
Treatment				
5.	Patients with a new diagnosis of OA who wish to take medication for joint symptoms should be offered a trial of acetaminophen.	2.	Patients with a new diagnosis of OA who wish to take medication for joint symptoms should be offered a trial of acetaminophen.	ACCEPTED
6.	Providers caring for patients with symptoms of hip or knee OA should recommend both of the following at least once in 2 years: a. exercise programs for persons with hip or knee OA; b. weight loss among persons with knee OA and a BMI >25.	3.	Providers caring for patients with symptoms of hip or knee OA should recommend both of the following at least once in 2 years: a. exercise programs for persons with hip or knee OA; b. weight loss among persons with knee OA and a BMI > = 25.	MODIFIED: Corrected typo in "b", which should read "greater than or equal to 25."
		a.		**"a" ACCEPTED**
		--		**"b" DROPPED due to low validity score.** Evidence of benefit is lacking for patients who already have OA. The success rate for weight reduction is also very low.
Follow-up				
7.	Patients receiving care for symptoms of OA should be seen in follow-up at least every 6 months.	--	Patients receiving care for symptoms of OA should be seen in follow-up at least every 6 months.	DROPPED due to low validity score

462

Chapter 18 - Dyspepsia and Peptic Ulcer Disease

		Indicator Proposed by Staff		Indicator Voted on by Panel	Comments/Disposition
		Dyspepsia: Diagnosis			
1.		Patients presenting with a new episode of dyspepsia should have the presence or absence of NSAID use noted in the medical record on the date of presentation.	1.	Patients presenting with a new episode of dyspepsia should have the presence or absence of NSAID use noted in the medical record on the date of presentation.	ACCEPTED
		Dyspepsia: Treatment			
2.		Patients prescribed empiric antiulcer treatment for dyspepsia who were not using NSAIDs within the previous month should have at least one of the following within 8 weeks:	2.	~~Patients prescribed empiric antiulcer treatment for dyspepsia~~ Dyspepsia patients whose **persistent and bothersome symptoms have not improved after 8 weeks of empiric** antiulcer treatment and who were not using NSAIDs within the previous month should have at least one of the following within ~~8 weeks~~ **one month:**	MODIFIED: Panelists wanted to be sure that severity was sufficient to justify action. An upper GI series is also an option.
		• documentation in medical record that symptoms have improved;		• ~~documentation in medical record that symptoms have improved;~~	ACCEPTED AS MODIFIED
		• endoscopy;		• endoscopy;	
		• *pylori* test.		• *h. pylori* test;	
				• **upper GI series.**	
3.		Patients with new dyspepsia who have any of the following "alarm" indicators on the date of presentation should have endoscopy performed within 1 month, unless endoscopy has been performed in the previous 6 months:	3.	Patients with new dyspepsia who have any of the following "alarm" indicators on the date of presentation should have endoscopy performed within 1 month, unless endoscopy has been performed in the previous 6 months:	MODIFIED: Clarifications added.
	a.	a. anemia;	a.	a. **new** anemia;	"a-e" ACCEPTED AS MODIFIED
	b.	b. early satiety;	b.	b. early satiety;	
	c.	c. significant unintentional weight loss (exceeding 15 pounds in the past 3 months);	c.	c. significant unintentional weight loss (exceeding 15 pounds in the past 3 months);	
	d.	d. guaiac-positive stool;	d.	d. guaiac-positive stool if **not on NSAIDs;**	
	e.	e. dysphagia;	e.	e. dysphagia;	
	--	f. over age 60.	--	f. over age 60 if **not on NSAIDs.**	"f" DROPPED due to low validity score

463

	Indicator Proposed by Staff		Indicator Voted on by Panel	Comments/Disposition
4.	Patients who are prescribed *H. pylori* eradication antibiotic treatment within 3 months after presentation for a new episode of dyspepsia should have one of the following noted in the medical record before start of antibiotic treatment: • prior positive test for *H. pylori*; • documentation of endoscopically confirmed ulceration of the duodenum at any time in the past.	--	Patients who are prescribed *H. pylori* eradication antibiotic treatment within 3 months after presentation for a new episode of dyspepsia should have one of the following noted in the medical record before start of antibiotic treatment: • prior positive test for *H. pylori*; • both a history of documented duodenal ulcer and absence of NSAID use.	**DROPPED due to low validity score.** Panelists were uncomfortable because guidelines in this area are changing rapidly.

Peptic Ulcer Disease: Prevention

	Indicator Proposed by Staff		Indicator Voted on by Panel	Comments/Disposition
5.	For patients with endoscopically documented PUD who have been noted to use NSAIDs within 2 months before endoscopy, the medical record should indicate, within 2 months before or 1 month after endoscopy, one of the following: • a reason why NSAIDs or aspirin will be continued; • advice to the patient to discontinue NSAIDs or aspirin.	4.	For patients with endoscopically documented PUD who have been noted to use NSAIDs **or aspirin** within 2 months before ~~endoscopy~~ **diagnosis**, the medical record should indicate, ~~within 2 months before or 1 month after endoscopy,~~ one of the following **at the time of diagnosis**: • a reason why NSAIDs or aspirin will be continued; • advice to the patient to discontinue NSAIDs or aspirin.	MODIFIED: Panelists wanted to allow for flexibility in manner of diagnosis. They also shortened the time frame. **ACCEPTED AS MODIFIED**

Peptic Ulcer Disease: Treatment

	Indicator Proposed by Staff		Indicator Voted on by Panel	Comments/Disposition
6.	Patients in whom peptic ulceration is confirmed on endoscopy should have antiulcer treatment for a minimum of 4 weeks.	5.	Patients in whom peptic ulceration is confirmed on endoscopy should have antiulcer treatment for a minimum of 4 weeks.	**ACCEPTED**
7.	Patients with endoscopically confirmed gastric or duodenal ulcer should have *H. pylori* testing within 3 months before or 1 month after endoscopy, unless the medical record, in the same time period, documents a past positive *H. pylori* test for which no *H. pylori* eradication treatment was given.	6.	Patients with endoscopically confirmed gastric ~~or duodenal~~ ulcer should have *H. pylori* testing within 3 months before or 1 month after endoscopy, unless the medical record, in the same time period, documents a past positive *H. pylori* test for which no *H. pylori* eradication treatment was given.	MODIFIED: Panelists did not think that H. pylori testing should be required for duodenal ulcers. **ACCEPTED AS MODIFIED**
8.	Eradication therapy for *H. pylori* should be offered within 1 month when all of the following conditions are met: • documentation of history of positive *H. pylori* test at any time in the past; • documentation of endoscopically confirmed ulceration of the duodenum at any time in the past.	7.	Eradication therapy for *H. pylori* should be offered within 1 month when all of the following conditions are met: • documentation of history of positive *H. pylori* test at any time in the past; • documentation of endoscopically confirmed **peptic** ulceration of the duodenum at any time in the past; • **no previous H. pylori eradication therapy.**	MODIFIED: Bullet added because previous therapy could be a contraindication. **ACCEPTED AS MODIFIED**

Indicator Proposed by Staff		Indicator Voted on by Panel	Comments/Disposition
Patients with a gastric ulcer confirmed by endoscopy should have one of the following: • a minimum of 3 biopsies during endoscopy; • follow-up endoscopy within 3 months.	8.	Patients with a gastric ulcer confirmed by endoscopy should have **at least** one of the following: • a minimum of 3 biopsies during endoscopy; • follow-up endoscopy within 3 months.	MODIFIED: Panelists wanted to clarify the intent of the indicator. ACCEPTED AS MODIFIED
Patients with endoscopically documented gastric ulcer who have follow-up endoscopy within 6 months should have one of the following at the follow-up endoscopy: • complete healing of the gastric ulcer noted; • a minimum of 3 biopsies of the ulcer.	9.	Patients with endoscopically documented gastric ulcer who have follow-up endoscopy within 6 months should have one of the following at the follow-up endoscopy: • complete healing of the gastric ulcer noted; • a minimum of 3 biopsies of the ulcer.	ACCEPTED
Patients with endoscopically documented PUD should be offered endoscopic treatment or surgery within the next 24 hours if either of the following are documented in the endoscopy note: a. continued oozing, bleeding, or spurting of blood; b. a visible vessel (or "pigmented protuberance").	10.	Patients with endoscopically documented PUD should be offered endoscopic treatment or surgery within the next 24 hours if either of the following are documented in the endoscopy note: a. continued oozing, bleeding, or spurting of blood; b. a visible vessel (or "pigmented protuberance").	ACCEPTED
Patients with a documented PUD complication who have had a positive *H. pylori* test within 3 months after the complication should be started on an *H. pylori* eradication regimen within 1 month of the positive test.	11.	Patients with a documented PUD complication who have had a positive *H. pylori* test (**by biopsy, breath test, or positive serology not previously treated**) within 3 months after the complication should be started on an *H. pylori* eradication regimen within 1 month of the positive test.	MODIFIED: Panelists specified acceptable methods of testing for H. pylori. ACCEPTED AS MODIFIED
Peptic Ulcer Disease: Follow-up			
Patients with endoscopically confirmed PUD whose symptoms of dyspepsia or documented ulcers recur within 6 months after eradication therapy for *H. pylori* should receive confirmatory testing for successful *H. pylori* cure by endoscopic biopsy or urease breath test within 1 month of symptom recurrence.	12.	Patients with endoscopically confirmed PUD whose symptoms of dyspepsia or documented ulcers recur within 6 months after eradication therapy for *H. pylori* should receive confirmatory testing for successful *H. pylori* cure by endoscopic biopsy or urease breath test within 1 month of symptom recurrence.	ACCEPTED
Patients with a history of PUD complications in the past year should have results of *H. pylori* testing documented in the medical record in the same time period.	13.	Patients with a history of PUD complications in the past year should have results of *H. pylori* testing documented in the medical record in the same time period.	ACCEPTED

Chapter 19 - Preventive Care

	Indicator Proposed by Staff		Indicator Voted on by Panel	Comments/Disposition
	Immunizations			
1.	For patients under age 50, notation of the date that a patient received a tetanus/diphtheria booster within the last ten years should be included in the medical record.	1.	For patients under age 50, notation of the date that a patient received a tetanus/diphtheria booster within the last ten years should be included in the medical record.	**INCLUDED BASED ON Q1 PANEL RATING**
2.	There should be documentation in the medical record that patients over the age of 50 were offered a tetanus/diphtheria booster after their 50th birthday.	2.	There should be documentation in the medical record that patients over the age of 50 were offered a tetanus/diphtheria booster after their 50th birthday **or in the last 10 years.**	MODIFIED: A booster is not needed if one has been received within the past 10 years. **ACCEPTED AS MODIFIED**
3.	Patients receiving medical attention for any wound should receive Td injection under either of the following conditions:	3.	Patients receiving medical attention for any wound should receive Td injection under either of the following conditions:	ACCEPTED
	a. For clean minor wounds, if the last Td booster was greater than 10 years;	a.	a. For clean minor wounds, if the last Td booster was greater than 10 years;	
	b. For other/dirty wounds, if the last Td booster was greater than 5 years.	b.	b. For other/dirty wounds, if the last Td booster was greater than 5 years.	
4.	All patients aged 65 and over should have been offered influenza vaccine in the past year.	4.	All patients aged 65 and over should have been offered influenza vaccine ~~in the past year~~ **annually or have documentation that they received it elsewhere.**	MODIFIED: The intent of indicator was clarified. **ACCEPTED AS MODIFIED**
5.	All patients under age 65 with any of the following conditions should have been offered influenza vaccination in the past year:	5.	All patients under age 65 with any of the following conditions should have been offered influenza vaccination ~~in the past year~~ **annually:**	MODIFIED: The intent of indicator was clarified. **ACCEPTED AS MODIFIED**
	a. Living in a nursing home;	a.	a. Living in a nursing home;	
	b. Chronic obstructive pulmonary disease;	b.	b. Chronic obstructive pulmonary disease;	
	c. Asthma;	c.	c. Asthma;	
	d. Chronic cardiovascular disorders;	d.	d. Chronic cardiovascular disorders;	
	e. Renal failure;	e.	e. Renal failure;	
	f. Immunosuppression;	f.	f. Immunosuppression;	
	g. Diabetes mellitus;	g.	g. Diabetes mellitus;	
	h. Hemoglobinopathies (e.g. sickle cell).	h.	h. Hemoglobinopathies (e.g. sickle cell).	

#	Indicator Proposed by Staff	#	Indicator Voted on by Panel	Comments/Disposition
6.	There should be documentation that all patients in the following groups and otherwise presenting for care were offered pneumococcal vaccine at least once: a. Patients aged 65 and older; b. Chronic cardiac or pulmonary disease; c. Diabetes mellitus; d. Anatomic asplenia; e. Persons over age 50 who are institutionalized.	6. a. b. c. d. e. --	There should be documentation that all patients in the following groups and otherwise presenting for care were offered pneumococcal vaccine at least once: a. Patients aged 65 and older; b. Chronic cardiac or pulmonary disease; c. Diabetes mellitus; d. Anatomic asplenia; e. Persons over age 50 who are institutionalized; f. Other immunocompromising conditions.	"a-e" ACCEPTED "f" PROPOSED BUT DROPPED BY Q2 PANEL due to disagreement on validity
7.	There should be documentation that all patients identified as being in the following high risk groups were offered hepatitis B vaccination within one year after identification of the risk, unless the patient has serologic evidence of immunity: a. Hemodialysis patients; b. Sexually active homosexual men; c. Household and sexual contacts of HBV carriers; d. Intravenous drug users; e. Persons with occupational risk ; f. Persons who have a history of sexual activity with multiple sexual partners in the past 6 months; g. Persons who have recently acquired another sexually transmitted disease.	7. a. b. c. d. e. f. g.	There should be documentation that all patients identified as being in the following high risk groups were offered hepatitis B vaccination within one year after identification of the risk, unless the patient has serologic evidence of immunity: a. Hemodialysis patients; b. Sexually active homosexual men; c. Household and sexual contacts of HBV carriers; d. Intravenous drug users; e. Persons with occupational risk; f. Persons who have a history of sexual activity with multiple sexual partners in the past 6 months; g. Persons who have recently acquired another sexually transmitted disease.	ACCEPTED

	Indicator Proposed by Staff		Indicator Voted on by Panel	Comments/Disposition
8.	All persons otherwise presenting for care in the following high risk groups should have documentation of measles immunization status: a. College students; b. Health-care workers; c. Day-care providers.	8. a. b. --	All persons otherwise presenting for care in the following high risk groups should have documentation of measles immunization status: a. College students; b. Health-care workers; c. Day-care providers	"a, b" ACCEPTED "c" DROPPED PRIOR TO PANEL
	Screening			
9.	There should be documentation of PPD reactivity status for all patients otherwise presenting for care who are identified as being in the following risk groups in the year following identification of the risk: a. Foreign born persons from countries of high TB prevalence (Asia, Africa, Latin America) who have been in the US less than 5 years; b. Injection drug users; c. Persons with immunosuppression; d. Residents of long-term care facilities such as nursing homes; e. Homeless persons; f. Health care workers.	9. a. b. c. d. e. f.	There should be documentation of PPD reactivity status for all patients otherwise presenting for care who are identified as being in the following risk groups in the year following identification of the risk: a. Foreign born persons from countries of high TB prevalence (Asia, Africa, Latin America) who have been in the US less than 5 years; b. Injection drug users; c. Persons with immunosuppression; d. Residents of long-term care facilities such as nursing homes; e. Homeless persons; f. Health care workers.	ACCEPTED
10.	All Mantoux tests read as positive or reactive should document both of the following: a. The presence of induration; b. The diameter of the induration in millimeters.	10. a. b.	All Mantoux tests read as positive or reactive should document both of the following: a. The presence of induration; b. The diameter of the induration in millimeters.	INCLUDED BASED ON Q1 PANEL RATING
11.	Mantoux tests should be read by a health professional or other trained personnel within 48-72 hours.	11.	Mantoux tests should be read by a health professional or other trained personnel within 48-72 hours.	INCLUDED BASED ON Q1 PANEL RATING
12.	Persons identified as having a newly positive or reactive PPD should have a chest radiograph performed within 1 month.	12.	Persons identified as having a newly positive or reactive PPD should have a chest radiograph performed within 1 month.	ACCEPTED

468

	Indicator Proposed by Staff		Indicator Voted on by Panel	Comments/Disposition
13.	Persons in the following risk groups who are identified as having TB infection (not disease) should be offered INH preventive therapy unless they have clear contraindications: a. Patients with diabetes mellitus; b. Patients with chronic renal failure; c. Recent exposure to a case of active TB; d. Recent conversion of PPD (documented negative test in the previous 2 years); e. Immunocompromised or chronic high dose corticosteroids; f. Injection drug users; g. Foreign born persons less than 35 years of age.	13. a. b. c. d. e. f. g.	Persons in the following risk groups who are identified as having TB infection (not disease) should be offered INH preventive therapy unless they have clear contraindications: a. Patients with diabetes mellitus; b. Patients with chronic renal failure; c. Recent exposure to a case of active TB; d. Recent conversion of PPD (documented negative test in the previous 2 years); e. Immunocompromised or chronic high dose corticosteroids; f. Injection drug users; g. Foreign born persons **from high prevalence countries** less than 35 years of age.	MODIFIED: Clarified the target population in "g". ACCEPTED AS MODIFIED
14.	If the initial PPD test on nursing home patients is negative, immediate retesting (two-step testing) should be performed.	14.	If the initial PPD test on nursing home patients is negative, ~~immediate~~ retesting (two-step testing) should be performed **within 2 weeks**	MODIFIED: Panelists did not feel that it was necessary to require immediate retesting. ACCEPTED AS MODIFIED
15.	Patients age 65 and older noted to have a hearing problem or complaint should be referred for a formal evaluation.	15.	Patients age 65 and older noted to have a hearing problem or complaint **without reversible cause or that persists despite treatment for reversible cause** should be ~~referred for a formal evaluation~~ **have formal evaluation for amplification offered or discussed.**	MODIFIED: Panelists wanted to exclude simple cases and clarify wording. ACCEPTED AS MODIFIED
16.	The medical record should include measurements of height and weight at least once.	16.	The medical record should include measurements of height and weight at least once.	INCLUDED BASED ON Q1 PANEL RATING
	Counseling			
17.	Patients otherwise presenting for care should receive counseling regarding the use of seat belts on at least one occasion.	17.	Patients otherwise presenting for care should receive counseling regarding the use of seat belts on at least one occasion.	INCLUDED BASED ON Q1 PANEL RATING

	Indicator Proposed by Staff		Indicator Voted on by Panel	Comments/Disposition
18.	Patients should be asked if they have ever been sexually active.	18.	Patients should be asked if they have ever been sexually active.	INCLUDED BASED ON Q1 PANEL RATING
19.	Patients under the age of 50, who have ever been sexually active, should be asked the following questions: a. if they currently have a single sexual partner; b. if they have had more than 2 sexual partners in the past 6 months; c. if they have a history of any STDs.	19. a. b. c.	Patients under the age of 50, who have ever been sexually active, should be asked the following questions: a. if they currently have a single sexual partner; b. if they have had more than 2 sexual partners in the past 6 months; c. if they have a history of any STDs.	INCLUDED BASED ON Q1 PANEL RATING
20.	Patients should be asked about current or past use of intravenous drugs at least once.	20.	Patients should be asked about current or past use of intravenous drugs at least once.	INCLUDED BASED ON Q1 PANEL RATING
21.	Patients who are sexually active and not in a monogamous relationship, have had more than 2 sexual partners in the past six months, have a history of STDs or have used intravenous drugs should be counseled regarding the prevention and transmission of HIV and other STDs.	21.	Patients who are sexually active and not in a monogamous relationship, have had more than 2 sexual partners in the past six months, have a history of STDs or have used intravenous drugs should be counseled regarding the prevention and transmission of HIV and other STDs.	INCLUDED BASED ON Q1 PANEL RATING
22.	Testing for HIV should have been offered in the past year to all persons in the following groups at increased risk for HIV infection: a. Those seeking treatment for sexually transmitted diseases (chlamydia, GC, syphilis, trichomonas, genital herpes, condyloma, or chancroid); b. Men who have sex with men; c. Past or present injection drug users; d. Persons who exchange sex for money or drugs; e. Women and men whose past or present sex partners were HIV-infected, bisexual, or injection drug users; f. Persons with a history of transfusion between 1978 and 1985.	22. a. b. c. d.	Patients with the following current HIV risk factors should have HIV testing offered or discussed at the visit in which the risk factor is noted: a. Having had sex with more than 2 male partners in the past 6 months; b. Injection drug use; c. Exchanging sex for money or drugs; d. Present sex partners are HIV-infected or injection drug users.	MODIFIED: Panelists reworded the indicator to clarify its intent. They separated current and past risk factors (see also new indicator #23) "a-d" ACCEPTED AS MODIFIED "e-f" DROPPED by panel without rating (moved to new indicator #23)

470

	Indicator Proposed by Staff		Indicator Voted on by Panel	Comments/Disposition
		23. (24)	Patients with the following past HIV risk factors should have HIV testing offered or discussed at the visit in which the past risk factor is noted (unless HIV status has been documented since the termination of the risk factor)	**PROPOSED AND ACCEPTED BY Q2 PANEL** Panelists felt that separating past risk factors clarified the intent of the indicators (see #22)
		a.	Past injection drug use;	
		b.	Having had sex with more than 2 male partners in a six month period;	
		c.	Exchanged sex for money or drugs in the past;	
		d.	Past sex partners were HIV-infected or injection drug users;	
		e.	History of transfusion between 1978 and 1985.	
23.	There should be documentation that patients' level of physical activity was assessed on at least one occasion.	--	There should be documentation that patients' level of physical activity was assessed on at least one occasion.	**DROPPED due to low validity score.** Panelists felt that there is insufficient evidence that provider counseling improves exercise rates.
		24. (25)	Patients over age 65 should be asked about hearing difficulties at least every 2 years.	**PROPOSED AND ACCEPTED BY Q2 PANEL.** Panelists felt that this is an important screening for this age group.

471

Chapter 20 - Vaginitis and Sexually Transmitted Diseases

	Indicator Proposed by Staff		Indicator Voted on by Panel	Comments/Disposition
	Vaginitis - Diagnosis		*Vaginitis - Diagnosis*	
1.	A sexual history should be obtained at the time of presentation from all women with a chief complaint of vaginal discharge. The history should include: a. Number of male partners in the previous 6 months; b. Absence or presence of symptoms in partners; c. Prior history of sexually transmitted diseases.	1.	A sexual history should be obtained at the time of presentation from all women with a chief complaint of vaginal discharge. The history should include: a. Number of male partners in the previous 6 months; b. Absence or presence of symptoms in partners; c. Prior history of sexually transmitted diseases.	INCLUDED BASED ON Q1 PANEL RATING
2.	In women presenting with a chief complaint of vaginal discharge, the practitioner should perform a speculum exam at the time of the initial presentation to determine if the source of the discharge is vaginal or cervical.	2.	In women presenting with a chief complaint of vaginal discharge, the practitioner should perform a speculum exam at the time of the initial presentation to determine if the source of the discharge is vaginal or cervical.	INCLUDED BASED ON Q1 PANEL RATING
3.	If three of the following four criteria are met, a diagnosis of bacterial vaginosis, or gardnerella vaginitis should be made: • pH greater than 4.5; • positive whiff test; • clue cells on wet mount; and • thin homogeneous discharge.	3.	If three of the following four criteria are met, a diagnosis of bacterial vaginosis, or gardnerella vaginitis should be made: • pH greater than 4.5; • positive whiff test; • clue cells on wet mount; and • thin homogeneous discharge.	INCLUDED BASED ON Q1 PANEL RATING
	Vaginitis - Treatment		*Vaginitis - Treatment*	
4.	Treatment for bacterial vaginosis should be with metronidazaole (orally or vaginally) or clindamycin (orally or vaginally) at the time of diagnosis.	4.	Treatment for bacterial vaginosis should be with metronidazaole (orally or vaginally) or clindamycin (orally or vaginally) at the time of diagnosis.	INCLUDED BASED ON Q1 PANEL RATING
5.	Treatment for *T. Vaginalis* should be with oral metronidazole, if the patient does not have an allergy to metronidazole or is not in first trimester of pregnancy at the time of diagnosis.	5.	Treatment for *T. Vaginalis* should be with oral metronidazole, if the patient does not have an allergy to metronidazole or is not in first trimester of pregnancy at the time of diagnosis.	INCLUDED BASED ON Q1 PANEL RATING
6.	Treatment for non-recurrent (< 3 episodes in the previous year) yeast vaginitis should be with topical 'azole' preparations (e.g. clotrimazole, butoconazole, etc.) or fluconazole at the time of diagnosis.	6.	Treatment for non-recurrent (< 3 episodes in the previous year) yeast vaginitis should be with topical 'azole' preparations (e.g. clotrimazole, butoconazole, etc.) or fluconazole at the time of diagnosis.	INCLUDED BASED ON Q1 PANEL RATING

	Indicator Proposed by Staff		Indicator Voted on by Panel	Comments/Disposition
	Cervicitis - Diagnosis		*Cervicitis - Diagnosis*	
7.	Routine testing for gonorrhea (culture) and chlamydia trachomatis (antigen detection), should be performed with the routine pelvic exam for women with multiple male sexual partners (more than 1 during the previous 6 months).	7.	Routine testing for gonorrhea (culture) and chlamydia trachomatis (antigen detection), should be performed with the routine pelvic exam for women with multiple male sexual partners (more than 1 during the previous 6 months).	INCLUDED BASED ON Q1 PANEL RATING
	Cervicitis - Treatment		*Cervicitis - Treatment*	
8.	Women treated for gonorrhea should also be treated for chlamydia at the time of presentation.	8.	Women treated for gonorrhea should also be treated for chlamydia at the time of presentation.	INCLUDED BASED ON Q1 PANEL RATING
	Urethritis - Diagnosis			
9.	If a sexually active male patient presents with penile discharge he should be tested for both chlamydia and gonorrhea at the time of presentation.	9.	If a sexually active male patient presents with penile discharge he should be tested for both chlamydia and gonorrhea at the time of presentation.	ACCEPTED
	Pelvic Inflammatory Disease (PID) - Diagnosis			
10.	Patients with the diagnosis of PID should receive all of the following at the time of diagnosis: a. Speculum exam; b. Bi-manual exam.	10. a b	Patients with the diagnosis of PID should receive all of the following at the time of diagnosis: a. Speculum exam; b. Bi-manual exam.	INCLUDED BASED ON Q1 PANEL RATING
11.	If a patient is given the diagnosis of PID, at least 2 of the following signs should be present on physical exam: • lower abdominal tenderness; • adnexal tenderness; and • cervical motion tenderness.	11.	If a patient is given the diagnosis of PID, at least 2 of the following signs should be present on physical exam: • lower abdominal tenderness; • adnexal tenderness; and • cervical motion tenderness.	INCLUDED BASED ON Q1 PANEL RATING
	Pelvic Inflammatory Disease - Treatment			
12.	Women with PID and any of the following conditions should receive parenteral antibiotics at the time of diagnosis: a. Pelvic abscess is present or suspected; b. Pregnancy; c. HIV infection; d. Uncontrolled nausea and vomiting; e. Lack of clinical improvement within 72 hours of beginning therapy.	12. a. b. c. d. e.	Women with PID and any of the following conditions should receive parenteral antibiotics at the time of diagnosis: a. Pelvic abscess is present or suspected; b. Pregnancy; c. HIV infection; d. Uncontrolled nausea and vomiting; e. Lack of clinical improvement within 72 hours of beginning therapy.	INCLUDED BASED ON Q1 PANEL RATING
13.	Duration of total antibiotic therapy for PID should be no less than 10 days (inpatient, if applicable, plus outpatient).	13.	Duration of total antibiotic therapy for PID should be no less than 10 days (inpatient, if applicable, plus outpatient).	INCLUDED BASED ON Q1 PANEL RATING
	Pelvic Inflammatory Disease - Follow-up			
14.	Patients receiving outpatient therapy for PID should receive follow-up contact within 72 hours of diagnosis.	14.	Patients receiving outpatient therapy for PID should receive follow-up contact within 72 hours of diagnosis.	INCLUDED BASED ON Q1 PANEL RATING

473

	Indicator Proposed by Staff		Indicator Voted on by Panel	Comments/Disposition
	Genital Ulcers - Diagnosis		*Genital Ulcers - Diagnosis*	
15.	All patients with genital herpes should be counseled on reducing the risk of transmission to a sexual partner.	15.	All patients with genital herpes should be counseled on reducing the risk of transmission to a sexual partner.	INCLUDED BASED ON Q1 PANEL RATING
16.	If a patient presents with the new onset of genital ulcers then all of the following should be offered at the time of presentation: a. Cultures for HSV b. Blood test for HIV c. Blood test for syphilis.	16. a. -- **b.**	If a patient presents with the new onset of genital ulcers then all of the following should be offered at the time of presentation: a. Cultures **or DFA for HSV** b. ~~Blood test for HIV~~ c. Blood test for syphilis.	MODIFIED: Panelists added DFA because it has greater specificity. **"a, c" ACCEPTED AS MODIFIED** **"b" DROPPED PRIOR TO PANEL.** Redundant with indicator #23.
	Genital Ulcers - Chancroid - Treatment		*Genital Ulcers - Chancroid - Treatment*	
17.	Patients with chancroid should be treated with azithromycin, ceftriaxone, or erythromycin (in the absence of allergy to these medications).	17.	Patients with chancroid should be treated with azithromycin, ceftriaxone, or erythromycin (in the absence of allergy to these medications).	INCLUDED BASED ON Q1 PANEL RATING
	Genital Ulcers - Chancroid - Follow-up		*Genital Ulcers - Chancroid - Follow-up*	
18.	Patients receiving treatment for chancroid should be re-examined within 10 days of treatment initiation to assess clinical improvement.	18.	Patients receiving treatment for chancroid should be re-examined within 10 days of treatment initiation to assess clinical improvement.	INCLUDED BASED ON Q1 PANEL RATING
	Genital Ulcers - Syphilis - Treatment		*Genital Ulcers - Syphilis - Treatment*	
19.	Patients with primary and secondary syphilis who do not have a penicillin allergy should be treated with IM-administered benzathine penicillin G.	19.	Patients with primary and secondary syphilis who do not have a penicillin allergy should be treated with IM-administered benzathine penicillin G.	INCLUDED BASED ON Q1 PANEL RATING
20.	If a patient has a primary ulcer consistent with syphilis, treatment for syphilis should be initiated before laboratory test results are available.	20.	If a patient has a primary ulcer consistent with syphilis, treatment for syphilis should be initiated before laboratory test results are available.	INCLUDED BASED ON Q1 PANEL RATING
	Genital Ulcers - Syphilis - Follow-up		*Genital Ulcers - Syphilis - Follow-up*	
21.	Patients with primary or secondary syphilis should be re-examined clinically and serologically within 6 months after treatment.	21.	Patients with primary or secondary syphilis should be re-examined clinically and serologically within 6 months after treatment.	INCLUDED BASED ON Q1 PANEL RATING
	Genital Warts - Diagnosis		*Genital Warts - Diagnosis*	
22.	Women with an initial diagnosis of HPV should have a speculum examination and a pap smear (if not performed during the preceding year).	22.	Women with an initial diagnosis of HPV should have a speculum examination and a pap smear (if not performed during the preceding year).	INCLUDED BASED ON Q1 PANEL RATING

	Indicator Proposed by Staff		Indicator Voted on by Panel	Comments/Disposition
	STDs (General) - Diagnosis		*STDs (General) - Diagnosis*	
23.	If a patient presents with an initial infection of any STD, HIV testing should be discussed and offered at the time of presentation.	23.	If a patient presents with an initial infection of any STD, HIV testing should be discussed and offered at the time of presentation.	INCLUDED BASED ON Q1 PANEL RATING
24.	If a patient presents with any STD, a non-treponemal test (VDRL or RPR) for syphilis should be performed at the time of presentation.	24.	If a patient presents with any STD, a non-treponemal test (VDRL or RPR) for syphilis should be performed at the time of presentation.	INCLUDED BASED ON Q1 PANEL RATING
	STDs (General) - Treatment			
25.	Sexual partners of patients with new diagnoses of gonorrhea, chlamydia, chancroid, and primary or secondary syphilis should be referred for treatment as soon as possible.	25.	Sexual partners of patients with new diagnoses of gonorrhea, chlamydia, chancroid, and primary or secondary syphilis should be referred for treatment as soon as possible.	INCLUDED BASED ON Q1 PANEL RATING

475

Chapter 21 - Urinary Tract Infection

	Indicator Proposed by Staff		Indicator Voted on by Panel	Comments/Disposition
	Diagnosis			
1.	In patients presenting with dysuria, presence or absence of fever and flank pain should be elicited.	1.	In patients presenting with dysuria, presence or absence of fever and flank pain should be elicited.	INCLUDED BASED ON Q1 PANEL RATING
2.	In women presenting with dysuria, a history of vaginal discharge should be elicited.	2.	In women presenting with dysuria, a history of vaginal discharge should be elicited.	INCLUDED BASED ON Q1 PANEL RATING
3.	Patients who present with dysuria and are started on antimicrobial treatment for urinary tract infection should have had a urinalysis or dipstick evaluation on the day of presentation.	--	Patients who present with dysuria and are started on antimicrobial treatment for urinary tract infection should have had a urinalysis or dipstick evaluation on the day of presentation.	DROPPED due to low validity score. Panelists felt there could be exceptions.
4.	A urine culture should be obtained for patients who have dysuria and any one of the following: a. "several" (three or more) infections in the past year; b. diabetes or immunocompromised state c. fever, chills and/or flank pain; d. suspected diagnosis of pyelonephritis; e. structural or functional anomalies of the urinary tract; f. a relapse of symptoms, if no culture previously obtained; g. a recent invasive procedure.	3. a. b. c. d. e. f. g.	A urine culture should be obtained for patients who have dysuria and any one of the following: a. "several" (three or more) infections in the past year; b. diabetes or immunocompromised state; c. fever, chills and/or flank pain; d. suspected diagnosis of pyelonephritis; e. structural or functional anomalies of the urinary tract; f. a relapse of symptoms, if no culture previously obtained; g. a recent invasive procedure.	INCLUDED BASED ON Q1 PANEL RATING
	Treatment			
5.	If a diagnosis of UTI (upper or lower tract) has been made, the patient should be treated with antimicrobial therapy.	4.	If a diagnosis of UTI (upper or lower tract) has been made, the patient should be treated with antimicrobial therapy.	INCLUDED BASED ON Q1 PANEL RATING
6.	Trimethoprim-sulfamethoxazole should be used as a first-line agent in women under age 65 with uncomplicated lower tract infection unless there is documented history of allergy or pregnancy	5.	Trimethoprim-sulfamethoxazole should be used as a first-line agent in women under age 65 with uncomplicated lower tract infection unless there is documented history of allergy or pregnancy	INCLUDED BASED ON Q1 PANEL RATING
7.	Treatment with antimicrobials for uncomplicated lower tract infections in women under age 65 should not exceed 7 days.	6.	Treatment with antimicrobials for uncomplicated lower tract infections in women under age 65 should not exceed 7 days.	INCLUDED BASED ON Q1 PANEL RATING
8.	At least 10 days of antimicrobial therapy should be prescribed for a suspected upper tract infection (pyelonephritis).	7.	At least 10 days of antimicrobial therapy should be prescribed for a suspected upper tract infection (pyelonephritis).	INCLUDED BASED ON Q1 PANEL RATING

	Indicator Proposed by Staff		Indicator Voted on by Panel	Comments/Disposition
9.	A patient with known or suspected upper tract infection who has uncontrolled vomiting in the office or ER should receive parentral antibiotics.	8.	A patient with known or suspected upper tract infection who has uncontrolled vomiting in the office or ER should receive parentral antibiotics.	INCLUDED BASED ON Q1 PANEL RATING
10.	Regimens of at least 7 days should be used for patients with complicated lower tract infections: that is, those with: a. diabetes, b. functional or structural anomaly of the urinary tract, c. symptoms for longer than 7 days, d. urinary tract infection in the past month, e. pregnancy.	9. a. b. c. d. e.	Regimens of at least 7 days should be used for patients with complicated lower tract infections: that is, those with: a. diabetes, b. functional or structural anomaly of the urinary tract, c. symptoms for longer than 7 days, d. urinary tract infection in the past month, e. pregnancy.	INCLUDED BASED ON Q1 PANEL RATING
	Follow-up			
11.	For upper tract infection a repeat culture should be obtained within 2 weeks of finishing treatment.	10.	For upper tract infection a repeat culture should be obtained within 2 weeks of finishing treatment.	INCLUDED BASED ON Q1 PANEL RATING
12.	For complicated lower tract infection, a repeat culture should be obtained within 2 weeks of finishing treatment.	11.	For complicated lower tract infection, a repeat culture should be obtained within 2 weeks of finishing treatment.	INCLUDED BASED ON Q1 PANEL RATING

Chapter 22 - Vertigo and Dizziness

	Indicator Proposed by Staff	Indicator Voted on by Panel	Comments/Disposition
	Diagnosis		
1.	Patients who present with vertigo should have all of the following documented at the time of initial presentation with symptoms: a. the duration of episodes; b. presence or absence of precipitation by head movements; c. presence or absence of any association with hearing loss or tinnitus,	1. Patients who present with vertigo should have all of the following documented at the time of initial presentation with symptoms: a. the duration of episodes; b. presence or absence of precipitation by head movements; c. presence or absence of any association with hearing loss or tinnitus,	ACCEPTED
2.	Patients who present with prolonged spontaneous vertigo should have documentation of risk factors for cerebrovascular disease at the time of presentation.	-- Patients who present with prolonged spontaneous vertigo should have documentation of risk factors for cerebrovascular disease at the time of presentation.	**DROPPED due to low validity score.** Panelists felt this was not a good measure of quality because there are many possible risk factors.
3.	Patients who present with disequilibrium should have all of the following documented at the time of initial presentation: a. presence or absence of diabetes; b. presence or absence of alcohol consumption; c. use of ototoxic medications; d. recent poor oral intake.	-- Patients who present with disequilibrium should have all of the following documented at the time of initial presentation: a. presence or absence of diabetes; b. presence or absence of alcohol consumption; c. use of ototoxic medications; d. recent poor oral intake.	**DROPPED due to low validity score.** Panelists felt that this documentation requirement is too stringent.
4.	Patients who present with presyncope should be asked about all of the following possible precipitants at the time of initial presentation: a. standing up; b. urination; c. exertion; d. emotional stress.	-- Patients who present with presyncope should be asked about all of the following possible precipitants at the time of initial presentation: a. standing up; b. urination; c. exertion; d. emotional stress.	**DROPPED due to low validity score:** Panelists preferred the way presyncope is addressed by indicator #7.
5.	Patients who present with vertigo should have documented an examination of tympanic membranes at the time of presentation.	-- Patients who present with vertigo should have documented an examination of tympanic membranes at the time of presentation.	**DROPPED due to low validity score.** The evidence of usefulness is insufficient to require this.
6.	Patients who present with recurrent positional vertigo should have documented the results of a Hallpike maneuver at the time of presentation.	-- Patients who present with recurrent positional vertigo should have documented the results of a Hallpike maneuver at the time of presentation.	**DROPPED due to low validity score.** The usefulness of Hallpike is not clear. The results are not likely to change management.
7.	Patients who present with presyncope should have all of the following documented at the time of presentation: a. orthostatic vital signs; b. heart examination.	2. Patients who present with presyncope should have all of the following documented at the time of presentation: a. orthostatic vital signs; b. heart examination.	ACCEPTED

#	Indicator Proposed by Staff		Indicator Voted on by Panel	Comments/Disposition
8.	Patients who present with disequilibrium should have documentation of visual acuity testing at the time of presentation.	--	Patients who present with disequilibrium should have documentation of visual acuity testing at the time of presentation.	**DROPPED due to low validity score.** The evidence of benefit is lacking.
9.	Patients who present with disequilibrium should have documentation of the following components of a neurological examination at the time of presentation: a. cerebellar exam; b. gait observation; c. Romberg testing.	--	Patients who present with disequilibrium should have documentation of the following components of a neurological examination at the time of presentation: a. cerebellar exam; b. gait observation; c. Romberg testing.	**DROPPED due to low validity score**
10.	Patients who present with vertigo and new neurological deficits should have MRI within 2 weeks of presentation.	--	Patients who present with vertigo and new neurological deficits should have MRI within 2 weeks of presentation.	**DROPPED due to low validity score**
11.	Patients who present with disequilibrium and unilateral hearing loss should have audiometry within 3 weeks of presentation.	--	Patients who present with disequilibrium and unilateral hearing loss should have audiometry within 3 weeks of presentation.	**DROPPED due to low validity score.** Acoustic neuroma is very rare.
12.	Patients who present with sudden presyncope and HR < 55 on exam should have an ECG at the time of presentation.	--	Patients who present with sudden presyncope and HR < 55 on exam should have an ECG at the time of presentation.	**DROPPED due to low validity score.** Panelists felt this was Too basic to be a quality indicator.
	Treatment		*Treatment*	
13.	Patients who present with torsional-vertical nystagmus on Hallpike testing should have the canalith repositioning procedure within 1 week of presentation.	--	Patients who present with torsional-vertical nystagmus on Hallpike testing should have the canalith repositioning procedure within 1 week of presentation.	**DROPPED due to low validity score.** The success of this procedure is very operator dependent.
14.	Patients who present with a diagnosis of Meniere's syndrome and have bothersome symptoms should be advised to follow a 1–2 gram sodium/day diet or be given a diuretic or both within one month of presentation.	--	Patients who present with a diagnosis of Meniere's syndrome **and have bothersome symptoms** should be advised to follow a 1–2 gram sodium/day diet or be given a diuretic or both within one month of presentation.	**DROPPED due to low validity score.** The group that would benefit is small.
15.	Patients who present with recurrent spontaneous vertigo and any risk factor for cerebrovascular disease should start aspirin or ticlopidine at the time of presentation or be referred to a neurologist within 2 weeks of presentation.	--	Patients who present with recurrent spontaneous vertigo and any risk factor for cerebrovascular disease should start aspirin or ticlopidine at the time of presentation or be referred to a neurologist within 2 weeks of presentation.	**DROPPED due to low validity score.** This indicator is relevant to a very small population.
16.	Patients who present with disequilibrium and decreased visual acuity should be referred to an ophthalmologist or optometrist within one month of presentation.	--	Patients who present with disequilibrium and decreased visual acuity should be referred to an ophthalmologist or optometrist within one month of presentation.	**DROPPED due to low validity score**